Manual Asymmetries *in* Motor Performance

Edited by
Digby Elliott
Eric A. Roy

CRC Press
Boca Raton New York London Tokyo

Manual Asymmetries *in* Motor Performance

Senior Editor: Paul Petralia
Editorial Assistant: Cindy Carelli
Project Editor: Carrie L. Unger
Marketing Manager: Susie Carlislie
Direct Marketing Manager: Becky McEldowney
Prepress: Carlos Esser
Cover Designer: Dawn Boyd

Library of Congress Cataloging-in-Publication Data

Elliott, Digby
Manual asymmetries in motor performance/ edited by Digby Elliott, Eric A. Roy.
p. cm.
Includes bibliographical references and index.
ISBN 0-8493-8999-2 (alk. paper)
1. Cerebral Dominance. 2. Motor Ability. 3. Laterility.
I. Elliott, Digby, 1950- . II. Roy, Eric A. (Eric Alexander), 1947- .
QP385.5.M26 1996
612.8′ 25--dc20
DNLM/DLC

96-98
CIP

International Standard Book Number 0-8493-8999-2
Library of Congress Card Number 96-98
Printed in the United States of America 1 2 3 4 5 6 7 8 9 0
Printed on acid-free paper

PREFACE

All animals show a preference for using one limb in activities such as feeding. It is only our human species which shows a consistent preference for the right, a preference which has been present for thousands of years as evidenced by the tools used by our hominid ancestors. This overriding bias toward the use of the right hand in most people has had a profound impact on society in many areas, including the design of tools and work environments and education-related activities such as handwriting. What is the reason for this right-hand bias? Some investigators have been interested in the evolutionary significance of this asymmetry. Others have focused on what this asymmetry reveals about the cerebral lateralization of cognitive and motor functions. Still others have addressed how best to measure this asymmetry and what these measures tell us about the processes involved in the control of hand movements.

Research dealing with manual asymmetries and how these asymmetries relate to cerebral organization thus cuts across a number of disciplines including neuropsychology, neurophysiology, kinesiology, and anthropology. As a consequence, empirical work in this general area is published in scientific journals with very different orientations and audiences. Our attempt in compiling this volume was to bring together under one cover a collection of chapters that could serve as a reference text or handbook for graduate students, researchers, and clinicians interested in cerebral asymmetry, motor control, and human handedness.

The authors contributing to this volume are all active researchers in the topic area they cover. The format followed by most authors has been to provide an initial overview of the research in their particular area, identifying some of the classic work. The authors then review the most recent findings in their topic area outlining his/her own research and, in some cases, presenting new empirical work. In having each author set their own research into a historical and contemporary context, our goal is to make the reader aware of the controversial issues, as well as the research strategies that have been employed to resolve these issues.

The volume is divided into four sections. Section I deals with the Biological and Anthropological Antecedents of Motor Asymmetry. In Chapter 1, Lesley Rogers and John Bradshaw develop the evolutionary antecedents of human handedness and asymmetries in motor control by examining Motor Asymmetries in Birds and Nonprimate Mammals. In the next chapter, Bradshaw and Rogers take us one step closer to the issues of manual asymmetry in contemporary humans in their review of Tool Use and the Evolutionary Development of Manual Asymmetry in early humans and nonhuman primates.

Section II of this volume addresses Human Handedness. In a chapter entitled The Measurement of Handedness and Its Relation to Neuropsychological Issues, Phil Bryden, Barbara Bulman-Fleming, and Valerie MacDonald provide a broad overview of the origins of human handedness and its relation to cerebral organization of cognitive functions such as language. As well as introducing a number of specific models of handedness, this chapter identifies the problems researchers face in the measurement of handedness and in relating asymmetries in both preference and performance to cerebral lateralization of function.

The next two chapters in this section focus on a key challenge to any comprehensive model of human handedness, the incidence of left handedness as well as cerebral organization in left-handers. In his chapter entitled Pathological Causes and Consequences of Left-Handedness, Stanley Coren makes a strong case for a genetically determined predisposition to be right-handed in humans with left-handedness resulting only as a consequence of neurological pathology. Michael Peters also discusses the ability of various models of handedness to explain left-handedness. He goes on to identify two types of left-handers on the basis of hand preference and performance differences in many everyday activities (i.e., Hand Preference and Performance in Left-Handers). Peters' chapter provides an excellent transition to Section III, which deals exclusively with Manual Performance Asymmetries.

Runa Steenhuis continues the discussion of the relation between preference and performance in both right-handers and left-handers in her chapter entitled Hand Preference and Performance in Skilled and Unskilled Manual Activities. In the next chapter, Digby Elliott and Romeo Chua review both performance and kinematic studies which have attempted to reveal the underlying left hemisphere processing advantages that lead to Manual Asymmetries in Goal-Directed Movement in Right-Handers. In a chapter entitled Putative Right Hemisphere Contributions to the Preparation of Reaching and Aiming Movements, Richard Carson goes on to demonstrate that while the left cerebral hemisphere enjoys an advantage when it comes to movement execution, the right hemisphere has a special role to play not only in evaluating the spatial aspects of the movement environment, but also in movement preparation.

In Section IV, the final section of this volume, three chapters examine The Implications of Asymmetric Motor Function. In a thought provoking chapter entitled Asymmetry in Bimanual Skills, Yves Guiard and Thierry Ferrand reject more traditional views of manual asymmetry in their examination of the complementary roles of the right and left hands in bimanual tasks. Their chapter provides a compelling framework for future research. Deborah Dewey then tackles the controversial topic of Manual Asymmetries in Children With Developmental Disabilities, and the relation between atypical cerebral specialization and developmental movement pathology. Eric Roy completes this section and the volume with a chapter entitled Hand Preference, Manual Asymmetries, and Limb Apraxia. The central question in this chapter is how handedness relates to disruptions in limb praxis in which the patient is unable perform a variety of hand gestures. Since apraxia in right-handers most often arises from damage to the left hemisphere, the hemisphere controlling the preferred right hand, some researchers have argued that handedness arises from praxis laterality. The fact that both hands are often affected in apraxia, however, raises some interesting questions about the relationship between apraxia and handedness which are addressed in this chapter.

As editors of this volume, we are indebted to a number of agencies and individuals who made our task easier. First, we thank the Natural Sciences and Engineering Research Council of Canada, a foundation which has funded much of our own work over the years.

We wish to acknowledge our colleagues and students at McMaster University and the University of Waterloo who read and commented on first drafts of many of the chapters in this volume. We owe thanks to Paul Petralia at CRC Press for his guidance and encouragement from the beginning of the project to the end.

We are particularly indebted to Mary Cleland, whose organizational and word processing skills allowed us to put together a final product almost on time. Without Mary, we would still be working on the volume.

Finally, we thank Elaine and Betty for their continued love and support in this and all the other projects that have occupied the majority of our time over the years.

EDITORS

Digby Elliott, Ph.D., is a Professor with the Department of Kinesiology at McMaster University in Hamilton, Ontario, Canada. In the 1994-1995 academic year, he received the McMaster Student Union Teaching Excellence Award for the Faculty of Social Science and the University at large.

Dr. Elliott received his B.Sc. (1978) and M.Sc. (1980) from the Department of Kinesiology at the University of Waterloo and his Ph.D. from the Department of Psychology (1983) at the University of Waterloo.

Dr. Elliott is a member of the Psychonomic Society, the North American Society for the Psychology of Sport and Physical Activity, and the Canadian Society for Brain, Behaviour and Cognitive Science. He is president-elect of the Canadian Society for Psychomotor Learning and Sport Psychology. From 1993 to 1996, he was a member of the Natural Science and Engineering Research Council of Canada, Animal Biology, Grant Selection Committee. He has served as a consulting editor for the *Journal of Motor Behavior* and reviews regularly for 16 other journals and 7 granting agencies.

Dr. Elliott has published over 80 scientific papers and was listed by Current Contents as one of the most productive authors in psychology between 1986 and 1990. He has published a number of book chapters and has co-edited a book on vision and motor control. His research interests include the visual control of voluntary movement, asymmetries in motor control, and cerebral organization and motor control in children and adults with Down's syndrome.

Eric A. Roy, C. Psych., is a Professor of Kinesiology and Psychology at the University of Waterloo, Waterloo, Ontario, Canada. He is also Director of the Centre for Habilitation Education and Research as well as Coordinator of the Neurobehavioural Assessment Unit. Dr. Roy also holds appointments at the University of Toronto as Professor of Rehabilitation Science and Speech Pathology and has research appointments at the Toronto Hospital and Sunnybrook Health Science Centre in Toronto, Ontario, Canada.

Dr. Roy received a B.Sc. in Kinesiology from the University of Waterloo in 1971, a M.P.E. in Human Performance from the University of British Columbia, Vancouver, British Columbia, Canada in 1973, and a Ph.D. in Psychology from the University of Waterloo in 1976. Dr. Roy received his license to practice Psychology from the College of Psychologists of Ontario in 1977.

Dr. Roy is a member of the International Neuropsychological Society, the Neuroscience Society, the National Academy of Neuropsychology, the Canadian Society for Brain, Behaviour and Cognitive Science, the Canadian Psychological Society, the Ontario Psychological Society, the North American Society for the Psychology of Sport and Physical Activity, and the Canadian Psychomotor Learning and Sport Psychology Society. He is a recipient of the first Doctoral Gold Medal Award from the University of Waterloo. He has also received awards as a Visiting Scientist from the Medical Research Council of Canada and as a Heritage Scholar from the University of Alberta, Edmonton, Alberta, Canada.

Dr. Roy has presented over 40 invited lectures to national and international meetings and approximately 30 guest lectures at universities and institutes. He has published one book and more than a hundred research papers and book chapters. The focus of Dr. Roy's research is on prehension, movement sequencing, limb gesturing, and how these movements are affected by aging, stroke, and neurodegenerative disorders, particularly Parkinson's and Alzheimer's diseases. He is also a licensed psychologist specializing in clinical neuropsychology and practices as an Associate with Charles Pierce Associates in Kitchener, Ontario, Canada. He is listed in the Canadian Register of Health Service Providers in Psychology and acts as a consultant to a number of legal and rehabilitation firms.

CONTRIBUTORS

John L. Bradshaw, Ph.D., D.Sc.
Department of Psychology
Monash University
Clayton, Victoria, Australia

M.P. Bryden, Ph.D.
Department of Psychology
University of Waterloo
Waterloo, Ontario, Canada

M. Barbara Bulman-Fleming, Ph.D.
Department of Psychology
University of Waterloo
Waterloo, Ontario, Canada

Richard G. Carson, M.Sc., Ph.D.
Department of Human Movement Studies
University of Queensland
St. Lucia
Brisbane, Queensland, Australia

Romeo Chua, M.Sc., Ph.D.
Laboratory for Perceptual-Motor Dynamics
Faculty of Physical Education and Recreation
University of Alberta
Edmonton, Alberta, Canada

Stanley Coren, Ph.D.
Department of Psychology
University of British Columbia
Vancouver, British Columbia, Canada

Deborah Dewey, Ph.D.
Department of Paediatrics
Alberta Children's Hospital
University of Calgary
Calgary, Alberta, Canada

Digby Elliott, M.Sc., Ph.D.
Department of Kinesiology
McMaster University
Hamilton, Ontario, Canada

Thierry Ferrand, M.S.
Movement and Perception
CNRS and University of the Mediterranean
Marseille, France

Yves Guiard, Ph.D.
Movement and Perception
CNRS and University of the Mediterranean
Marseille, France

Valerie MacDonald, Ph.D.
Health Services Association of the South Shore
Bridgewater, Nova Scotia, Canada

Michael Peters, Ph.D.
Department of Psychology
University of Guelph
Guelph, Ontario, Canada

Lesley J. Rogers, D. Phil., D.Sc.
Department of Physiology
The University of New England
Armidale, New South Wales, Australia

Eric A. Roy, Ph.D., C. Psych.
Department of Kinesiology
University of Waterloo
Waterloo, Ontario, Canada

Runa E. Steenhuis, Ph.D., C. Psych.
Psychological Services
University Hospital Campus
London Health Services Centre
London, Ontario, Canada

CONTENTS

Section I

Biological *and* Anthropological Antecedents *of* Motor Asymmetry

Chapter 1

Motor Asymmetries in Birds and Nonprimate Mammals

Lesley J. Rogers and John L. Bradshaw

CONTENTS

1. INTRODUCTION

Lateralization of brain function is known for a range of animal species and for many different behaviors. In general, the pattern of lateralization is similar to that found in humans. This chapter covers lateralizations in animal species other than primates. The emphasis is on motor function, but various possible influences of perceptual lateralization on motor function are also discussed. Some mention is made of the development of lateralization and environmental influences on this process, but this aspect of the topic has been reviewed elsewhere in more detail (Rogers and Adret, 1993; Bradshaw and Rogers, 1993; Rogers, 1991, 1995).

We begin with an example of motor lateralization that operates internally and is not directly evident by observing the behavior of the whole animal, namely, bird song. Then we move on to motor lateralities that are clearly evident in behavior of intact animals, such as turning or circling biases and limb preferences. Some of these motor asymmetries are present in individuals without any tendency for these individuals to be lateralized in a consistent direction. Other examples of motor asymmetries are present in individuals,

0-8493-8999-2/96/$0.00+$.50

and there is also a consistent bias in the direction of the lateralization for the group or population. The latter category indicates hemispheric specialization.

It is frequently assumed that consistent hemispheric specialization is more important than directionally random lateralization at the level of the individual only, but this might be a human-centered view. Many researchers have sought the equivalence of human handedness in animals. While it is important to recognize the differences between individual lateralizations and lateralization caused by consistent hemispheric specialization, the distinction is rather irrelevant for the functioning of an individual brain. In this respect, it may be important to be lateralized, for whatever reason and in either direction, but not important that all individuals are lateralized in the same direction. Moreover, it is often assumed that lateralization at the individual level only represents learned preferences by the individuals, whereas hemispheric specialization is a more fundamental aspect of a species, determined by genetic selection. This distinction is not necessarily correct. Evolutionary processes may select for a lateralized brain, irrespective of the direction of lateralization. Having a lateralized brain, irrespective of the direction of lateralization, may confer a selective advantage. Furthermore, evolutionary selection would not exclude the influence of learning on the development of lateralization by the individual. Not even hemispheric specialization need be exclusively encoded in the genome. For example, the hemispheric specialization ultimately established for controlling many visual functions of the chick is determined by light stimulation of the embryo. We will elaborate on the way in which the orientation of the chick embryo in the egg restricts light stimulation to the right eye only and establishes at least some of the lateralized functions, as well as structural asymmetries in the brain.

2. LATERALIZATION OF MOTOR MECHANISMS IN VOCAL PRODUCTION

Asymmetry for motor control of vocalizations appeared very early in evolution. In fact, the lateralizations for perception and production of song in birds and of speech in humans may well have followed long evolutionary trajectories from a common ancestor. Of course, the distinctly different neural and anatomical structures used for song and speech production might suggest separate evolution of analogous structures in the more recent past of birds and primates, but evidence of lateralization of neural control of vocalization by the frog, *Rana pipiens* (Bauer, 1993), suggests that homologous differences might well come about by separate forms of elaboration on a basic pattern of lateralization which was already present in amphibia. The left hemisphere is specialized to control the production of vocalization in the frog, in most avian species so far investigated, and in primates, including humans. To our knowledge, nothing is known about possible lateralization of vocal control in reptiles, though, given the findings for amphibia and birds, we can easily predict the likely situation in reptiles.

2.1 FROGS

The dominance of the left hemisphere in *R. pipiens* was demonstrated by lesioning the tracts leading from the vocal centers on the left or right side of the brain and then attempting to elicit an alarm vocalization by clasping the frog behind its forelimbs at regular intervals over a period of 6 weeks (Bauer, 1993). Vocalization frequency and quality were reduced significantly more by the lesions placed in the left side than the right side. It remains to be seen whether other vocalizations, for example those used in mating, are lateralized similarly and whether this lateralization is present in other anuran species.

2.2 BIRDS

There is a large amount of information on the lateralization of song in birds. Most species of songbird examined exhibit dominance of the left side of the brain for control of singing (Nottebohm, 1980). Of nine species so far investigated, only one species, the zebra finch, has right-side dominance (Williams, 1990; Williams, Crane, Hale, Esposito, and Nottebohm, 1992), and two species have no dominance (Suthers, 1990).

The first studies reporting left-hemispheric dominance for the control of song production involved sectioning the nerves that innervate the left and right sides of the vocal apparatus, the syrinx, of male chaffinches, *Fingilla coelebs* (Nottebohm, 1970, 1971, 1972). Sectioning the nerve on the left side results in loss of most of the components of song, subsong, and calling, whereas sectioning the equivalent nerve on the right side has very little effect on these vocalizations. Similar results have been found for several other species of songbird, including the canary (Nottebohm, 1977), and two species of sparrow (Lemon, 1973; Nottebohm and Nottebohm, 1976). Cutting the left nerve of adult-male canaries has a dramatic effect on song; the bird performs all of the beak and body movements as if it were singing, but utters only faint clicks or an occasional, brief syllable. Cutting the right nerve causes no more than a 10% loss of syllables, noticeable only on sound spectrographs.

Left-side dominance appears to be the most common pattern of asymmetry for control of song production, but, as mentioned above, there is one known example of the reverse pattern. In the zebra finch, *Taeniopygia guttata*, sectioning the right nerve has a greater effect on vocal behavior than sectioning the left (Williams et al., 1992).

Birds vocalize by expelling air over the elastic membranes of the syrinx and modulating the tension in the muscles of the syrinx. In songbirds, the syrinx consists of two parts, one in each bronchus, and each is innervated separately (Nottebohm, 1972). In most songbird species, the left and right sides of the syrinx act largely as independent sound sources for the production of most vocalizations, although to a much lesser extent both sides of the syrinx may jointly contribute to some syllables (Nowicki and Capranica, 1986).

The dominance of the left side of the syrinx has been demonstrated by placing a plug in the bronchus on either the left or right side. In canaries, plugging the left side degrades the song, whereas plugging the right has no significant effect (Hartley and Suthers, 1990). Consistent with this functional lateralization, the musculature on the left side of the syrinx of the canary is larger than that on the right side (Nottebohm, 1971, 1977).

In another species, the brown thrasher (*Toxostoma rufum*), both sides of the syrinx contribute almost equally to song production. The muscles that control song by regulating the airflow through each side of the syrinx can act independently (Goller and Suthers, 1995). The latter authors referred to this independent action as lateralization, but it is not lateralization in the generally accepted sense of the term, or as we use it here. One side does not dominate the other or act in a manner entirely different from the other — only the timing is different on each side. Other muscles of the syrinx that control the phonetic structure of the vocalizations are active in parallel on both sides of the syrinx irrespective of which side is generating the sound. This bilateral motor pattern is therefore coupled with the unilateral system for controlling airflow.

The nerves which supply the musculature of the syrinx branch off from the hypoglossal nerves (also known as the XII cranial nerves) on each side, originating from nuclei on either side of the hindbrain (nXII in Figure 1.1). The motor neurons which innervate the syrinx have their cell bodies in the motor nucleus nXII, close to the motor neurons which control expiration of air from the air sac system (Wild, 1994). This anatomical proximity may indicate a single functional unit for producing song both by modulation of the muscles of the syrinx and by expiration of air over the membranes of the syrinx. As yet, there is no evidence of lateralized control of the left and right sets of abdominal expiratory muscles, but as Wild (1994) suggests, this is not inconceivable because separate abdominal air sacs on each side of the body provide air to the bronchus in each side of the syrinx. Each might therefore act independently to expel air over the syringeal membranes to produce song.

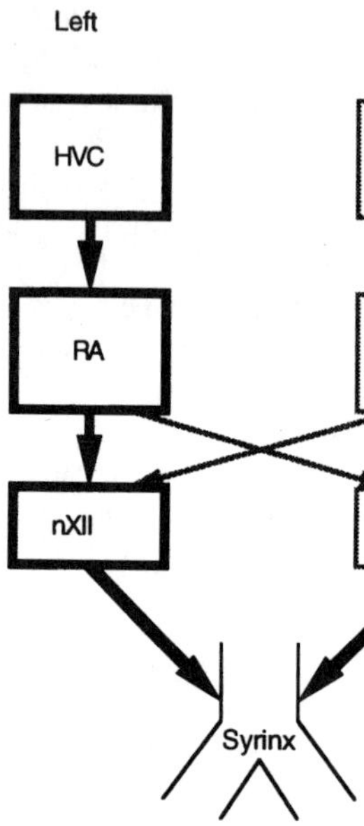

Figure 1.1 A simplified representation of the motor system involved in song production in the canary is presented. The two of the nuclei, HVC, known as the "higher vocal center," and RA, nucleus robustus archistriatalis, are located in the forebrain. The nucleus nXII which gives rise to the hypoglossal nerve is in the hindbrain. A branch of the hypoglossal nerve supplies the muscular on one side of the syrinx, the left side being larger. The motor control system on the left side is dominant. Note, however, the minor crossing-over pathway from each RA to its contralateral nXII. The function of these contralateral projections is not known. The other forebrain nuclei involved in song perception and learning are not included (see Konishi, 1994, and Vicario, 1994, for more details).

Opening and closing of the beak also affects the song produced and this motor component of singing might likewise be under lateralized control (Wild, 1994), although there has been no investigation of this so far.

The asymmetrical control of song can be traced to centers in the forebrain which control the output of the motor neurons to the syrinx. First, the left-side dominance, where present, can be traced to the nucleus robustus archistriatalis (RA), located in the caudal region of the forebrain, and sending direct projections to the nXII. Although some of these projections cross the midline to innervate the nXII on the contralateral side, by far the majority project from RA to nXII on the same side (Figure 1.1).

Lesioning the left RA of the canary causes a greater disruption of singing than lesioning the right RA (Nottebohm, Stokes, and Leonard, 1976). Without a left RA the bird sings with a reduced frequency range of the song fundamental. Lesions of either side lead to a reduction in the number of syllables of song. Therefore, asymmetry is present, but not absolute.

The main source of neurons which project to each RA is the higher vocal center (HVC) in the roof of the forebrain on the same side. Lateralization is present also at this higher order of neural control. The neurons in HVC seem to have both sensory and motor functions (McCasland and Konishi, 1981), and the motor ones, at least, are lateralized. Lesions of the left HVC of the canary disrupt song more than lesions of the right HVC (Nottebohm, 1977). After the left HVC has been lesioned, canaries retain the ability to produce no more than one of their syllables of song, the rest of the song being a monotonous, simple succession of notes. After the right HVC has been lesioned, the song is either totally unaffected or only marginally affected.

Thus, in most species of songbird studied so far, there is an entire system of left-side dominance for the motor control of singing. Both RA and HVC receive auditory inputs (Konishi, 1994; Vicario and Yohay, 1993), which must be important for their role in the motor control of song (Margoliash et al., 1994). However, the mechanisms by which these auditory inputs affect song production, and whether they too are lateralized, is not yet known. Nevertheless, it is known that the most effective stimulus for activating the neurons in HVC is the bird's own song (McCasland and Konishi, 1981; Margoliash and Fortune, 1992) and the same is true for RA (Vicario, 1994). The bird's own song is more effective than the songs of conspecifics (Vicario, 1994). This suggests that the perceptual input to these motor nuclei provides auditory feedback used in the motor control of song, but it is also possible that motor processes influence perceptual processing in the same way (Vacario, 1994).

The perception of song involves lateralized processes, but it is not limited to the left side of the brain, at least on the auditory input side of the system. Unilateral lesions placed in the input side of the auditory system (in the left or right nucleus ovoidalis) affect song perception in a lateralized manner. Following the placement of a lesion in the left nucleus ovoidalis, which removes auditory input to the left HVC, a zebra finch is unable to discriminate between two familiar songs, an ability which the intact bird possesses. Following placement of the lesion in the right nucleus ovoidalis (removing input to the right HVC), the zebra finch retains its ability to distinguish two whole songs, but has an impaired ability to detect a missing harmonic in a syllable of a song (Cynx, Williams, and Nottebohm, 1992). Thus, as Nottebohm et al. (1990) suggest, the left hemisphere of the zebra finch may be better at discriminating between stimuli in a "holistic" sense, whereas the right hemisphere is better at making discriminations which require analysis of components of the song. It must be mentioned again that the zebra finch is, so far, the odd species out in lateralization of the motor mechanisms for song (the right hemisphere controls singing), but these experiments demonstrate, although the motor control of vocal production is lateralized in such a way that one side dominates, that song perception is lateralized without exclusive dominance. It seems that song perception involves differentially specialized but cooperative use of both hemispheres. Somewhere in the interconnected system from perceptual input to motor output, dominance is manifested. In other words, the perception of song requires cooperation between differential processing that occurs in equivalent nuclei on the left and right sides of the brain, whereas the production of song depends on dominance from one side only.

It should also be noted that it is only during the reproductive season that songbirds sing such as the canary. In spring, the level of the hormone testosterone rises, and the sizes of the nuclei used in singing increase, by the addition of new neurons, at the same time that the musculature of the syrinx increases in size, also in response to the testosterone. Thus, it becomes possible for the bird to sing (Nottebohm 1987, 1989). New neurons are added to the song nuclei in both hemispheres and, presumably, only at this time does one of the hemispheres assume dominance. After the reproductive season, neurons are lost from the song nuclei and they shrink in size. It is not known whether the song system of the canary has any functional role outside of the reproductive period or whether it is lateralized at such times. Given the ability of the right hemisphere to assume control of song following lesioning of the left side, it may be that the lateralization for song in the intact bird develops and subsides along with the seasonal fluctuations in testosterone levels.

Nottebohm (1989) has suggested that the avian brain, unlike all other vertebrate brains, may have retained the ability to make large numbers of new neurons in adulthood so that the size of the brain can be kept small, recruiting certain neurons only when needed and losing them afterwards. There might be a sort of time sharing of neurons in the different functional systems of the avian brain. In this way, neural capacity would be enhanced while the brain is kept small. In addition to this, lateralization of function might enhance the neural capacity by freeing one side to perform other functions. Perhaps this explains the rather unusual arrangement in which the main motor nuclei for song, RA and HVC, receive auditory input (Vicario, 1994). On the side of the brain in which these nuclei play no functional role in producing song, they may be more involved in processing the song of other birds or the bird's own song, particularly during the song-learning phase.

This plasticity of the song system is not shared by other known lateralities in the adult avian brain. For example, there is asymmetry of function and structure in the visual system of adult pigeons, *Columba livia*, which may develop under the influence of hormones and light exposure but does not fluctuate in adulthood (see below).

2.3 RODENTS

Specialization of the left hemisphere for processing species-specific vocalizations also occurs in mice (Ehret, 1987), just as it does in Japanese macaque monkeys (see Chapter 2). Ehret tested lactating mice with a choice between two ultrasonic sounds, one resembling the distress calls of mice pups and the other a neutral signal. When tested with the left ear plugged (reduced input to the right hemisphere) or no plugs in the ears, the mouse approached the speaker emitting the distress calls, presumably in attempt to retrieve the "pups." By contrast, when the right ear was plugged (reduced input to the left hemisphere) the mouse, apparently unable to discriminate between the two sounds, approached the speakers at random. This apparent specialization of the left hemisphere was for species-specific calls only, because mice trained to discriminate between two artificial ultrasounds performed equally well with either ear plugged.

Lateralized perception and processing of auditory stimuli has also been shown in the rat (Fitch, Brown, O'Connor, and Tallal, 1993). In this case, the lateralization was shown using pure tone sequences, rather than the species-specific vocalization. Adult male rats with the left ear plugged showed better ability to discriminate tone sequences than those with the right ear plugged, indicating dominance of the left hemisphere. The lateralization was stronger in males and enhanced by handling. Left hemispheric advantage for discriminating temporal acoustic features is characteristic of humans also (Divenyi and Efron, 1979).

It is not yet known whether the lateralization of vocal perception in mice or rats has any associated motor asymmetries for vocal production. However, lateralization of the production of vocalization has been demonstrated in another rodent, the Mongolian gerbil (*Meriones unguiculatus*). The courtship vocalizations produced by male gerbils are controlled by a nucleus in the left side of the hypothalamus (Holman and Hutchison,

1993). There is a positive correlation between the rate of production of an androgen-sensitive courtship vocalization and the volume of a region in the left side of the hypothalamus, the sexually dimorphic region known as the pars compacta nucleus. No such correlation exists for the same area on the right side. The authors were led to suggest that gonadal hormones are required to expose the asymmetric relationship in adult male gerbils. Treatment with gonadal hormones increases the size of the nuclei on both the left and right sides in males and females (there is no asymmetry in size), but only in males and only for the nucleus on the left side is there a significant correlation between size and calling rate during sexual interactions (Holman and Hutchison, 1991). Similarly, the volume of HVC in the songbird correlates with the size of the song repertoire of canaries, and that of the left HVC correlates more strongly with song repertoire than that of the right (Nottebohm, Kasparian, and Pandazis, 1981).

The hypothalamus is the region controlling the motor response of copulation in rodents, and this too is lateralized, as determined by the differential effects of implanting estradiol into the left and right sides of the hypothalamus (Nordeen and Yahr, 1982). Hence, there may be a lateralized relationship between the androgen-sensitive asymmetries for production of courtship vocalization and performance of sexual behavior in rodents.

2.4 DOGS

Lateralized processing of vocalizations has also been demonstrated in dogs. The demonstrated laterality involves acoustic processing by the right hemisphere. In humans, the left hemisphere plays the main role in language perception and speech production, but the right hemisphere is known to have a lesser role in language perception. It does analyze some aspects of heard speech (e.g., voicing and contrasts). As in humans and monkeys, the right hemisphere of the dog acts to discriminate between voicing contrasts, such as "gu" and "ku" sounds. Adams, Molfese, and Betz (1987) demonstrated this by recording auditory evoked responses from the left and right hemispheres of 15-week-old collie dogs as they listened to the sounds. It remains to be seen whether, as with humans, the left hemisphere of dogs is specialized for processing other aspects of (human) speech and for the species-specific vocalizations, and whether the production of vocalizations is similarly lateralized.

2.5 GENERAL ISSUES OF LATERALIZED VOCAL CONTROL

To summarize so far, the present state of knowledge on vocal production in frogs, songbirds, mice, and dogs indicates a general, although not exclusive, pattern of left hemispheric dominance for vocal production, but not for vocal perception. Unfortunately, none of these studies have provided information about the degree of dominance of the left hemisphere, nor would such information be possible from, at least, those studies involving unilateral lesioning of the brain. Therefore, we cannot say whether the degree of asymmetry in the motor mechanisms involved in vocal production is equivalent to that of, for example, handedness in humans or, perhaps more appropriately, of other motor asymmetries in the same or more closely related species. One does, however, glean the impression that in those species with left hemispheric dominance for the motor control of song, the lateralization is consistent across all individuals so far studied, and so may be of an equivalent dimension to that of handedness in humans. The lateralization of many more individuals in each species of songbird would have to be studied before this could be ascertained.

The reverse dominance for control of song by the zebra finch presents a problem for the general hypothesis outlined above. If the laterality of song production came about by gradual evolutionary elaboration on a left hemispheric dominance already present in the amphibia, the right hemisphere dominance of the zebra finch is difficult to explain. Perhaps this exception disproves the rule, or perhaps there is something unusual about the development of the zebra finch. All of the nuclei used for singing are present in the left and right hemispheres of songbirds irrespective of whether singing is controlled by the left or right hemisphere, or by both hemispheres. Those nuclei in the hemisphere not used to control singing in lateralized species are merely inactive for song production although not for perception. It is possible to activate the song control system in the nondominant hemisphere by removing them from suppression by the dominant hemisphere. For example, following lesioning of the left HVC of the canary, singing is resumed, although not so perfectly, in the next season (when the sex hormone levels rise again). As for the other hemisphere, the new song is controlled by the right HVC, RA, and nXII, since sectioning the right hypoglossal nerve prevents the birds from singing (Nottebohm, 1977). Therefore, the hemispheric specialization in songbirds is not absolute and depends on interhemispheric interaction, as well as hormonal condition. Both sides of the songbird brain have the full complement of nuclei used for singing and furthermore there are no known subcellular asymmetries, such as differences in cell size or synaptic density (Nottebohm, 1981). Either side can assume dominance depending on the context and on the species. It is only in humans, or possibly higher primates, that the functional lateralizations for vocal behavior are associated with specialized asymmetries in structure and are less readily reversed in adulthood, although in young humans damage to one hemisphere can reverse dominance. The neural pathways that can be used for speech, for example, are at first present in both hemispheres, and it is only with maturation that those in one hemisphere are no longer designated for performing this function. The avian brain differs only to the extent that it retains its plasticity in adulthood (Nottebohm, 1981).

3. CIRCLING AND TURNING BEHAVIOR

The motor asymmetries associated with vocal production are not manifest in the behavior of intact individuals. They can be revealed only by unilateral surgical intervention. Lateralities in turning behavior are, on the other hand, easily assessed, although the context in which they are assessed influences the results and adds complexity to the interpretation. In general, it appears that circling or rotational behavior performed in a familiar or nonstressful environment is lateralized for individuals, but there is no preferred direction at the group or population level (i.e., no equivalent of handedness in humans). However, when the context of testing is more demanding and when lateralized sensory systems and cognitive processes must be used, population biases in turning or rotation emerge. Examples of the latter are discussed in the section on lateralization of perceptual systems to follow. Turning in birds is covered also in that section.

3.1 FISH

Reist, Bodaly, Fudge, Cash, and Stevens (1987) have reported that whitefish, *Coregonus* sp., have more superficial scars on the left side of the body. These scars are attributed to lampreys. The lateral bias suggests that the whitefish is better able to remove lampreys from its right side by rubbing them against surfaces or that the lampreys have a lateral bias that leads them to attach to the left side of the whitefish more readily. This population bias might possibly reflect a bias for turning or a side preference.

More recent evidence shows that the fish *Girardinus falcatus* exhibits a significant population bias to turn right when first presented with the shape of a simulated predator (Cantalupo, Bisazza, and Vallortigara, 1995a). On subsequent presentations of the stimulus, there is a shift towards turning leftward. No such population bias of turning during escape behavior was found in another species of fish, *Jenynsia lineata*, although individuals of this species had turning preferences, half of them to the right and half to the left (Bisazza, Cantalupo, and Vallortigara, 1995).

Individual turning preferences have been found also in male siamese fighting-fish, *Betta splendens*, during lateral threat displays to a mirror or courtship displays when presented with a female of the species (Cantalupo, Bisazza, and Vallortigara, 1995b). Fighting fish perform the agonistic and courtship displays by turning broadside to the stimulus, and the bias was found in terms of consistency of side turned towards the stimulus, duration of presenting that side, and frequency of presenting that side. There is no population bias.

Turning in a T-maze has been scored using the freshwater fish, *Oreochromis niloticus*, and 20% of the group tested had a significant preference to turn right, 30% to turn left, and the rest had no preference (Gonçalves and Hoshino, 1990a). In this species, there is a significant correlation between the direction of turning in the T-maze and the direction of turning away from an agonistic encounter with a conspecific (Gonçalves and Hoshino, 1990b), suggesting that the same motor asymmetries are expressed in both tests.

3.2 RODENTS

Rats caged in the laboratory turn in circles or rotate spontaneously at night when they are most active, or in the daytime if they are injected with the stimulant amphetamine (Glick and Cox, 1978; Glick and Shapiro, 1985). Most individuals prefer to rotate consistently in the same direction. This motor asymmetry is persistent. Although rats can be trained to rotate in the opposite direction to their spontaneous preference, they revert to the original, preferred direction within 3 weeks following the cessation of training (Zimmerberg, Stumpf, and Glick, 1978).

Collins (1985) measured rotation of swimming direction in mice by placing them in a 12 in. plastic container half filled with water. In this context, they are likely to be performing under stress. Nevertheless, he obtained similar results to the rats tested in the home cage: some rotated in one direction, some in the other, and a lesser number of mice had no preference.

The direction of rotating correlates with neurochemical asymmetries in the dopaminergic pathways of the nigrostriatal basal ganglia system (Jerussi and Glick, 1976). The rat has lower levels of dopamine on the side ipsilateral to the direction of turning. Unilateral destruction of the dopaminergic system in the substantia nigra by injection of 6-hydroxy-dopamine results in a predictable rotation to the side of the lesion (Morgan, Nomikos, and Huston, 1993; Robinson and Becker, 1981).

Although the neural pathways used in rotating behavior are relatively well characterized, it is not known exactly what functional mechanisms are involved. Rotational preference may be determined by lateralized perceptual processes (see below) or a form of motor dominance of limb usage in stepping. A detailed analysis of rotating behavior by Ziegler and Szechtman (1990) describes different styles of rotation and concludes that bias of leg usage is not the explanation for rotating; the direction of rotating is independent of motor asymmetries of the hindlimbs.

The earliest studies of rotational behavior reached the general conclusion that, although most rats display a preferred direction of rotation, the distribution of clockwise and counterclockwise preferences is random. In other words, it was considered that no population bias for lateralization existed (Glick and Cox, 1978). However, Glick and Ross (1981) found an overall 55% right-side bias in a group of Sprague-Dawley-derived rats, and Robinson (1985) found a slight population bias to circle to the right in a group of female rats (around 57%). By contrast, males of two other strains displayed a leftward bias (60%), indicating that sex hormones may have an influence (Robinson, 1985). There is evidence that activity of the nigrostriatal dopamine system is modulated by the circulating sex hormones (Becker, Robinson, and Lorenz, 1982), but the effect is to modulate the rate rather than the direction of rotation.

Turning preferences can be measured in other contexts. For example, left or right side turning can be measured in a T-maze. Using this testing procedure, Castellano, Diaz-Palerea, Rodriguez, and Barroso (1987) found a stronger population lateralization for a right-side bias in male Sprague-Dawley rats (69% right-biased, 17% left-biased, and 14% without a bias). The dopamine levels of the nigrostriatal system influence the turning preferences in the T-maze also (Zimmerberg, Glick, and Jerussi, 1974). However, these neurochemical asymmetries in the motor control regions are probably modified by the perceptual or cognitive demands of the particular tests used to measure turning or rotation (see below). The influence of the task on emotional behavior might also influence the expression of the individual lateral biases for rotating determined by the dopamine levels in the nigrostriatal system. Denenberg (1981, 1984) has shown that the right hemisphere of the rat is specialized to control affective behavior. This form of lateralization is present as a population bias. In certain contexts, it may therefore interact with the individual lateralization of turning determined by the nigrostrial dopamine levels to cause a population bias in rotating.

Conversely, rats that circle to the right might differ from those that circle to the left in some more general aspects of behavior. In fact, right-rotating rats fail to learn to escape from a foot-shock and instead become "helpless," whereas left-circling rats avoid the foot-shock (Carlson and Glick, 1989). Affective behavior and the direction of rotation are linked in some way.

The asymmetry in dopamine systems of the mesencephalon is already present in neonatal rats and to a greater degree than in older rats (Rodriguez, Martin, and Santana, 1994). There is a gradual decline in the degree of asymmetry at the individual level with increasing age up to 60 days. A significant population bias for higher levels of dopamine on the left side occurred on day 30 only. Thus, one might expect changes in functional lateralities with age and a transient population bias on day 30.

Newborn rats display asymmetry of tail posture after they are released from being held with the tail and head in a line (Ross, Glick, and Meiback, 1981). Female pups were found to have a population bias of 62% to the right, and males had no significant bias. As adults, the same rats were tested for rotation and a tail posture was found to correlate with the direction of rotation. The direction of tail posture, as for rotation, varies from strain to strain and between the sexes, but the correlation between tail posture and rotational direction is consistent (Denenberg, 1984; Denenberg, Rosen, Hofmann, Gall, Stockler, and Yutzey, 1982). Thus, tail posture might be a convenient measure to correlate with the changing laterality in dopamine levels in the developing neonate.

3.3 OTHER MAMMALIAN SPECIES

By contrast to circling in rodents, which in most studies has either a weak population bias for turning to the right or no population bias, the direction of turning or circling in other mammalian species is biased consistently in the same direction across individuals.

Ridgeway (1986) noted that dolphins in tanks and aquariums have a marked preference to swim counterclockwise and to favor the right eye. Ridgeway suggested that the dolphins might have dominance of the right eye. The counterclockwise preference for circling was confirmed by Sobel, Supin, and Myslobodsky (1994), who sampled 13 dolphins, *Tursiops truncatus*, in a pool and found that 85% of them swam consistently in the counterclockwise direction. Only during social interactions was the direction of this stereotyped swimming altered. (Informal observations by one of the authors indicate that humans also tend to walk around large enclosed spaces in a counterclockwise direction.)

Turning biases are indicated in some species of baleen whales by the distributions of barnacle encrustations (Mathews, 1978). There are fewer barnacles on the right side, possibly related to the observation that these species are also observed to swim near the bottom of the ocean with their right side downwards. As for dolphins, this is a bias present in the population as well as in individuals.

Side preferences apparently also occur in elephants, as indicated by more wear of one tusk than the other. The bias might be toward consistently more wear of the right tusk, although this needs to be confirmed (Warren, 1980).

Ungulates also exhibit turning biases at the population level. The presence of a greater number of scars, caused by aggressive encounters with conspecifics, on the right side of the skin of impala, *Aepyceros melampus*, indicates a turning bias during attacking or avoiding. Either the attacking individual is more successful with a left-side turn or the attacked individual turns broadside to present its right-side to the aggressor. Alternatively, both motor acts may occur within the same agonistic encounter. It is interesting to note that both forms of laterality would be for turning to the left side.

Domestic cows show a left-side preference for lying down (Uhrbrock, 1969; Wagnon and Rollin, 1972) provided that they are chewing (Grant, Colenbrander, and Albright, 1990). This posture may optimize the positioning of the rumen, which is placed asymmetrically in the body cavity. Such forms of side bias, though perhaps secondary to structural asymmetries in the viscera, could be scored in wild ungulates with relative ease.

4. LATERALITY OF LIMB USE

There have been many studies of preferences in use of the forelimbs to reach for food in rodents, some in cats and dogs, and only a few in marsupials. To our knowledge, there has been no investigation of hind-limb preferences in any species (other than birds, which are a special case), despite the fact that useful comparisons could be made between fore- and hind-limb use within the same subject.

4.1 RODENTS

When reaching for food, the majority of rats and mice prefer to use one forelimb consistently. This preference is referred to as "pawedness." In general, within a group of rodents there are equal numbers of individuals that are right-pawed and left-pawed, and a lesser number are ambidextrous. That is, there is no population bias equivalent to handedness in humans.

Collins (1975) has tested mice with a task that requires them to reach into a cylindrical tube attached to the front wall of the cage to obtain a food reward. Individuals of an inbred strain were found to be either strongly left-pawed or strongly right-pawed, and only few used both paws relatively equally. Thus, almost half the population was found to be lateralized in one direction and half in the other, and the females were more strongly lateralized than the males. The paw preferences were consistent over weeks and even months (Collins, 1985). Signore, Nosten-Bertrand, Chaoui, Roubertoux, Marchland, and Perez-Diaz (1991) have used the same procedure to test over 300 male and female mice of a variety of inbred strains and found the same results, but other strains tested by Betancur, Neveu, and Le Moal (1991) have been found to be only weakly lateralized. In the latter strains, the females were more strongly lateralized than the males.

In the tests described so far, the tube was placed in the center of the cage front so that each forelimb could be used with equal ease. Other mice were tested in conditions that made use of one or the other of the forelimbs more difficult by locating the feeding tube next to either the right or left wall of the cage. The distribution of paw preferences in the population was influenced by these external biases. With the tube next to the right wall, more mice were found to be left-paw preferent and vice versa, although a residual of approximately 10% retained the original paw preference. These results illustrate that environmental factors influence paw preference.

Genetic factors also influence the degree of lateralization, but not paw preference. It is possible to select genetically lines of mice for stronger or weaker lateralization, but not for more right-pawedness or left-pawedness per se (Collins, 1991).

The selection for a line of mice that is strongly lateralized ("high" line) was carried out by testing for paw preference, selecting animals that showed strong paw preferences, and then inbreeding them. This procedure was repeated over generations. Selection for the weakly lateralized line ("low" line) involved choosing mice that were ambidextrous and then inbreeding them. Significant line differences emerged by the third generation (Collins, 1991), and continued to increase with each subsequent generation. After 11 generations, each line was allowed to continue to breed at random within the line. The significant differences between the lines remained for at least a further 16 generations, showing that the determinants of the degree of lateralization were remarkably stable within each of the selected lines.

There is a relationship between paw preference and the corpus callosum (Schmidt, Manhăes, and de Moraes, 1991). In a strain of mice in which 20% of the pups are born with a very small corpus callosum, there is a significant left-paw bias (78%) at the population level. Hence, population lateralization emerges when there is a defect in the development of the corpus callosum. In other strains of mice, defects of the corpus callosum have a variety of different effects. Ward, Tremblay, and Lassonde (1987) reported that a smaller corpus callosum is associated with weaker paw preference in mice of the strain 129/J, but not in those of the strain BALB/cCF. Organization of the corpus callosum is also affected by the strength of lateralization of paw use (Cassells, Collins, and Wahlsten, 1990).

The complete absence of a corpus callosum weakens lateralization of paw preference. Gruber, Waanders, Collins, Wolfer, and Lipp (1991) tested a strain of mice which lacks the corpus callosum and found most of them to be ambilateral. This result supports Denenberg's (1981) hypothesis that the corpus callosum mediates lateralization by allowing one hemisphere to inhibit the other.

Other regions of the brain must also be involved in determining paw preferences, and several regions of the brain differ in size according to the degree of pawedness. Lipp, Collins, and Nauta (1984) measured asymmetry in cortical thickness in several regions of the cortex in the "high" and "low" lines of mice and selected over 11 generations for strong or weak degrees of paw preference. Individuals of the "high" line had larger asymmetries in four regions of the cortex than did the "low" line. In addition, the two lines could be differentiated by the asymmetries in the volume of the hippocampus, but no significant difference was found between the weights of the left and right halves of the brain in either of the lines (Cassells, Collins, and Wahlsten, 1990). However, overall brain weight does differ between the lines. Mice of the strongly lateralized line have heavier brains than mice of a weakly lateralized line (Ward and Collins, 1985).

The reasons for the difference in brain weight are unknown, but as the authors point out, it cannot be assumed that the causes are entirely genetic because the effect of selecting for strongly and weakly lateralized lines may have produced two groups which manipulate objects in their environment to different degrees. For example, the strongly lateralized line may interact more with the environment and so experience "environmental enrichment," a state which is known to alter cortical thickness and asymmetry (reviewed by Diamond, 1988).

Lateralized behavior may also be passed on from generation to generation by a process of learning. We have discussed the influence of physical bias in the environment on paw preference. Mice can learn lateralized behavior by observation (Collins, 1988). A "teacher" mouse was trained to open a door either on the right or the left side of a cage to obtain a food reward. Five mice watched the teacher from cubicles behind a barrier. Male, but not female, observers that had watched the teacher open a door on the left side performed sinistrally, whereas those that had watched the teacher open a door on the right side performed dextrally. Thus, observation learning may contribute to lateralized motor preferences. Possible influences of this kind on paw preferences have not yet been tested.

Pawedness can develop in response to reward. Weakly lateralized (ambilateral) rats rewarded by intracranial self-stimulation in the lateral hypothalamus for reaching into a feeder tube were found to shift their paw preference to use the paw contralateral to the stimulated side of the hypothalamus (Hernandez-Mesa and Burĕs, 1985). Paw preference of strongly lateralized individuals is not affected by this procedure. The authors concluded that because the reward affects integration of sensory and motor elements, motor asymmetries occur as a consequence of asymmetries in motivational and attentional mechanisms (also see below).

The tests described so far for pawedness in mice and rats have involved use of the paw to grasp food. Another form of unilateral paw use occurs in the Mongolian gerbil: the gerbil adopts a tripedal stance and holds one forelimb in the air, much like the pointing behavior of some hunting dogs. The paw is, therefore, not used to manipulate an object. Clark, Robertson, and Galef (1993) have scored limb preferences for this behavior, and the data presented in their paper show a left bias at the population level for males and right bias for females, although this was not clearly stated as such by the authors. Evidence was, however, given for an effect of uterine position adopted by the fetus (being next to males or females) and hence testosterone level on these preferences. For example, males that had been positioned next to females *in utero* are more right-limb preferent than males that had been positioned next to males and vice versa for females. A female positioned next to males is exposed to a higher testosterone level via the shared placental circulation. The preferred paw correlates with the eye that opens first, as we will discuss below.

4.2 BIRDS

Many species of parrots and cockatoos have strong preferences for using one foot for feeding (see Harris, 1989, for a comprehensive review of footedness in parrots). As the bias is present at a population level, the parrots are said to have "footedness." Most species examined so far are left-footed, but there are exceptions.

Friedman and Davis (1938) reported left-footedness for manipulating food objects in several species of African parrots, scored in captivity when feeding. The samples sizes in this study were, however, very small, but reanalysis of their data revealed that, of the 15 species which they listed, 7 had significant footedness. Six species were significantly left-footed and only one species, *Tanygnathus megalorhynochos*, was significantly right-footed (Rogers 1980).

Australian cockatoos and parrots also have footedness for manipulating food objects (Rogers 1981, 1989). A strong bias for left-footedness has been found in eight of the nine species, with an exception in the crimson rosella, *Platycercus elegans*, which showed right-footedness. Cannon (1983) has reported right-footedness in two other species of this genus, the eastern rosella, *Platycercus eximius*, and the pale-headed rosella, *Platycercus adscitus*. The reason why some species of parrot are right-footed while the majority are left-footed is not known. It may relate to the type of food eaten. When the parrot feeds by holding the food object in one foot, it also uses the beak to manipulate the food object, and it turns the head to view the food with the eye that is on the same side as the foot holding the food. If parrots have lateralization of visual perception, visual requirements may be associated with the limb used for holding food.

In parrots, only those species that feed while perched in trees use the prehensile-footed style — not those that feed predominantly on the ground. Nos and Camerino (1984; cited in Harris, 1989) studied five species of South American parrots and found that footedness was stronger when the parrots were perched above ground than when they fed on the ground. These researchers observed very few individuals from each species, but most were left-footed.

Footedness for manipulation of food objects also occurs in other avian species. Vince (1964) studied foot use of the great tit, *Parus major*, during feeding, by giving them a variety of food objects. The foot used to stabilize the bird against the perch was scored. Individuals showed significant foot preferences, but there was no population bias. Of the nine birds tested, three were strongly right-footed; two were less strongly right-footed; and four were strongly left-footed. The birds were also tested with objects of food tied to a length of string hanging in a glass cylinder. The great tits retrieved these objects by pulling up a loop of string with the beak, holding it with one foot, and pulling it again. A foot preference was found for each individual, but as before there was no population bias. A population bias of footedness has been found, however, for goldfinches, *Carduelis carduelis*, tested on a task requiring them to manipulate doors and catches using the beak and a foot in order to obtain a food reward (Ducker, Luscher, and Schultz, 1986). All the birds preferred to use the right foot.

Walker (1980) has stated a general hypothesis that preferential use of a limb occurs only in those species that use their limbs for manipulative tasks. Thus, footedness may occur only in those avian species that use their feet in feeding. Pigeons, for example, do not manipulate food objects with their feet, and Güntürkün, Kesch, and Delius (1988) have reported the absence of footedness in pigeons tested by sticking a piece of tape on the tip of the beak and scoring the foot used in the first attempt to remove it. No bias in foot use was found, at either the population or individual level. The lack of footedness in pigeons tested on this task is species rather than task specific because they tested a small number of parrots on the same task and found the preferred foot used to remove the tape was consistent with their footedness for manipulation of food objects.

Some individual pigeons do, however, display footedness in other situations. Davies and Green (1991) investigated foot use in pigeons during taking off for flight and landing. They tested the birds in a flight tunnel and scored foot use using frame-by-frame analysis of videotapes of these behaviors. Some individuals showed footedness for landing, although not for taking off. No population bias of footedness was found. The authors proposed that footedness may occur in landing as it is a more stressful maneuver, requiring fine visuomotor control. By contrast, removing a piece of sticking tape from the beak is not likely to be so stressful. Grooming movements are used and therefore the response may be entirely under proprioceptive control.

Budgerigars have also been tested for foot use in removing a piece of sticking tape from the beak (Rogers and Workman, 1993). They were chosen for the study because they are parrots, but they do not use their feet when feeding. Like the pigeons tested on this task, the budgerigars showed no foot preference either at the population level or as individuals. This supports the hypothesis that laterality occurs only when the feet are used to manipulate objects.

Chickens (*Gallus gallus*) do not use their feet to pick up and manipulate food or other objects, but they frequently scratch the ground when searching for food and may manipulate food objects against the substrate. Though both feet are used in ground-scratching, there is a significant tendency to initiate a bout of scratching with the right foot (Rogers and Workman, 1993). Moreover, the latter researchers found that when 10-day-old chicks were tested on the task requiring removal of sticking tape from the beak, an even stronger right-foot bias occurs (84%). Thus, active use of the feet in any manner for feeding or searching for food may lead to footedness in birds.

4.3 OTHER MAMMALS

As there have been few investigations of paw preferences in nonprimate mammals other than rodents, the other mammalian species will be considered under one heading.

Several studies have found a nonrandom distribution for use of the left and right paws by dogs and cats. Cole (1955) trained 60 cats to reach into a glass tube to obtain a piece of meat. If an individual used the same paw for 75% or more of the reaches, it was considered to have a paw preference, and 58% of the cats met this criterion; the remainder were ambidextrous. Of the cats which showed pawedness, 34% were right-pawed and 66% left-pawed (i.e., 20 and 38% of the total population, respectively). Another study of limb use in 16 cats found significant preferences in all of the subjects: 6 were right-pawed and 10 were left-pawed (Forward, Warren, and Hara 1962). In this study, the cats were tested on three different tasks, each requiring reaching for food from containers or obtaining food by moving a block aside. Paw preference was consistent across tasks for all subjects, indicating "pawedness."

Contrary to these results showing a predominance of left-paw preference over right-paw preference in cats, Tan, Yaprak, and Kutlu (1990) found a bias for right-paw preference. A further study by Tan and Kutlu (1991) using a larger sample size (109 cats, of which 63 were females and 46 were males) and a task requiring the cats to reach for food through a small hole in the middle of one wall of a cage, found that 50% were right-pawed, 40% were left-pawed, and 10% were ambidextrous. Thus, compared to the study by Cole (1955), a much higher proportion of these cats showed pawedness, but there was no significant difference between the proportions of left- and right-pawed individuals. In fact, the distribution of pawedness in this study is similar to that obtained for pawedness in mice and rats. However, a population bias did emerge when the sexes were examined separately. Although the distribution of paw preference for males did not differ from that of the entire population, significantly more females were right-pawed rather than left-pawed (54% of females were right-pawed and 36% were left-pawed; the proportion of ambidextrous individuals was the same as for males, 10%). Furthermore, significantly more females than males were strongly right-pawed. In a more recent study from the same laboratory, it was found that all of nine males were left preferent and all of 13 females were right preferent (Tan, 1993). In other words, cats might show a "right shift" in females. A similar pattern of right shift in females has been reported for lower primates and humans (Annett, 1985; Ward, Milliken, and Stafford, 1992).

The exact nature of the task may be another variable influencing choice of paw used. Moving targets, for example, may elicit responses controlled by a different hemisphere than stationary targets. In fact, moving targets appear to reveal left-pawedness. A left-paw bias has been found in cats tested using swiping movements to catch a piece of dangling string, 14 out of 17 cats having a left-paw preference (Burgess and Villablanca, 1986). Similarly, a more comprehensive study conducted by Fabre-Thorpe, Fagot, Lorincz, Levesque, and Vauclair (1993) found a bias for left-paw preference in cats trained to reach out for a moving spot of light. It should be noted that these were all male cats, a factor which may strengthen the left preference. Most of the cats showing lateralized limb use were left-paw preferent, but half of the subjects tested were ambidextrous. The lateralized cats had a faster reaction time than the ambidextrous ones and were more accurate. This important result suggests that lateralization of limb use may confer a functional advantage for limb speed and accuracy of limb use. It would be worth investigating other nonprimate mammals for similar effects.

A consistent right-paw preference occurs in dogs. Tan (1987) investigated forepaw use in a sample of 28 dogs by closing their eyes with sticking plaster and then scoring paw use in attempts to remove the plaster. The distribution of paw preference was 57% right-pawed, 18% left-pawed, and 25% ambidextrous. By extrapolation from the data for cats, the significant right-paw bias in the total sample may have depended on the preponderance of females in the sample, as there were 19 females and only 9 males in the sample. Furthermore, the result could have been influenced by arousal level, because this task would clearly have been stressful for the dogs. More studies on dogs using extra control procedures are needed to clarify these issues.

Moreover, environmental factors that may influence the development of pawedness in cats and dogs have been barely studied. It is known that once a paw preference has been established, it is maintained persistently even when the test imposes difficulties on use of the preferred paw (Warren, Cornwell, Webster, and Pubols, 1972). Forcing cats to use the nonpreferred paw in certain manipulative tasks does not affect spontaneous paw preference in other situations.

Limb use has only been studied in a limited number of species of marsupials, and this is unfortunate given that many species of marsupials have well-developed hands, some even with opposable thumbs. Megirian, Weller, Martin, and Watson (1977) investigated wild-caught Australian brush-tailed possums, *Trichosurus vulpecula*, reaching into a narrow feeding tube to obtain a food reward. Of the 78 possums they tested, 40 preferred to use the left forepaw, 35 preferred the right, and 3 were ambidextrous. Even with extreme paralysis of the preferred limb, the possums persisted in trying to use that limb.

There has been another brief mention of handedness in marsupials for koalas. Smith (1979) reported a 59% left-hand preference in koalas feeding on leaves, but the data are somewhat unreliable because although 140 observations were made, the study included 113 koalas, and no mention was made of whether the observations were for repeated data on individuals.

Further information on hand use in marsupials would make an interesting comparison with hand use in primates, particularly since many have similar feeding habits in similar environmental niches.

5. LATERALIZATION OF PERCEPTUAL SYSTEMS AND INFLUENCES ON MOTOR BEHAVIOR

Motor behavior may be lateralized without concomitant hemispheric specialization for perceptual processing, or lateralization of perceptual processing may lead to the lateralization of motor function.

5.1 BIRDS

As mentioned above, there is asymmetry in the organization of the visual system of the pigeon. The tectofugal visual system on the left side is more developed than that on the right side (Güntürkün and Melsbach, 1992; Melsbach, Hahman, Waldmann, Wörtwein, and Güntürkün, 1991). There are a number of known structural asymmetries in the tectofugal pathway; for example, the nucleus rotundus on the left side receives almost equal numbers of projections from the left and right optic tecta, whereas the nucleus rotundus on the right side receives inputs almost only from the right optic tectum (Figure 1.2). This means that the dominant left tectofugal system (to the left hemisphere) integrates information from both eyes, whereas the right one deals with information almost exclusively from the contralateral visual field (Güntürkün and Melsbach, 1992). The right eye is better able to discriminate grain from pebbles (Güntürkün, 1985, 1993) and recall memory of complex visual patterns presented along with hundreds of conflicting patterns (von Fersen and Güntürkün, 1990). This form of lateralization in the avian brain is present in adulthood, and unlike that for song, it is not influenced by hormonal condition in adulthood and does not change over time.

Until they are three weeks of age young chicks, *G. gallus*, also have structural asymmetry in the visual projections to the forebrain. In this case it is known to be present in the thalamofugal visual system (Adret and Rogers, 1989; Rogers and Sink, 1988; and summarized in Bradshaw and Rogers, 1993, and Rogers, 1995). Also, in this system there are more projections to the forebrain from the left side of the thalamus, stimulated by inputs from the right eye (see Figure 1.2).

Like pigeons, chickens learn to peck at grain scattered on a background of small pebbles in fewer pecks when they are using the right eye rather than the left (Mench and Andrew, 1986; Zappia and Rogers, 1987) and, when using the right eye, they have better acquisition and recall of a pattern discrimination task in an operant-conditioning situation (Gaston and Gaston, 1984). The left eye has superior performance on visual searching tasks that rely on topographical cues (Rashid and Andrew, 1989) and in recognizing other individual chicks — a familiar cagemate from a stranger (Vallortigara and Andrew, 1994). In general, the lateralized perceptual functions of the chick can be summarized as follows: the right eye system is specialized for categorizing stimuli and the left eye system for attending to the details of each individual stimulus. Consistent with this, chicks using the right eye respond to large changes in a visual imprinting stimulus, whereas those using the left eye respond to small changes in the stimulus (Vallortigara and Andrew, 1991).

Lateralized processing of perceptual information and memory storage has now been described for the food-storing bird, the marsh tit, *Parus palustris* (Clayton and Krebs, 1994a). As in chickens, the two-eye systems encode different types of memory that allow them to find hidden seeds. When the tits are allowed to store food using only the left eye and are tested later using the same eye, they retrieve food located at the correct spatial position even though other aspects of the stimulus are changed (Clayton and Krebs, 1994b). When they are allowed to store and then retrieve using the right eye only, they retrieve from a site with incorrect spatial cues but with all the other cues correct. That is, exactly as in the chick, the marsh tit attends to topographical cues only when using the left eye and uses texture, size, brightness, and other cues to recognize food objects with the right eye.

The perceptual asymmetries are known to influence some motor behaviors of the chick. Depending on its age, the chick opts to view an imprinting stimulus or other attractive stimuli with a preferred eye (Dharmaretnam and Andrew, 1994). On day 8, they choose to look at an imprinting stimulus or a hen with the right eye and on day 11 with the left eye. A less attractive stimulus (e.g., a small light) is viewed by the other eye in each case. This change in eye preference has been explained in terms of shifts in hemispheric dominance, as there is considerable evidence indicating that the left hemisphere (largely right eye) is dominant during the first week of posthatching life, and the right hemisphere assumes dominance temporarily around days 10 to 12 (Andrew, 1991; Rogers, 1986). Thus, motor movements of the head may be determined by perceptual asymmetries.

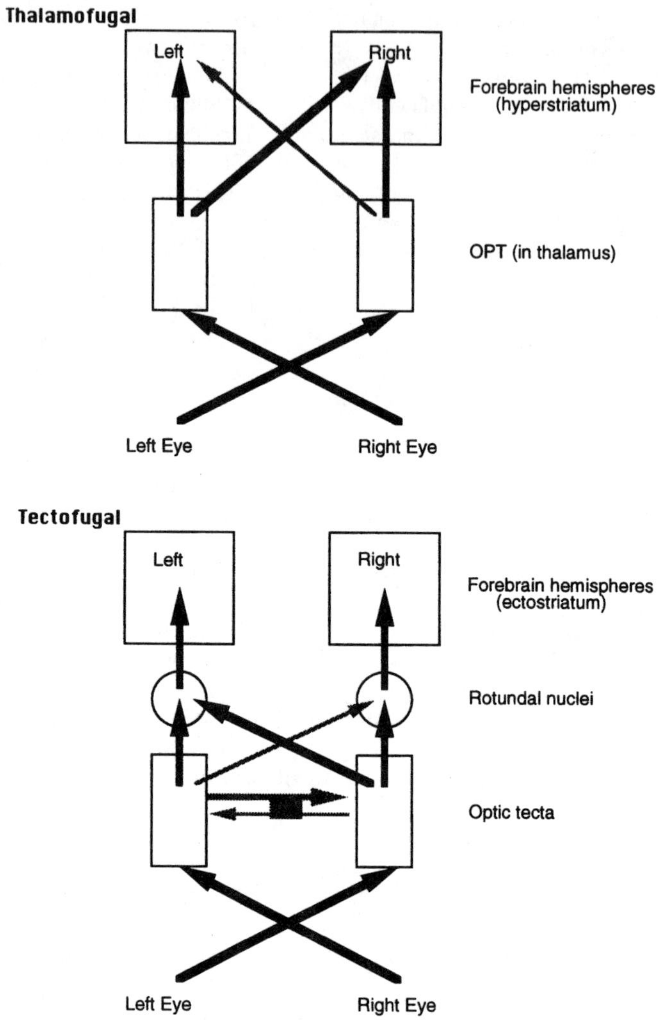

Figure 1.2 The tectofugal and thalamofugal visual systems in the avian brain are presented. The asymmetry in the thalamofugal system has been demonstrated in the chick: note that there are fewer projections from the right nucleus opticus principalis (OPT) of the thalamus to the left side of the forebrain than from the left OPT to the right side of the forebrain. The asymmetry in the tectofugal system has been demonstrated in the adult pigeon: note that there are more projections from the right optic tectum to the left nucleus rotundus than from the left optic tectum to the right nucleus rotundus. TC refers to the tectal commissure, and there is evidence that there are more projections from the left tectum to the right than vice versa.

Direction of turning may be similarly influenced by perceptual biases. A chick presented with an imprinting stimulus (a red ball) behind a barrier (a grid through which it can see the ball) chooses to detour to its left side to reach the ball, thereby keeping sight of the object with the right eye (Regolin, Pagni, and Vallortigara, personal communication, Jan. 1995). When the red ball is replaced by an unfamiliar blue ball, the chick chooses to detour in the opposite direction, keeping the ball in view of the left eye.

Chicks also display a preferred direction for turning or circling for courtship or copulating behavior. Following treatment with testosterone, a young chick circles a stuffed model of a crouching chick, which elicits copulation, in the counterclockwise direction, thus viewing the stimulus with its left eye (Workman, personal communication). This motor bias might be driven by lateralization of processing perceptual information because the mechanisms that control attack and copulation are lateralized in the forebrain (Rogers, Zappia, and Bullock, 1985). Paradoxically, the copulation can be elicited from testosterone-treated chicks using the right eye and not the left, whereas the chicks prefer to circle so that they view the model with the left eye. However, Workman did not measure the behavioral outcome of the courtship circling. It is possible that circling is maintained by viewing with the subordinate eye, leaving the right eye for use just prior to the act of copulation. In zebra finches, the courting male approaches the female so that she is seen by his right eye, as in chicks (Workman and Andrew, 1986).

The fact that chickens show right-footedness to initiate ground-scratching when searching for food correlates with the specialization of the right eye for making decisions about food vs. nonfood. Scratching of the ground is used to expose grains of food or insects, and the eye on that side connects to the neural systems that can make more rapid or accurate decisions about whether to peck or not.

The pigeon has the same lateralization of eye use for categorization of visual stimuli as does the chicken, and this is present at the population level, but it does not have footedness at the population level. As pigeons do not use the feet to scratch the ground while feeding, we suggest that a population bias for footedness (in both feeding and nonfeeding tasks) in avian species may develop secondarily to lateralization of visual functions at the perceptual level. Therefore, laterality of limb use may occur only in species which must coordinate eye and foot use in feeding or some other behavior. In other words, if the feet are used in feeding, laterality of foot use may occur as a result of the constraints placed upon the motor act by lateralization of perceptual or cognitive processes used to recognize and categorize food objects.

5.2 RODENTS

Turning preferences in other species as well as in chicks might also be influenced by eye preferences, rather than being exclusively determined by asymmetries in the dopamine levels in the nigrostriatal systems on the left and right sides of the brain (see above). It should be noted, however, that turning preferences in many strains of rodents, at least, are not strongly biased at a population level, unlike the turning choices described for chicks. Individual eye dominances may influence turning, but at least in the contexts in which the turning preferences of rodents have been measured, no overall effect of lateralized perception has an influence. This is so despite the fact that the same strains of rodents have hemispheric specialization for many functions (Denenberg, 1984; and summarized in Bradshaw and Rogers, 1993).

At the hemispheric level, rats have a consistent direction of lateralization for certain functions. By ablating either the left or right hemisphere of rats, it has been possible to demonstrate that activity levels are elevated in the handled rats following removal of the right hemisphere and not the left (Denenberg, Garabanati, Sherman, Yutzey, and Kaplan, 1978). Unilateral ablation or unilateral inactivation of a hemisphere by spreading depression has also revealed hemispheric specialization for the preferred direction of moving off in the open field (Sherman, Garbanati, Rosen, Yutzey, and Denenberg, 1980), for control of emotional behavior (Denenberg, 1984). Rats are similar to humans in terms of their superior ability to recognize sequentially presented visual stimuli by the left hemisphere and simultaneously presented stimuli by the right hemisphere (Bianki, 1988).

These lateral specializations have now been demonstrated in monocular testing, made possible by the fact that the optic nerves of rodents decussate almost completely (Lund, 1965). In this respect, and because they have laterally placed eyes, rodents are more similar to many species of birds than to mammals such as cats, monkeys, and humans. Monocular testing provides inputs almost exclusively to the contralateral hemisphere, although thereafter the ipsilateral processes may be involved because rodents have a corpus callosum connecting the left and right hemispheres. (This structure is not present in birds.) Even when rodents are tested binocularly, stimuli presented in the lateral, monocular field provide input to the contralateral hemisphere only.

Mittleman, Whishaw, and Robbins (1988) tested the reaction time of rats trained to hold their noses in a central hole in response to a light inside being switched on. A light cue was then presented on either the left or right side and the rat was required to move its head to the lighted side in order to receive a food reward. Their reaction time was shorter when the light was on their right side, indicating superior performance of the left hemisphere.

Monocular testing of rats in the Morris swim maze test has also revealed lateralization with a group bias. Adelstein and Crowne (1991) tested female Sprague-Dawley rats on this spatial learning task, and found that they performed better when using the right eye than when using the left. Their performance was measured in terms of latency to find the hidden escape platform using spatial cues and area over which the rat searched for the platform. This result would suggest left hemispheric specialization for performing this task, contradicting earlier evidence for spatial ability being a specialization of the right hemisphere in rats (Denenberg, 1984) as well as other mammalian species and birds (see above and review by Bradshaw and Rogers, 1993). In fact, another study using a different strain (Purdue/Wistar) of rat has found superior performance in the swim maze by handled, male rats using the left eye compared to those using the right eye (Cowell, Waters, and Denenberg, personal communication, Feb. 1995), and lesions of the parietal cortex in the right hemisphere result in greater performance deficits than do lesions of the left (Crowne, Novotny, Maier, and Vitols, 1992). Although these discrepancies remain unresolved, there is no question that the monocular visual fields of rats are specialized for processing different visual information and thus have different influences on motor responses. Unfortunately, to our knowledge there has been no published report of circling by rats tested in the swim maze, but a recent study by Patrech and Rogers (unpublished data) has found a directional bias for swimming in female Wistar-Kyoto rats during the acquisition of a task using visual cues in the swim maze: the rats swam past the visual cues in a clockwise direction. This might be considered as turning rather than circling. Unlike circling in the home cage, there may be a group bias for turning preference in the swim maze (i.e., either a predominance of rats with clockwise or counterclockwise turning preferences, but not equal representation of both preferences within the population), the preferred direction of turning being determined by use of spatial or other visual cues. Perhaps the absence of a group bias for the direction of circling in the home cage or in an open field occurs because no or fewer visual demands are made in these situations. The same would be true of Collins' (1985) apparatus for scoring circling of swimming in mice; a plastic container 12 in. in diameter does not compare to a much larger swim maze in which the animal is using spatial and visual cues. Only in contexts not requiring use of visual cues might the direction of turning be controlled entirely by the nigrostriatal system with its asymmetrical dopamine levels (see above). In fact, circling behavior in a featureless or a familiar environment is likely to be a form of displacement behavior, controlled by internal mechanisms rather than being guided by external cues. Involvement of higher cortical influences in other testing contexts may impose lateralization at a population level. In other words, we suggest that turning biases at a group level are more likely to occur if rats are tested with specific visual demands such as those already described for testing chicks. It is possible that some of the apparent species differences in individual vs. population biases for turning might be explained by relative differences in use of vision between tasks and species.

Perceptual processes are known to influence paw preferences in mice. These include inputs in the visual, somatosensory, and possibly also the olfactory systems.

Visual processes have been found to influence paw-preferences in mice, but only during the learning phase of a paw-preference test (Barnéoud, Bronchti, and Van der Loos, 1994). Application of an opaque contact lens to one or the other eye of mice trained to reach into a tube for food had no effect on paw-preference, but, after application of the monocular occluder before training, the mice learned to use the paw ipsilateral to the open eye. The latter group contained fewer ambidextrous mice than found following binocular training (Collins, 1985). The imposed lateralization of vision leads to pawedness. Information from one eye is processed primarily by the contralateral hemisphere, the same hemisphere that controls the paw ipsilateral to that eye. Apparently, acquisition of this task requires visuomotor coordination controlled by the same hemisphere, and this establishes the link between the eye and its ipsilateral paw.

Paw preference for "pointing" in gerbils (see above) may also be determined by visual processes during development. Clark, Robertson, and Galef (1993) have found a correlation between the paw preferred and the eye that opens first. In gerbils, eye opening is desynchronized by one or two days, somewhat longer than in rats or mice, and females open the right eye first, whereas males open the left eye first. Correlating with the order of eye opening, females prefer to point with the right paw and males with the left. As the pointing was measured at 60 days of age and eye opening occurs at around 14 days of age, one conclusion to be reached from these results is that early visual experience influences the development of paw preferences. Testosterone levels *in utero* also appear to play a role, since both first eye open and paw preference depends on the position of the pup in the uterus. Females that have been flanked by two males have a greater tendency to open the left eye first and later to point with the right paw, and vice versa for males (Clark, Robertson, and Galef, 1993). Thus, testosterone and early visual experience may interact to determine limb (paw) preference.

Paw preference may also be determined by lateralization of the whisker-to-barrel somatosensory pathway. Barnéoud and Van der Loos (1993) have shown that paw preference can be influenced by an asymmetry in the pattern of whiskers on either side of the muzzle. These researchers have bred two strains of mice with asymmetry of the whiskers, one with supernumerary whiskers on the right side, and the other with the same on the left side. This peripheral asymmetry connects to asymmetrical arrangement of the barrels in the somatosensory cortex (Tobet, Roca, and Crandall, 1993). The inbred strains of mice were tested for paw preferences for reaching into a tube, and compared to another inbred strain without asymmetry of the whiskers (Barnéoud and Van der Loos, 1993). Left- and right-paw preferent individuals were equally represented in this control strain. The strain with more whiskers on the right side had a higher proportion of left-paw preferent individuals than the control strain, and the strain with more whiskers on the left side had more right-paw preferent individuals. Within each of these lines, there were some individuals that expressed asymmetry of the whisker pattern opposite to that for which the particular line had been selected. These individuals were ambidextrous. This latter result indicates that there is some degree of linkage between pawedness and "whiskeredness," but the asymmetry in somatosensory input could have an important influence on the development of paw preference in the selected lines of mice. Thus, visual and somatosensory perception both determine paw preference. The relative importance of each of these perceptual systems is not known, nor is it known how important these systems are compared to olfactory perception.

Olfaction is an important, if not dominant, sense of rodents, and it can guide reaching for food and grasping it with a paw. In fact, one study has shown that the latter behaviors are disrupted to a greater extent by preventing olfactory perception rather than by preventing visual perception (Whishaw and Tomie, 1989). It is possible that olfaction also may exert a lateralized influence on paw preference. The volume of the olfactory bulb is larger on the right side (Heine and Galaburda, 1986), and ablation of the left olfactory bulb has a greater effect on the detection of a stress-inducing odor than ablation of the right (Dantzer, Tazi, and Bluthé, 1990). It is difficult to reconcile those two apparently contradictory results, although larger size may not necessarily mean better detection. Lateralization of olfactory perception occurs in humans also; for example, *n*-butanol is detected with greater sensitivity when the nostril ipsilateral to the preferred hand is used (Youngentob, Kurtz, Leopold, Mozell, and Hornung, 1982), and odor recognition is impaired to a greater extent by lesions to the right temporal or orbitofrontal cortex than the left (Jones-Gotman and Zatorre, 1993). Irrespective of the direction of lateralization, lateralization clearly exists in the olfactory system of the rat. Given that each olfactory bulb projects its ipsilateral hemisphere, olfactory cues detected by the left nostril would guide the right paw and vice versa. Thus, there may be left-right paw differences in accuracy or delay in reaching that occur under olfactory guidance. The link between olfactory input and motor output may occur via neural projections from the olfactory bulb to the prefrontal cortex, although this is not known (Cinelli, Ferreyra-Moyano, and Barragan, 1987). From their results showing that skilled limb use by rats is under olfactory guidance, Whishaw and Tomie (1989) have speculated that forelimb movement for reaching may have initially been under olfactory control, and that it was only later in evolution supplanted by visual control. In primates, vision appears to be the predominant sense used for reaching, and hand preferences may change with different visual demands for reaching.

For example, marmosets use one hand for simple reaching for stationary food objects and the other hand for moving targets (Hook-Costigan and Rogers, 1996). Nevertheless, the predominance of the olfactory, visual, or proprioceptive system in any species is likely to depend on the task and food-type presented. Under certain testing conditions, for example, marmosets may use their well-developed olfactory abilities (Epple et al., 1993), and rats may depend to a greater extent on vision and proprioceptive inputs. Evolutionary theories should also take into account that paws and hands are used for purposes other than feeding, and skilled limb guidance may have evolved for these functions as much as for reaching for and grasping of food.

Moreover, the lateralization of visual perception and visually guided behaviors in birds might indicate that skilled limb use evolved from a common ancestor of both birds and mammals. If so, that ancestor could have used predominantly vision to guide reaching. In other words, the ability of rats to use olfactory guidance for reaching may be a recent specialization of the species.

6. EXPERIENCE, HORMONES, AND LATERALIZATION

We have mentioned previously the close association in gerbils between the eye that opens first and the paw used to point (Clark, Robertson, and Galef, 1993). It is possible that the one to two days of monocular visual experience at a sensitive period of development provides the basis for the subsequent development of lateralizations, both perceptual and motor. A series of experiments with light exposure of the chick embryo underpin this suggestion.

For the last few days before hatching, the chick embryo is oriented in the egg so that the left eye, but not the right, is occluded by the chick's body (Rogers, 1986). The monocular experience received by the chick embryo determines the asymmetry in the visual projections from thalamus to forebrain (Rogers and Bolden, 1991; Rogers and Sink, 1988), and also the lateralization for categorizing food from nonfood, as well as for control of attack and copulation behavior (Rogers, 1982; Zappia and Rogers, 1987). Incubating eggs in darkness removes all of these asymmetries, and by manipulating the embryo so that the left eye is exposed to light and the right eye is occluded by an eye-patch, it is possible to reverse the direction of both the structural (Rogers and Sink, 1988) and functional (Rogers, 1990) lateralities. As yet, there has been no attempt to see whether motor asymmetries, such as those for turning or preferred use of the right foot in ground-scratching, are reversed similarly by exposing the left, instead of the right eye to light. However, the technique of reversed eye exposure to light would be an excellent way of determining the association between perceptual and motor asymmetries.

In pigeons, the asymmetry in the tectofugal visual system is also determined by light exposure of the embryo. Güntürkün (1990, 1993) found no asymmetry in the size of the cells in the optic tecta of pigeons incubated and raised in darkness, whereas the cells of layer 13 are larger on the right side in pigeons exposed to light as embryos. Thus, in two avian species, light influences lateralization.

The sex hormones also influence the development of asymmetry in birds. Elevated testosterone or estrogen levels during the sensitive period when the chick embryo responds to light prevents the development of asymmetry in the visual projections (Rogers and Rajendra, 1993; Schwarz and Rogers, 1992). Details of this effect of hormones have been covered elsewhere (Rogers, 1995). It will suffice to say here that light exposure and sex hormone levels interact to determine lateralization of visual function in the chick.

Similar interactions between sex hormones and visual experience appear to occur in the gerbil and presumably other species that open one eye before the other. Rabbits, for example, have been reported to open the right eye first (Narang, 1977), and handled rat pups to open the left eye first (Smart, Tonkiss, and Massey, 1986). Handling itself may alter hormonal state, as it is generally considered to be stressful. Handling unmasks in rats a preference to move off in a leftward direction when placed in an open field (Denenberg, 1981). Together with sex hormones, handling influences the development of the corpus callosum. For example, the size of the corpus callosum is larger in rat pups that have been handled and exposed to testosterone (Denenberg, Fitch, Schrott, Cowell, and Waters, 1991). Thus lateralization is affected, because the corpus callosum modulates lateral differences between the hemispheres.

The corpus callosum and other brain structures develop both prior to as well as after birth, and stress during gestation in rats is known to affect the development of lateralization. Wakshlak and Weinstock (1990) found that stressing rats during fetal development causes a left bias in directional preference but that handling reverses this effect.

Further elucidation of early environmental influences on the development of both perceptual and motor lateralities should assist our understanding of individual and species differences in laterality. The process of developing lateralization clearly involves complex interactions between genetic, hormonal, and environmental influences, and changing associations between different perceptual and motor lateralizations that depend on age, sex, and experiential factors.

Now that so many examples of lateralization have been reported for different species, it is clear that lateralization of perceptual and motor systems occurs throughout the various genera, and that the development of lateralization is subject to various environmental influences, and in many cases, to hormonal influences.

REFERENCES

Adams, C.L., Molfese, D.L., and Betz, J.C. (1987). Electrophysiological correlates of categorical speech perception for voicing contrasts in dogs. *Dev. Neurophysiol.*, 3, 175.

Adelstein, A. and Crowne, D.P. (1991). Visuospatial asymmetries and interocular transfer in the split-brain rat. *Behav. Neurosci.*, 105, 459.

Adret, P. and Rogers, L.J. (1989). Sex difference in the visual projections of young chicks: a quantitative study of the thalamofugal pathway. *Brain Res.*, 478, 59.

Andrew, R.J. (1991). The nature of behavioral lateralization in the chick. In R.J. Andrew (Ed.), *Neural and Behavioral Plasticity: The Use of the Domestic Chick as a Model.* Oxford University Press, Oxford, p. 536.

Annett, M. (1985). *Left, Right, Hand and Brain: The Right Shift Theory.* Hillsdale, N.J., Erlbaum.

Barnéoud, P. and Van der Loos, H. (1993) Direction of handedness linked to hereditary asymmetry of the sensory system. *Proc. Natl. Acad. Sci., U.S.A.*, 90, 3246.

Barnéoud, P., Bronchti, G., and Van der Loos, H. (1994). Vision influences paw-preference in mice. *Behav. Brain Res.*, 62, 157.

Bauer, R.H., (1993). Lateralization of neural control for vocalization by the frog (*Rana pipiens*). *Psychobiology*, 31, 243.

Becker, J.B., Robinson, T.E., and Lorenz, K.A. (1982). Sex differences and estrous cycle variations in amphetamine-elicited rotational behavior. *Eur. J. Pharmacol.*, 80, 65.

Betancur, C., Neveu, P.J., and Le Moal, M. (1991). Strain and sex differences in the degree of paw preference in mice. *Behav. Brain Res.*, 45, 97.

Bianki, V.L. (1988). *The Right and Left Hemispheres: Cerebral Lateralization of Function. Monographs in Neuroscience, Vol. 3*, New York, Gordon and Breach.

Bisazza, A., Cantalupo, C., and Vallortigara, G. (1995). Lateral asymmetries during escape behavior in a species of teleost fish (*Jenynsia lineata*). Submitted.

Bradshaw, J.L. and Rogers, L.J. (1993). *The Evolution of Lateral Asymmetries, Language, Tool Use, and Intellect.* San Diego, Academic Press.

Burgess, W.J. and Villablanca, J.R. (1986). Recovery of function after neonatal or adult hemispherectomy in cats. II. Limb bias and development, paw usage, locomotion and rehabilitative effects of exercise. *Behav. Brain Res.*, 20, 1.

Cannon, C.E. (1983). Descriptions of foraging behavior of eastern and pale-headed rosellas. *Bird Behav.*, 4, 63.

Cantalupo, C., Bisazza, A., and Vallortigara, G. (1994). Preliminary evidence of lateral asymmetries in lower vertebrates. *Boll. Zool.*, Supp., 28.

Cantalupo, C., Bisazza, A., and Vallortigara, G. (1995a). Lateralization of a predator-evasion response in a teleost fish (*Girardinus falcatus*). *Neuropsychologia*, 33(12), 1637.

Cantalupo, C., Bisazza, A., and Vallortigara, G. (1995b). Eye use during aggressive and courtship behavior in the siamese fighting-fish (*Betta splendens*). *Physiolog. Behav.*, in press.

Carlson, J.N. and Glick, S.D. (1989). Cerebral lateralization as a source of interindividual differences in behavior. *Experimentia*, 45, 788.

Cassells, B., Collins, R.L., and Wahlsten, D. (1990). Path analysis of sex difference, forebrain commissure area and brain size in relation to degree of laterality of selectively bred mice. *Brain Res.*, 529, 50.

Castellano, M.A., Diaz-Palarea, M.D., Rodriguez, M., and Barroso, J. (1987). Lateralization in male rats and dopaminergic system: evidence of right-side population bias. *Physiol. Behav.*, 40, 607.

Cinelli, A.R., Ferreyra-Moyano, H., and Barragan, E. (1987). Reciprocal functional connections of the olfactory bulbs and other olfactory related areas with the prefrontal cortex. *Brain Res. Bull.*, 19, 639.

Clark, M.M., Robertson, R.K., and Galef, B.G., Jr. (1993). Intrauterine position effects on sexually dimorphic asymmetries of mongolian gerbils: testosterone, eye opening, and paw preference. *Dev. Psychobiol.*, 26, 185.

Clayton, N.S. and Krebs, J.R. (1994a). One-trial associative memory: Comparison of food-storing and nonstoring species of birds. *Anim. Learn. Behav.*, 22(4), 366.

Clayton, N.S. and Krebs, J.R. (1994b). Memory for spatial and object-specific cues in food-storing and non-storing birds. *J. Comp. Physiol.*, 174, 371.

Cole, J. (1955). Paw preference in cats related to hand preference in animals and man. *J. Comp. Physiol. Psychol.*, 48, 137.

Collins, R.L. (1975). When left-handed mice live in right-handed worlds. *Science*, 18, 181.

Collins, R.L. (1985). On the inheritance of direction and degree of asymmetry. In S.D. Glick (Ed.), *Cerebral Lateralization in Nonhuman Species* New York, Academic Press, 41.

Collins, R.L. (1988). Observational learning of a left-right behavioral asymmetry in mice (*Mus musculus*). *J. Comp. Psychol.*, 102, 222.

Collins, R.L. (1991). Reimpressed selective breeding for lateralization of handedness in mice. *Brain Res.*, 564, 194.

Crowe, D.P., Novotny, M.F., Maier, S.E., and Vitols, R. (1992). Effects of unilateral parietal lesions on spatial localization in the rat. *Behav. Neurosci.*, 106, 808.

Cynx, J., Williams, H., and Nottebohm, F. (1992). Hemispheric differences in avian song discrimination. *Proc. Natl. Acad. Sci. U.S.A.*, 89, 1372.

Dantzer, R., Tazi, A., and Bluthé, R-M. (1990). Cerebral lateralization of olfactory-mediated affective processes in rats. *Behav. Brain Res.*, 40, 53.

Davies, M.N.O. and Green, P.R. (1991). Footedness in pigeons, or simply sleight of foot? *Anim. Behav.*, 42, 311.

Denenberg, V.H. (1981). Hemispheric laterality in animals and the effects of early experience. *Behav. Brain Sci.*, 4, 1.

Denenberg, V.H. (1984). Behavioural asymmetry. In N. Geschwind and A.M. Galaburda (Eds.), *Cerebral Dominance: The Biological Foundations*, Cambridge, MA, Harvard University Press, 114.

Denenberg, V.H., Fitch, R.H., Schrott, L.M., Cowell, P.E., and Waters, N.S. (1991). Corpus callosum: interactive effects of infantile handling and testosterone in the rat. *Behav. Neurosci.*, 105, 562.

Denenberg, V.H., Garbanati, J.A., Sherman, G., Yutzey, D.A., and Kaplan, R. (1978). Infantile stimulation induces brain lateralization in rats. *Science*, 201, 1150.

Denenberg, V.H., Rosen, G.D., Hofmann, M., Gall, J., Stockler, J., and Yutzey, D.A. (1982). Neonatal postural asymmetry and sex differences in the rat. *Dev. Brain Res.*, 2, 417.

Dharmaretnam, M. and Andrew, R.J. (1994). Age- and stimulus-specific use of right and left eyes by the domestic chick. *Anim. Behav.*, 48, 1395.

Diamond, M.C. (1988). *Enriching Heredity: The Impact of the Environment on the Anatomy of the Brain.* New York, The Free Press.

Divenyi, P.L. and Efron, R. (1979). Spectral vs. temporal features in dichotic listening. *Brain Lang.*, 7, 375.

Ducker, G., Luscher, C., and Schultz, P. (1986). Problemlöseverhalten von Stieglitzen (*Carduelis carduelis*) bei "manipulativen" Aufgaben. *Zool. Beitr.*, 23, 377.

Ehret, G. (1987). Left hemisphere advantage in the mouse brain for recognizing ultrasonic communication cells. *Nature*, 325, 249.

Epple, G., Belcher, A.M., Küderling, I., Zeller, U., Scolnick, L., Greenfield, K.L., and Smith III, A.B. (1993). Making sense out of scents: species differences in scent glands, scent marking behavior, and scent-mark composition in the Callitrichidae. In A.B. Ryland (Ed.), *Marmosets and Tamarins: Systematics, Behavior, and Ecology* Oxford, Oxford University Press, 123.

Fabre-Thorpe, M., Fagot, J., Lorincz, E., Levesque, F., and Vauclair, J. (1993). Laterality in cats: paw preference and performance in a visuomotor activity. *Cortex*, 29, 15.

Fersen, L. von and Güntürkün, O. (1990). Visual memory lateralization in pigeons. *Neuropsychologia*, 28, 1.

Fitch, R.H., Brown, C.P., O'Connor, K., and Tallal, P. (1993). Functional lateralization for auditory temporal processing in male and female rats. *Behav. Neurosci.*, 107, 844.

Forward, E., Warren, J.M., and Hara, K. (1962). The effects of unilateral lesions in sensorimotor cortex on manipulation by cats. *J. Comp. Physiol. Psychol.*, 55, 1130.

Friedman, H. and Davis, M. (1938). "Left-handedness" in parrots. *Auk*, 80, 478.

Gaston, K.E. and Gaston, M.G. (1984). Unilateral memory after binocular discrimination training: Left hemisphere dominance in the chick? *Brain Res.*, 303, 190.

Glick, S.D. and Cox, R.D. (1978). Nocturnal rotation in normal rats: Correlation with amphetamine-induced rotation and effects of nigrostriatal lesions. *Brain Res.*, 150, 149.

Glick, S.D. and Ross, D.A. (1981). Right-sided population bias and lateralization of activity in normal rats. *Brain Res.*, 205, 222.

Glick, S.D. and Shapiro, R.M. (1985). Functional and neurochemical mechanisms of cerebral lateralization in rats. In S.D. Glick (Ed.), *Cerebral Lateralization in Nonhuman Species*, New York, Academic Press, 158.

Goller, F. and Suthers, R.A. (1995). Implications for lateralization of bird song from unilateral gating of bilateral motor patterns. *Nature*, 373, 63.

Gonçalves, E. and Hoshino, K. (1990a). Behavioral lateralization in the freshwater fish, Oreochromis niloticus. Abstract translated from the *Annals of the 5th Annual Meeting of the Federation of Brazilian Societies for Experimental Biology* (FESBE), p. 25.

Gonçalves, E. and Hoshino, K. (1990b). Lateralized behavior of Nile tilapia in natural conditions. Abstract translated from the *Annals of the 5th Annual Meeting of the Federation of Brazilian Societies for Experimental Biology* (FESBE), p. 423.

Grant, R.J., Colenbrander, V.F., and Albright, J.L. (1990). Effect of particle size of forage and rumen cannulation upon chewing activity and laterality in dairy cows. *J. Dairy Sci.*, 73, 3158.

Gruber, D., Waanders, R., Collins, R.L., Wolfer, D.P., and Lipp, H-P. (1991). Weak or missing paw lateralization in a mouse strain (I/LnJ) with congenital absence of the corpus callosum. *Behav. Brain Res.*, 46, 9.

Güntürkün, O. (1985). Lateralization of visually controlled behavior in pigeons. *Physiol. Behav.*, 34, 575.

Güntürkün, O. (1990). Embryonale Orientierung als Ontogenetischer Auslöser für Visuelle Lateralization. In D. Frey (Ed.), *Bericht über den 37. Kongress der Deutschen Gesellschaft für Psychologie in Kiel 1990, Band 1* Verlag für Psyschologie, 51.

Güntürkün, O. (1993). The ontogeny of visual lateralization. *Germ. J. Psychol.*, 17, 276.

Güntürkün, O. and Melsbach, G. (1992). Asymmetric tecto-rotundal projections in pigeons: Cues to the origin of lateralized binocular integration. In N. Elsner and D.W. Richter (Eds.), *Rythmogenesis in Neurons and Networks*, Proceedings of the 20th Göttingen Neurobiology Conference, Vol. 20.

Güntürkün, O., Kesch, S., and Delius, J.D. (1988). Absence of footedness in domestic pigeons. *Anim. Behav.*, 36, 602.

Harris, L.J. (1989). Footedness in parrots: three centuries of research, theory, and mere surmise. *Can. J. Psychol.*, 43, 369.

Hartley, R.J. and Suthers, R.A. (1990). Lateralization of syringeal function during song production in the canary. *J. Neurobiol.*, 21, 1236.

Heine, O. and Galaburda, A.M. (1986). Olfactory asymmetry in the rat brain. *Exp. Neurol.*, 91, 392.

Hernandez-Mesa, N. and Burěs. (1985). Lateralized rewarding brain stimulation affects forepaw preference in rats. *Physiol. Behav.*, 34, 495.

Holman, S.D. and Hutchinson, J.B. (1991). Lateralized action of androgen on development of behavior and brain sex differences. *Brain Res. Bull.*, 27, 261.

Holman, S.D. and Hutchinson, J.B. (1993). Lateralization of a sexually dimorphic brain area associated with steroid-sensitive behavior in the male gerbil. *Behav. Neurosci.*, 107, 186.

Hook-Costigan, M. and Rogers, L.J. (1996). Lateralization of hand, mouth and eye use in the common marmoset (*Callithrix jacchus*). *Folia Primatol.*, in press.

Jerussi, T.P. and Glick, S.D. (1976). Drug-induced rotation in rats without lesions: behavioral and neurochemical indices of a normal asymmetry in nigrostriatal function. *Psychopharmacology*, 47, 249.

Jones-Gotman, M. and Zatorre, R.J. (1993). Odor recognition memory in humans: role of right temporal and orbitofrontal regions. *Brain Cognit.*, 22, 182.

Konishi, M. (1994). An outline of recent advances in bird song neurobiology. *Brain Behav. Evol.*, 44, 279.

Lemon, R.E. (1973). Nervous control of the syrinx of white-throated sparrows (Zonotrichia albicollis), *J. Zool.*, 171, 131.

Lipp, H-P., Collins, R.L., and Nauta, W.J.H. (1984). Structural asymmetries in brains of mice selected for strong lateralization. *Brain Res.*, 310, 393.

Lund, R.D. (1965). Uncrossed visual pathways of hooded and albino rats. *Science*, 149, 1506.

Margolaish, D. and Fortune, E.J. (1992). Temporal and harmonic combination-sensitive neurons in the zebra finch's HVc. *J. Neurosci.*, 12, 4309.

Margoliash, D., Fortune, E.S., Sutter, M.L., Yu, A.C., Wren-Hardin, B., and Dave, A. (1994). Distributed representation in the song system of oscines: evolutionary implications and functional consequences. *Brain Behav. Evol.*, 44, 247.

Mathews, L.J. (1978). *The Natural History of the Whale*. London, Weidenfeld and Nicholson.

McCasland, J.S. and Konishi, M. (1981). Interactions between auditory and motor activities in an avian song control nucleus. *Proc. Natl. Acad. Sci., U.S.*, 78, 7815.

Megirian, D., Weller, L., Martin, G.F., and Watson, C.R.R. (1977). Aspects of laterality in the marsupial *Trichosurus vulpecula* (brush-tailed possum). *Ann. N. Y. Acad. Sci.*, 299, 197.

Melsbach, G., Hahmann, U., Waldmann, C., Wörtwein, G., and Güntürkün, O. (1991). Morphological asymmetries of the optic tectum of the pigeon. In N. Elsner and H. Penzlin (Eds.), *Synapse-transmission-modulation*, Stuttgart, Thiem, 553.

Mench, J.A. and Andrew, R.J. (1986). Lateralization of a food search task in the domestic chick. *Behav. Neural Biol.*, 46, 107.

Mittleman, G., Whishaw, I.Q., and Robbins, T.W. (1988). Cortical lateralization of function in rats in a visual reaction time task. *Behav. Brain Res.*, 31, 29.

Morgan, S., Nomikos, G., and Huston, J.P. (1993). Behavioral analysis of asymmetries induced by unilateral 6-OHDA injections into the substantia nigra. *Behav. Neural Biol.*, 60, 241.

Narang, H.K. (1977). Right-left asymmetry of myelin development in epiretinal portion of rabbit optic nerve. *Nature*, 266, 855.

Nordeen, E.J. and Yahr, P. (1982). Hemispheric asymmetries in the behavioral and hormonal effects of sexually differentiating mammalian brain. *Science*, 218, 391.

Nottebohm, F. (1970). Ontogeny of bird song. Science, 167, 950.

Nottebohm, F. (1971). Neural lateralization of vocal control in a Passerine bird. I. Song. *J. Exp. Zool.*, 177, 229.

Nottebohm, F. (1972). Neural lateralization of vocal control in a passerine bird. II. Sub-song, calls, and a theory of vocal learning. *J. Exp. Zool.*, 179, 35.

Nottebohm, F. (1977). Asymmetries in neural control of vocalization in the canary. In S. Harnard, R.W. Doty, L. Goldstein, J. Jaynes and G. Krauthamer (Eds.), *Lateralization in the Nervous System*. New York, Academic Press, 23.

Nottebohm, F. (1980). Brain pathways for vocal learning in birds: a review of the first 10 years. In J.M. Sprague and A.N. Epstein (Eds.), *Progress in Psychobiology,* New York, Academic Press, 85.

Nottebohm, F. (1981). Laterality, seasons and space govern the learning of a motor skill. *Trends Neurosci.*, 4, 104.

Nottebohm, F. (1987). Plasticity in adult avian central nervous system: possible relation between hormones, learning, and brain repair. In V.B. Mountcastle, F. Plum and S.R. Geiger (Eds.), *Handbook of Physiology V; Section I. The Nervous System*, Maryland, American Physiological Society, 85.

Nottebohm, F. (1989). From bird song to neurogenesis. *Sci. Am., Feb.*, 55.

Nottebohm, F., Alvarez-Buylla, A., Cynx, J., Kirn, J., Ling, C-Y., Nottebohm, M., Sutter, R., Tolles, A., and Williams, H. (1990). Song learning in birds: The relation between perception and production. *Phil. Trans. R. Soc. London Ser. B*, 329, 115.

Nottebohm, F. and Nottebohm, M.E. (1976). Left hypoglossal dominance in the control of canary and white-crowned sparrow song. *J. Comp. Physiol.*, 108, 171.

Nottebohm, F., Kasparian, S., and Pandazis, C. (1981). Brain space for a learned task. *Brain Res.*, 213, 99.

Nottebohm, F., Manning, E., and Nottebohm, M.E. (1979). Reversal of hypoglossal dominance in canaries following unilateral syringeal denervation. *Comp. Physiol.*, 134, 227.

Nottebohm, F., Stokes, T.M., and Leonard, C.M. (1976). Central control of song in the canary, *Serinus canarius*. *J. Comp. Neurol.*, 165, 457.

Nowicki, S. and Capranica, R.R. (1986) Bilateral syringeal interaction in vocal production of an oscine bird sound. *Science*, 231, 1297.

Rashid, N. and Andrew, R.J. (1989). Right hemisphere advantage for topographical orientation in the domestic chick. *Neuropsychologia*, 27, 937.

Reist, J.D., Bodaly, R.A., Fudge, R.J.P., Cash, K.J., and Stevens, T.V. (1987). External scarring of whitefish, *Coregonus nasus* and *C. clupeaformis* complex, from the western Northwest Territories, Canada. *Can. J. Zool.*, 65, 1230.

Ridgeway, S.H. (1986). Physiological observation on dolphins' brains. In R.J. Schusterman, J.A. Thomas and F.G. Wood (Eds.), *Dolphin Cognition and Behavior: A Comparative Approach* , Hillsdale, N.J., Erlbaum, 31.

Robinson, T.E. (1985). Variation in the pattern of behavioral and brain asymmetries due to sex differences. In S.D. Glick (Ed.), *Cerebral Lateralization in Nonhuman Species* , New York, Academic Press, 185.

Robinson, T.E. and Becker, J.B. (1981). Variation in lateralization: selected examples do not a population make. *Brain Sci.*, 4, 34.

Rodriguez, M., Martin, L., and Santana, C. (1994). Ontogenic development of brain asymmetry in dopaminergic neurons. *Brain Res. Bull.*, 33, 163.

Rogers, L.J. (1980). Lateralization in the avian brain. *Bird Behav.*, 2, 1.

Rogers, L.J. (1981). Environmental influences on brain lateralization. *Behav. Brain Sci.*, 4, 35.

Rogers, L.J. (1982). Light experience and asymmetry of brain function in chickens. *Nature (London)*, 297, 223.

Rogers, L.J. (1986). Lateralization of learning in chicks, *Adv. Study Behav.*, 16, 147.

Rogers, L.J. (1989). Laterality in animals. *Int. J. Comp. Psychol.*, 3, 5.

Rogers, L.J. (1990). Light input and the reversal of functional lateralization in the chicken brain. *Behav. Brain Res.*, 38, 211.

Rogers, L.J. (1991). Development of lateralization. In R.J. Andrew (Ed.), *Neural and Behavioral Plasticity: The Use of the Domestic Chick as a Model*, Oxford, Oxford University Press, 507.

Rogers, L.J. (1995). *The Development of Brain and Behavior in the Chicken*. Wallingford, Oxon, CAB International.

Rogers, L.J. and Adret, P. (1993). Developmental mechanisms of lateralization. In H.P. Zeigler and H-J Bischof (Eds.), *Vision, Brain, and Behavior in Birds,* Cambridge, MA., MIT Press, 227.

Rogers, L.J. and Bolden, S.W. (1991). Light-dependent development and asymmetry of visual projections. *Neurosci. Letters*, 121, 63.

Rogers, L.J. and Rajendra, S. (1993). Modulation of the development of light-initiated asymmetry in chick thalamofugal visual projections by oestradiol. *Exp. Brain Res.*, 93, 89.

Rogers, L.J. and Sink, H.S. (1988). Transient asymmetry in the projections of the rostral thalamus to the visual hyperstriatum of the chicken, and reversal of its direction by light exposure. *Exp. Brain Res.*, 70, 378.

Rogers, L.J. and Workman, L. (1989). Light exposure during incubation affects competitive behavior in domestic chicks. *Appl. Anim. Behav. Sci.*, 23, 187.

Rogers, L.J. and Workman, L. (1993). Footedness in birds. *Anim. Behav.*, 45, 409.

Rogers, L.J., Zappia, J.V., and Bullock, S.P. (1985). Testosterone and eye-brain asymmetry for copulation in chickens. *Experientia*, 1, 1447.

Ross, D.A., Glick, S.D., and Meibach, R.C. (1981). Sexually dimorphic brain and behavioral asymmetries in the neonatal rat. *Proc. Natl. Acad. Sci., U.S.*, 78, 1958.

Schmidt, S.L., Manhaeš, A., and de Moraes, V.Z. (1991). The effects of total and partial callosal agenesis on the development paw preference performance in the BALB/cCF mouse. *Brain Res.*, 545, 123.

Schwarz, I.M. and Rogers, L.J. (1992). Testosterone: a role in the development of brain asymmetry in the chick. *Neurosci. Letters*, 146, 167.

Sherman, G.F., Garbanati, J.A., Rosen, G.D., Yutzey, D.A., and Denenberg, V.H. (1980). Brain and behavioral asymmetries for spatial preferences in rats. *Brain Res.*, 192, 61.

Signore, P., Nosten-Bertrand, M., Chaoui, M., Roubertoux, P.L., Marchland, C., and Perez-Diaz, F. (1991). An assessment of handedness in mice. *Physiol. Behav.*, 49, 701.

Smart, J.L., Tonkiss, J., and Massey, R.F. (1986). A phenomenon: Left-biased asymmetrical eye-opening in artificially reared rat pups. *Dev. Brain Res.*, 28, 134.

Smith, M. (1979). Behaviour of the koala, *Phascolarctos cinereus* Goldfuss, in captivity, I. Non-social behavior. *Aust. Wildlife Res.*, 6, 117.

Sobel, N., Supin, A.Ya., and Myslobodsky, M.S. (1994). Rotational swimming tendencies in the dolphin (*Tursiops truncatus*). *Behav. Brain Res.*, 65, 41.

Suthers, R.A. (1990). Contributions to birdsong from the left and right sides of the intact syrinx. *Nature*, 347, 473.

Tan, Ü. (1987). Paw preferences in dogs. *Int. J. Neurosci.*, 32, 825.

Tan, Ü. (1993). Distribution of paw preference in mongrel and tortoise-shell cats and the relation of hemispheric weight to paw preference: Sexual dimorphism in paw use and its relation in hemispheric weight. *Int. J. Neurosci.*, 70, 199.

Tan, Ü. and Kutlu, N. (1991). The distribution of paw preference in right-, left-, and mixed pawed male and female cats: The role of a female right-shift factor in handedness. *Int. J. Neurosci.*, 59, 219.

Tan, Ü., Yaprak, M., and Kutlu, N. (1990). Paw preference in cats: Distribution and sex differences. *Int. J. Neurosci.*, 50, 195.

Tobet, S.A., Roca, A.L., and Crandall, J.E. (1993). Cellular organization in rat somatosensory cortex: Effects of sex and laterality. *Exp. Neurol.*, 121, 65.

Uhrbrock, R.S. (1969). Bovine laterality. *J. Gen. Psychol.*, 115, 77.

Vallortigara, G. and Andrew, R.J. (1991). Lateralization of response by chicks to change in a model partner. *Anim. Behav.*, 41, 187.

Vallortigara, G. and Andrew, R.J. (1994). Differential involvement of right and left hemisphere in individual recognition in the domestic chick. *Behav. Process.*, 33, 41.

Vicario, D.S. (1994). Motor mechanisms relevant to auditory-vocal interactions in songbirds. *Brain Behav. Evol.*, 44, 265.

Vicario, D.S. and Yohay, K.H. (1993). Song-selective auditory input to a forebrain vocal control nucleus in the zebra finch. *J. Neurobiol.*, 24, 488.

Vince, M.A. (1964). Use of the feet in feeding by the Great Tit, *Parus major. Ibis*, 106, 500.

Wagnon, K.A. and Rollin, W.C. (1972). Bovine laterality. *J. Anim. Sci.*, 35, 486.

Wakshlak, A. and Weinstock, M. (1990). Neonatal handling reverses behavioral abnormalities induced in rats by prenatal stress. *Physiol. Behav.*, 48, 289.

Walker, S.F. (1980). Lateralization of function in the vertebrate brain: A review. *Br. J. Psychol.*, 71, 329.

Ward, R. and Collins, R.L. (1985). Brain size and shape in strongly and weakly lateralized mice. *Brain Res.*, 328, 243.

Ward, R., Tremblay, L., and Lassonde, M. (1987). The relationship between callosal variation and lateralization in mice is genotype-dependent. *Brain Res.*, 424, 84.

Ward, J.P., Milliken, G.W., and Stafford, D.K. (1992). Patterns of lateralized behavior in prosimians, In J.P. Ward (Ed.), *Current Behavioral Evidence of Primate Asymmetry*, New York, Springer, 43.

Warren, J.M. (1980). Handedness and laterality in humans and other animals. *Physiol. Psychol.*, 8, 351.

Warren, J.M., Cornwell, P.R., Webster, W.G., and Pubols, B.H. (1972). Unilateral cortical lesions and paw preferences in cats. *J. Comp. Physiol. Psychol.*, 81, 410.

Whishaw, I.Q. and Tomie, J-A. (1989). Olfaction directs skilled forelimb reaching in the rat. *Behav. Brain Res.*, 32, 11.

Wild, J.M. (1994). The auditory-vocal-respiratory axis in birds. *Brain Behav. Evol.*, 44, 192.

Williams, H. (1990). Bird song. In R.P. Kesner and D.S. Olton (Eds.), *Neurobiology of Comparative Cognition*, Hillsdale, NJ, Erlbaum, 77.

Williams, H., Crane, L.A., Hale, T.K., Esposito, M.A., and Nottebohm, F. (1992). Right-side dominance for song control in the zebra finch. *J. Neurobiol.*, 23, 1006.

Workman, L. and Andrew, R.J. (1986). Asymmetries of eye use in birds. *Anim. Behav.*, 34, 1582.

Youngentob, S.L., Kurtz, D.B., Leopold, D.A., Mozell, M.M., and Hornung, D.E. (1982). Olfactory sensitivity: Is there laterality? *Chem. Senses*, 7, 11.

Zappia, J.V. and Rogers, L.J. (1987). Sex differences and reversal of brain asymmetry by testosterone in chickens. *Behav. Brain Res.* 23, 261.

Ziegler, M.G.M. and Szechtman, H. (1990). Relation between motor asymmetry and direction of rotational behavior under amphetamine and apomorphine in rats with unilateral degeneration of the nigrostriatal dopamine system. *Behav. Brain Res.*, 39, 123.

Zimmerberg, B., Glick, S.D., and Jerussi, T.P. (1974). Neurochemical correlate of a spatial preference in rats. *Science*, 185 623.

Zimmerberg, B., Stumpf, A.J., and Glick, S.D. (1978). Cerebral asymmetry and left-right discrimination. *Brain Res.*, 140, 194.

Chapter 2

Tool Use and the Evolutionary Development of Manual Asymmetry

John L. Bradshaw and Lesley J. Rogers

CONTENTS

1. INTRODUCTION

Until quite recently, humans were regarded as unique not only in terms of possessing consciousness, language, and tool use, but also as exhibiting asymmetries at a population level. While individuals in many species may display "handedness," or its homologs, analogs, or correlates, only humans, it was believed, shared the same preferential direction of asymmetry across the greater majority of individuals. Indeed the unique human possession of consciousness, language, praxis, and tool use was thought to be causally related to our manual and brain asymmetries, our predominant dextrality, and left-hemispace specialization for speech and fine manipulative control (Bradshaw and Rogers, 1993). That there may be causal connections between some or all such phenomena is now beyond reasonable doubt. However, it is also now beyond reasonable doubt that humans are *not* unique in possessing consciousness, language, tool use, or population-level asymmetries (see Chapter 1). A systematic attempt to explain newly-emerging evidence of primate handedness was first made by MacNeilage, Studdert-Kennedy, and Lindblom (1987, 1991). However, as we shall see, they do not account for the equally recent and significant evidence of far more ancient asymmetries, probably homologous to our own, in lower vertebrates.

0-8493-8999-2/96/$0.00+$.50

2. ASYMMETRIES IN THE PRIMATE VISUAL MODALITY

It is of course among the primates, especially the hominoids (apes and humans; for recent taxonomic considerations, see Andrews, 1992), that close parallels with human lateralization are both likely and significant. At a cognitive level, most of the visual studies have focused on face processing. This faculty ranks second, for us, to language in complexity and cultural significance (the recognition of individuals and of emotions, as well as nonverbal communication); in the nonhuman primates, given the complex social dynamics of chimpanzee (and many species of monkey) existence, it probably takes pride of place. Ifune, Vermeire, and Hamilton (1984) presented videotapes of monkeys, people, animals, and scenery to eight split-brain rhesus monkeys (*Macaca mulatta*); stimuli presented via the right eye to the right hemisphere elicited considerably more emotional expressions than when the left hemisphere was stimulated instead. We know of course that in humans the right hemisphere mediates many aspects of face processing (Benton, 1990; Sergent, Ohta, and MacDonald, 1992). Later, Hamilton and Vermeire (1985, 1991) found a strong right hemisphere superiority in (monkey) face discrimination, with a left hemisphere (i.e., right visual field) superiority for judgments of slope in a task where humans show a similar pattern of results (Mehta and Newcombe, 1991). Morris and Hopkins (1993) presented a series of photographically-combined composite human faces (one side smiling, the other side with a neutral expression) to three chimpanzees, after training them to indicate which of two normal faces displayed a smile. With pairs of composite faces where one member had the smile on the left half (side) of the composite, and the other member had it on the right, all three animals, just like humans in similar circumstances (Mattingley, Bradshaw, Phillips, and Bradshaw, 1993) consistently chose the composites where the smile lay to the left. At a *motor* level, Hauser (1993) found that free-living rhesus monkeys begin to display facial expressions earlier on the left side of the face, just as we do. Indeed, human subjects perceived composites of monkey faces created by pairing the left half (as "owned," not as viewed) with its mirror-reversed duplicate (i.e., ⌊ ⌋) as more expressive than composites made from ЯR pairings. Thus, as with humans, the right hemisphere seems preferentially to control facial expression; just as described in Chapter 1 in the contexts of chick and rat, it also has been reported (Fagot and Vauclair, 1994) to play a critical role in the processing of novelty by baboons (*Papio papio*). Therefore, shorter left than right visual half-field response times were found for novel (but not familiar) combinations of composite stimuli by six animals.

Recently, language-trained chimpanzees have been investigated in a number of studies designed to determine the possible role of lateralized communicatory mechanisms. Inevitably, subject numbers have been small in every case, making it difficult to generalize from the findings. Hopkins and Morris (1989) investigated lateralization for visuospatial processing in two such intact animals (*Pan troglodytes*) with presentations to one or the other visual field. The visual discrimination task involved the location of a short line within a geometrical form with a computer joystick response, and a left field (right hemisphere) superiority (reaction time) was observed. When priming was employed in a reaction time task with *meaningful* symbols used in chimpanzee-language experiments for interspecies (i.e., with humans) communication, *left* hemisphere activation apparently occurred in the two or three chimpanzees studied, whereas *nonmeaningful* symbols produced *bilateral* activation (Hopkins, Morris, and Savage-Rumbaugh, 1991; Hopkins, Morris, Savage-Rumbaugh, and Rumbaugh, 1992).

Visual lateralization in humans may also be indicated by eye dominance. Eye dominance refers to the consistent choice of a particular eye in tasks demanding the use of only one eye. Humans show a 65 to 70% right eye preference, measured in tasks such as sighting through a telescope or by determining the eye which dominates in binocular rivalry tasks (Porac and Coren, 1981). As shown in humans, an image remains visible for a longer time in the dominant eye and fades faster in the nondominant eye (Porac and Coren, 1982); objects appear to be larger when seen with the dominant eye (Coren and Porac, 1976); an image presented to the dominant eye is less likely to be suppressed by presenting a different image to the other eye (Sohmiya and Sohmiya, 1985); and judgments of apparent direction in egocentric localization are displaced towards the dominant eye (Porac and Coren, 1986). Sighting eye dominance shows a stronger relationship to language lateralization than does hand-use in writing (Bryden, 1988; Strauss and Goldsmith, 1987). Thus, eye dominance is somehow associated with specialization of the contralateral hemisphere for language: individuals who are left-eye dominant may make greater use of the right hemisphere and show superior ability to decode nonverbal cues (Domangue, 1984). Also, right-handed human males show greater verbal task accuracy during left-eye viewing and greater spatial task accuracy during right-eye viewing (Ádám, Szilagyi, and Lang, 1992).

Eye dominance does not appear to depend on peripheral differences between the eyes, such as in refractive index or functioning within the retina, but rather it seems to be associated with central processing (Porac and Coren, 1981). It is possible that the nature of the visual input to each side of the brain varies according to the eye used, as the crossed optic nerves from the nasal region of the retina have larger diameters and conduct faster than do the uncrossed fibers from the temporal retina (Bishop, Jeremy, and Lance, 1953), while lower sensitivity thresholds have been demonstrated for the temporal hemiretinae. To some extent, therefore, each eye sends a different input to each hemisphere, and so eye dominance may reflect lateralization of information processing.

There have not been many studies of eye dominance in primates, and the tasks used have been much simpler than those used for humans. Also, there has been no attempt to assess any potential influence of motor lateralization, such as the adoption of lateralized postures, on the eye preferences measured in monocular viewing tasks used. However, there are indications that primates show eye dominance as humans do. Cole (1957) has tested eye dominance in a small sample of macaques (*Macaca nemestrina*) by scoring the eye used in monocular sighting down a tube which had been baited with food. Out of the seven animals tested, five were right-eye preferent, one was left-eye preferent, and the other used binocular sighting. The same method was used by Kruper, Boyle, and Patton (1966) to test eye preference in *M. mulatta*; of the 19 subjects tested, 14 showed a significant preference for one eye, and 11 for use of the left eye. Smith (1970) devised a method for measuring eye dominance which involved differential training of each eye to respond to a red or green colored light by pressing a lever up or down for a food reward. Only one rhesus monkey was tested, and when presented with a conflict situation, it showed left-eye dominance. Eye preference has recently been measured in the small-eared bushbaby, *Otolemur garnetti*, by scoring monocular eye use for viewing a variety of stimuli through a grid (Rogers, Ward, and Stafford, 1994). The six subjects tested showed left-eye dominance for viewing the tester and for viewing food. The eye preference did not correlate with handedness for food reaching or holding in the same individuals. When the subjects viewed more arousing stimuli (e.g., their babies held in the tester's hand), the eye preference changed to either no preference or a weaker left-eye preference. Thus, eye preference may change with the nature of the stimulus viewed and/or the state of arousal of the subject. Common marmosets, *Callithrix jacchus*, also have a preferred eye for viewing food, but they choose the right eye (Hodgkinson and Rogers, 1994). Again, there was absolutely no correlation between handedness and eye preference. So far there are insufficient data to draw any conclusions about left and right eye preferences across species, but it may prove an interesting comparison with motor lateralities in the same individuals.

3. ASYMMETRIES IN THE PRIMATE AUDITORY MODALITY

Studies of auditory lateralization in nonhuman primates have a longer history and are more extensive than the visual studies. Dewson (1977) forced seven cynomolgus macaques (*Macaca fascicularis*) to form conditioned associations between acoustic and visual stimuli in an operant nonspatial auditory discrimination task, pressing a red panel to a pure tone and a green one to noise. Four animals with lesions in the left superior temporal gyrus (corresponding to Wernicke's receptive speech area in humans) performed very poorly, while two with damage to the right superior temporal cortex and one with damage to the primary auditory area of the left hemisphere showed no deficits. These differential laterality effects depended upon the occurrence of a variable delay between the auditory and the visual stimuli.

Pohl (1983, 1984) studied four baboons (*Papio cynocephalus*) in an auditory gap-detection task, in which it was hoped that such temporal resolution would be analogous to certain forms of consonant discrimination by humans. Humans have a right ear (left hemisphere) advantage. Of course, such material is meaningful only to humans. The animals also discriminated pure tones and three-tone musical chords in a task where humans might be expected to show a left ear (right hemisphere) advantage. The same three animals showed a clear left ear advantage (the fourth gave a clear right ear advantage) to the chords and the auditory gap-detection task. The small number of subjects and the lack of control over potential meaningfulness (see below) results in the need for caution in interpreting these findings too closely.

In an early study, but now in the context of a monkey's ability to discriminate species-specific vocalizations, (i.e., meaningfulness), Petersen, Beecher, Zoloth, Moody, and Stebbins (1978), found that all five Japanese macaques (*Macaca fuscata*) showed a significant right ear (left hemisphere) advantage in monaurally discriminating between two classes of species-specific "coo" sounds and not to other classes of sound (see also Petersen, Beecher, Zoloth, Green, Marler, Moody, and Stebbins, 1984, and Beecher, Peterson, Zoloth, Moody, and Stebbins, 1979). Moreover, macaques from a different species (*Macaca nemestrina* and *Macaca radiata*) to whom the *fuscata* sounds were not species-specific or, therefore, presumably significant, failed to show these asymmetries. Recently, Hauser, and Andersson (1994) reported that 61 out of 80 free-ranging adult rhesus monkeys (*M. mulatta*) favored the right ear (left hemisphere) in orienting towards species-specific vocalizations, with the reverse asymmetries for heterospecific calls. Infants failed to demonstrate such asymmetries, indicating the need for maturation and/or experience with species-typical calls for the asymmetries to manifest. Conclusions such as the above would suggest that left hemisphere lateralization may reflect processing of a communicatory significant nature, rather than merely an underlying specialization for sequential, analytic, time-dependent processing, though Bradshaw and Nettleton (1981) have presented contrary views.

Heffner and Heffner (1984, 1986) again trained Japanese macaques to discriminate between two subtypes of species-specific "coo" vocalizations. Five animals then received a unilateral left-temporal ablation in regions including the area equivalent to Wernicke's area in humans, a major language area, and five others a corresponding lesion on the right. Left but not right side lesions resulted in impaired performance.

In humans, the right hemisphere is thought to contribute to the discrimination of voicing contrasts (e.g.,/ba-pa/). Morse, Molfese, Laughlin, Linnville, and Wetzel (1987) presented rhesus monkeys with such stimuli. Electrophysiological indices showed that a late component of the average evoked response recorded over the temporal region of the right hemisphere of all 15 monkeys discriminated categorically between stimuli, just as occurs with humans.

4. MORPHOLOGICAL ASYMMETRIES OF THE PRIMATE BRAIN

Gross anatomical asymmetry of the human brain is visible even to the naked eye (Geschwind and Levitsky, 1968). The anterior portion of the right hemisphere and the posterior portion of the left protrude further and are wider than their counterparts (Bear, Schiff, Saver, Greenberg, and Freeman, 1986; Galaburda, LeMay, Kemper, and Geschwind, 1978; Weinberger, Luchins, Morihisa, and Wyatt, 1982), especially in dextrals and males. These effects may produce permanently visible impressions or petalias on the inner surface of the skull, and can be used in inferring brain structure (and, therefore, possible function) even in fossil material. Asymmetries in the periSylvian (speech related) cortex are prominent (Galaburda, 1984; LeMay, 1985). Thus, the Sylvian fissure separating the temporal from the frontoparietal regions is longer in the left hemisphere and continues further in a horizontal direction on that side before tending upwards (Rubens, Mahowald, and Hutton, 1976; Yeni-Komshian and Benson, 1976), especially in dextrals (Hochberg and LeMay, 1975; LeMay and Culebras, 1972). In consequence, the planum temporale, a major structure in the temporal speech areas, is larger on the left (Geschwind and Levitsky, 1968; Geschwind and Galaburda, 1985; Rubens et al., 1976; Witelson and Pallie, 1973). Just as in cats, dogs, and rabbits (Kolb et al., 1982), magnetic resonance imaging in humans also shows that the overall volume of the right hemisphere is larger than that of the left (Kertesz, Polk, Black, and Howell, 1990).

Many of these anatomical asymmetries also appear to some extent in Old World monkeys, suggesting their presence in a common ancestor. Thus, Cain and Wada (1979) found that six out of seven adult baboons (*Papio* spp.) possessed longer frontal poles on the right, the seventh showing no asymmetry.

LeMay, Billig, and Geschwind (1982) measured the endocranial casts of a considerable number of individuals and species of apes, as well as New and Old World monkeys. As in humans, the right frontal and left occipital poles were more prominent than their counterparts in chimpanzees and gorillas, but not in orang-utans. Old World monkeys showed similar though smaller effects; in the New World species the only significant effect was one of left occipital petalia. According to Holloway and de La Coste-Lareymondie (1982), who reviewed their earlier work on petalial asymmetries in a large number of living and extinct hominoids, *Gorilla* showed the greatest left occipital petalia, *Pan paniscus* an intermediate level, and *Pan troglodytes* and *Pongo pygmaeus* were symmetrical in this respect. Living and fossil *Homo* species (*Homo erectus* and *Homo sapiens neanderthalensis*) and two species of *Australopithecus* (*Australopithecus africanus* and *Australopithecus robustus*) showed fully modern patterns of asymmetrical frontal and occipital petalias, patterns which exceeded those of *Gorilla*. The hominid pattern seems therefore to date back to at least 3 million years.

Using more modern and sensitive three-dimensional techniques, Falk et al. (1990) succeeded in demonstrating frontal petalias similar to our own in rhesus monkeys, *M. mulatta*. Cheverud et al. (1990) extended these findings with rhesus monkeys to include some evidence for occipital petalias of the human pattern also.

Turning to the Sylvian fissure, Yeni-Komshian and Benson (1976) found that chimpanzees have longer fissures on the left, though not as markedly as in humans. Rhesus monkeys showed no such asymmetries, a conclusion echoed by LeMay and Geschwind (1975), who while finding such asymmetries in all three species of great ape failed to find them in either New or Old World monkeys. However, Heilbroner and Holloway (1988), with better controls and techniques, found that of two species of Old World and three of New World monkeys, only one of the latter had an overall length of the left Sylvian fissure that failed to exceed that of the right — and even then it did so if measurements were restricted to the anterior portion. They also noted that while macaques showed no Sylvian asymmetries posterior to the central sulcus, it is this region in humans, in the vicinity of the language-mediating temporal planum (a structure absent in other primates) that is most asymmetrical. This region may therefore have evolved shortly before the divergence of hominids from pongids.

5. MORPHOLOGICAL ASYMMETRIES OF THE LIMBS

5.1 HUMAN STUDIES

Schell, Johnston, Smith, and Paolone (1985) found that among 116 dextral white adolescents, biepicondylar breadth of the humerus was significantly larger on the right arm, consequent perhaps upon hypertrophy due to preferred use. Garn, Mayor, and Shaw (1976), though, found that the total cross-sectional length and cortical area of the second metacarpal was larger on the right irrespective of hand preference. Similarly, Plato, Wood, and Norris (1980) found that the total midshaft length, width, cross-sectional area, and cortical area of the second metacarpal bone was longer in the right hands of both dextrals and sinistrals, even though it only achieved significance in the former. Macho (1991) studied the femora of a large population of southern Africans; most dimensions (except anteroposterior diameter of proximal shaft, bicondylar width and collo-diaphyseal angle) were larger on the *left*, regardless of handedness, suggesting preferential use of the left leg for weight bearing and the right for other tasks, (e.g., kicking and foot overlapping). The fact that the left leg is generally longer and heavier with an asymmetry that increases during development, together with the fact that the right arm is longer from an early age, led Peters (1988) to suggest that stance and posture during active foot use, perhaps as a consequence of patterns of ongoing manual *activity*, may help determine lower limb asymmetries. Indeed, in many activities, foot roles are determined by what the hands are doing, as in the stance adopted while throwing. In this respect, foot roles are complementary and ofter subordinate to hand roles. If, however, we find that foot preferences relate to hand preferences in tasks where such complementarity is unlikely, then we may argue that the lateral specialization determining foot preferences cannot reside in the machinery guiding hand preferences, but must operate at a higher level. Foot preferences, moreover, are not dissociable from *leg* preferences, unlike the situation in the upper limb where writing places more emphasis upon hand and wrist movements than is the case in tasks such as throwing and kicking. In both limbs, there is the problem of role differentiation; in hands, the preferred hand realizes the goal of the movement, while the other hand lends support, a situation which may be particularly salient in natural bimanual activities. The same applies with respect to foot preferences; purposeful movements of one leg or foot cannot be performed in isolation from the other. Peters recommends that we define the preferred lower limb as the one used to manipulate or to lead as in jumping, the nonpreferred limb being the one used for support and postural stability. A good test for foot preference is ball work, though it should be noted that it combines two actions, fine manipulatory skill ("dribbling") and the ballistic application of force (kicking). Dextrals tend to prefer the right leg in these tasks (though just as with hand preferences in boxing, the left footed player may have the advantage of surprise). According to Peters, the right foot is also preferred for lifting objects, a task which when performed during standing forces a clear division of functional roles between limbs. The right foot is also the better *performer* in lifting, maneuvering, and manipulating objects; it performs better in tapping tasks, and in coordinated tapping of a simple rhythm where one foot makes one tap for every two of the other, performance is better when the right foot takes the faster beat. The same is found with hands.

5.2 NONHUMAN PRIMATE STUDIES

Falk, Pyne, Helmkamp, and DeRousseau (1988) recorded a number of forelimb dimensions of 150 rhesus monkeys (*M. mulatta*). Seven of the ten assessed dimensions were larger on the right, especially ulnar length and size of the olecranon process, length of the supracondylar ridge, and diameter of the humerus. Subsequently, Helmkamp and Falk (1990) studied developmental and gender aspects of these asymmetries in 76 male and 61 female rhesus monkeys of various ages. Males showed a consistently decreasing asymmetry with increasing age, while with females these effects reversed.

6. ASYMMETRIES OF HAND USE

6.1 PRELIMINARY CONSIDERATIONS

While the possession of two equally "dextrous" hands may be thought to permit maximal efficiency and flexibility, complex manual behaviors may nevertheless be more efficient with some degree of manual specialization. However, the most skillful hand is not always the one chosen, and in a complex task of several components there may be a switching of hand preferences between components or even a change in patterns of asymmetry as a function of practice.

Nonhuman primate studies have tended to rely on tests of the sort designed to be used with human infants (Harris and Carlson, 1992) — possibly a suboptimal approach. While asymmetries may appear pronounced at an individual level, it is certainly true that population-level primate asymmetries in hand preference or performance, denied until very recently, are usually weaker and more variable than our own; they tend to be more task dependent and more subject to chance and extraneous factors, for example, asymmetrical location of the manipulandum or incentive, initial posture, or behavior stereotypes. Other problems include differences or inadequacies in testing procedures, task complexity, statistical treatment, (small) number of subjects, lack of control of subjects' age, sex or practice levels, naturalistic vs. artificial settings or observations, prior experience, failure to distinguish between hand preference and performance, whether the task is routine or novel (when asymmetries may possibly be more evident), etc., (see Fagot and Vauclair, 1991; Fragaszy and Adams-Curtis, 1993; and Hopkins and Morris, 1993). Indeed Hopkins and Morris distinguish between *ambiguous* hand preferences, where there are inconsistencies *within* a specific task, and *ambidextrous* effects, where inconsistencies occur *between* tasks, and observe that we should try to take account of the animals' "intent" when grabbing an object (e.g., to eat it, carry it away, or break it open, as hand specializations may well differ between such circumstances).

Sometimes the two measures of hand preference and performance can be usefully combined. Thus, Hörster and Ettlinger (1985) reviewed their records of 237 rhesus monkeys that were initially trained on a particular tactile discrimination task. They fell into three almost equal groups of left-handed, right-handed, and ambilateral individuals. The last group attained performance criterion with the fewest trials, followed by the left-handers and then the right-handers. While conclusions could be drawn that bihemispheric involvement helps, or that one hemisphere is somehow faster or more efficient in such tasks than the other, it is instead possible that one or other group of individuals was simply smarter than the other, rather than that the differences occurred at an interhemispheric level. Moreover, as Ettlinger (1988) observed, forcing monkeys to use the nonpreferred hand might have meant that restriction of the preferred hand would have indirectly impeded performance of the other hand more than restriction of the nonpreferred hand. Hopkins, Washburn, Berke, and Williams (1992) studied 35 rhesus monkeys that were manipulating a joystick in response to two computerized tasks; there were no significant hand preference asymmetries at a population level, though individuals were strongly lateralized one way or another. However, right preferent animals mastered the task much faster than left preferent animals, even though both groups ultimately reached the same overall level of performance, (i.e., the asymmetries were *transient*). The authors go on to ask whether in human terms the task should be viewed as left-hemisphere sequential, or right-hemisphere visuospatial, or indeed whether the two groups, left and right handers, perhaps solved the task via different hemispherically appropriate strategies. Finally, Marchant and Steklis (1986) found that five chimpanzees *performed* bar presses more quickly with the right than the left hand, although hand *preferences* were quite inconsistent; two individuals preferred the right hand, two preferred the left, and one was ambidextrous.

6.2 RIGHT-HAND PERFORMANCE SUPERIORITIES IN NONHUMAN PRIMATES

Apart from the studies discussed above, only a handful of studies have found right-hand performance superiorities and almost none a left-hand performance superiority. Preilowski, Reger, and Engele (1986) required rhesus monkeys to produce isometric pressures of specific durations between the fingertips under various spatial and temporal constraints. Under the more difficult conditions, the right hand was significantly superior. Hopkins, Washburn, and Rumbaugh (1989) studied two rhesus monkeys and three chimpanzees in a computerized tracking task involving a display and a joystick. The right hand proved to be the faster one in all five subjects and was also the preferred hand. Since subjects were at times required to use the left hand, the right-hand performance superiorities were likely independent of preference or practice. Finally, Fagot, Bard, and Fort (1992) found that infant chimpanzees have stronger and longer lasting gripping responses with the right hand, although they found that right hand bias was stronger in nursery reared chimps, possibly suggesting an influence of their human care-givers (Bard, Hopkins, and Fort, 1990).

6.3 RIGHT-HAND PREFERENCES IN NONHUMAN PRIMATES

Costello and Fragaszy (1988) reported that of 419 acts of prehensile grip with one hand by six capuchin monkeys, 66% were right handed while 34% were left handed. Masataka (1990) observed hand preferences in 31 individuals of various capuchin species in food collection from the ground. Of these, 81% showed marked and statistically significant right hand preferences and only 7% were ambilateral. Kuhl (1988) had juveniles of various macaque species discriminate between pairs of speech sounds with a reasonably complex manual response. In this continuous speeded task, all subjects over 10 years of age preferred responding with the right hand, irrespective of the hand used for feeding. Fagot (1993) studied four infant Guinea baboons (*P. papio*) from birth. Initial manual preferences were all right handed, though changes often occurred later in development. Indeed Vauclair and Fagot (1987) found in a field situation that ten adult and eight juvenile baboons showed no population-level asymmetries, even though the strength of individual hand preferences was stronger in the adults.

Turning to gorillas (*Gorilla gorilla*), Fischer, Meunier, and White (1982) found that all four females displayed a very marked right hand preference for grasping, though this may have stemmed from their consistent use of the left hand to cradle an infant (see below). Similarly Lockard (1984) observed that five out of seven mobile gorillas in a naturalistic outdoor setting showed a right-hand preference for foraging and manipulation. Schaller (1963) reported that all of eight mountain gorillas preferred the right hand for chest beating displays. With respect to locomotion, Heestand (1987) noted that of 70 captive apes (*Gorilla*, *Pongo*, *Pan* and *Symphalangus/Hylobates*), all species led off with the right limb when terrestrially locomoting, irrespective of variable hand preferences during feeding. Hopkins, Bennett, Bales, Lee, and Ward (1993) extended this finding to the bonobo or pygmy chimpanzee (*Pan paniscus*). Stafford, Milliken, and Ward (1990) studied 19 individuals of various *Symphalangus/Hylobates* species in detail. They found no asymmetries in use of the leading limb in *arboreal* brachiation, but adult females were strongly right-hand preferent for food reaching, especially the *older* females, while asymmetries were nonsignificant for males and subadult females. Indeed, increasing tendencies towards a right-hand preference for food reaching with increasing age in females is characteriztic (see below) of lemurs (Forsythe and Ward, 1988; Ward, Milliken, Dodson, Stafford, and Wallace, 1990). Developmental changes with increasing age (see also Lehman, 1980, and Vauclair and Fagot, 1987) and stronger lateralization in females were also reported by Bard et al. (1990) in nursery-reared chimpanzees. Eight out of ten used their right hand in hand-to-mouth, self-calming behavior (see also Hopkins and Bard, 1993, where the effect was found to be stronger with females). Hopkins (1993) cites a recent study by Arguente, Ely, and King showing a right-hand preference in environmental manipulation by chimpanzees but not squirrel monkeys. We shall return in the next section to Hopkins' own findings of right-hand food-reaching preferences in chimpanzees and orang-utans, but might at this point note the study of Morris, Hopkins, and Bolser-Gilmore (1993) who found a right-hand preference for fine motor tasks requiring manual dexterity in two language-trained chimpanzees. With only two animals, conclusions are difficult; it is also not clear whether it is the task, or the language-training, or both which are operative. However, the authors review evidence that such tasks may be more sensitive to highly consistent (as found here) hand preferences than grosser reaching or feeding responses. Shafer (1993) also found a strong right-hand preference among 47 zoo-maintained gorillas for performance of fine motor tasks, especially among males; gorillas, of course, spend more time upright and bipedal than any other nonhuman primate. Finally, Hopkins, Bard, Jones, and Bales (1993) found a right-hand preference for throwing, especially with males and from a bipedal posture, in chimpanzees, while Hopkins and Bennett (1994) found that right-hand-preferring chimpanzees (35) approached and touched objects significantly faster than non-right-handed individuals (14); 49 animals were studied.

6.4 LEFT-HAND PREFERENCES IN NONHUMAN PRIMATES

Rogers and Kaplan (1994) observed that semiwild orang-utans tended to use the left hand to touch the face or head, provided that the fingers were flexed and a part of the face was manipulated (e.g., as in cleaning the nose, an eye, or the teeth). Dimond and Harries (1984) note the common occurrence of face touching (which cannot simply be attributed to local skin irritation) in primates, especially apes, again with a left-hand preference (cf. Suarez and Gallup, 1986; Kaplan and Rogers, 1994).

Box (1977) observed four male and four female common marmosets (*Callithrix jacchus*) for spontaneous hand usage in various behavioral categories. Only for taking food from a bowl and holding food was there a left-hand preference. Matoba, Masataka, and Tanioka (1991) confirmed these findings recently, but it has not been confirmed by Hodgkinson and Rogers (1994). Deuel and Schaffer (1987) and Kawai (1967) similarly report left-hand preferences by macaques in catching moving bait, and King, Landau, Scott, and Berning (1987; see also King and Landau, 1993) report that squirrel monkeys prefer to catch live gold fish with the left hand. Hauser et al. (1991) found that with 277 rhesus monkeys the left hand was greatly preferred for lifting the lid of a chow dispenser; the lid was then held open with the right, and chow was selected with the left. By contrast,

Annett and Annett (1991: lowland gorillas) and Byrne and Byrne (1991: mountain gorillas) found no population asymmetries in food-related behaviors in apes. Nevertheless, Olson, Ellis, and Nadler (1990) report that all of six gibbons (*Hylobates lar*) showed a left-hand preference, and 10 out of 12 gorillas a right-hand preference for extracting food attached to mesh high up in the animal's midsagittal plane. It is possible that these opposing asymmetries may reflect the gorilla's terrestrial and the gibbon's arboreal habitat; the latter may impose more spatial (right hemisphere) demands, though note that Rogers and Kaplan (1994) found that while some individual orang-utans showed hand preferences for manipulating food, there was no group bias or handedness, despite the species being highly arboreal. This study was of rehabilative orangutans living in their natural environment, and therefore with ample experience of arboreality and manipulation (see Kaplan and Rogers, 1994). By comparison, Hopkins (1993) found a right-hand population preference in nine captive orang-utans and 40 chimpanzees for food reaching from an upright (but not a quadruped) posture. Comparing his findings with those of Olson et al. (above), Hopkins notes that the latters' gorillas showed the biggest right hand bias, followed by Hopkins' chimpanzees and then the orangutans. He observes that if bipedalism were the sole operative factor, gorillas, being the least bipedal, should have shown the weakest effects. However, gorillas use their feet for holding objects, etc., during feeding *less* than chimpanzees, and so are in fact more reliant upon their hands. Hopkins further noted that fine digit control in food holding occurred more during upright bipedal reaching, with a more gross cupping configuration adopted with a quadrupedal posture, which may further contribute to right-hand preferences during bipedal stances.

In a recent study of a large number of wild chimpanzees, Marchant and McGrew (1994) have found no significant hand preferences in a variety of contexts of touching and manipulation. It should be noted, however, that they did not discriminate between the manipulations requiring different degrees of finger flexion or examine age or sex differences. Stronger handedness may well emerge if these factors are examined, as Rogers and Kaplan (1994) found that individual orang-utans showed stronger handedness with increasing age, and the left-handedness for face-touching was present only for touching with fine-finger manipulation.

Left-hand preferences in food related behaviors are reported in numerous studies with prosimians of various species (Masataka, 1989; Ward, Milliken, and Stafford, 1993), especially when a postural adjustment is required from an initially awkward stance, in younger animals and in males. This may partly stem from a right forelimb preference for postural support. Thus, MacNeilage et al. (1987, 1988, 1991) argue that left-hand reaching preferences in prosimians, whose ancestors were probably vertical clingers and leapers, led to two complimentary specializations: a left-hand (right-hemisphere) *perceptuomotor* specialization for unimanual predation, and a left hemisphere (right hand) specialization for whole-body postural organization. According to McNeilage et al., with the advent of quadrupedalism which freed the upper limb from clinging, the right side of the body became the operative side for forceful interactions with the environment during invasive foraging, manipulative, and practiced acts. Finally, they argue that left hemisphere specialization for whole-body postural organization became associated with vocal control and language. However, we would disagree on the grounds of the clear evidence (Bradshaw and Rogers, 1993, and above) of widespread perceptual and cognitive asymmetries in primates, birds, and rodents. We suggest that perceptual asymmetries preceded motor asymmetries.

Turning now to behaviors that are more complex than reaching for food, Watanabe and Kawai (1993) found a left hand preference by Japanese macaques (*M. fuscata*) for washing sweet potatoes and especially wheat (which was harder to do). Westergaard

(1991) observed the tool using behavior of five capuchins and four macaques. The task involved using a probe as a dipping tool to obtain food. In both groups, all but one showed a significant hand preference, and again in all but one it was for the left. (We shall see below that these left-hand preferences seem not to extend to chimpanzees in dipping or other forms of tool-using behavior.) In a yet more complex haptic-discrimination task, Fagot, Drea, and Wallen (1991) found 21 out of 29 rhesus monkeys preferred the left hand, especially when hanging from a vertical three-point posture. Indeed lateralization may be stronger with more complex behaviors (Fagot and Vauclair, 1991). In both gorillas (Fagot and Vauclair, 1988a) and baboons (Fagot and Vauclair, 1988b), simple reaching was not associated with hand asymmetries, whereas in a difficult manipulo-visuo-spatial adjustment task, strong left-hand superiorities occurred in both species, indicating a right-hemisphere involvement. A similar involvement is also invoked by Vauclair and Fagot (1993). Eight baboons, using a joystick, had to track and hit a randomly moving target. The four animals initially tested with the left hand outperformed the four initially tested with the right hand in terms of shortness and efficiency of resultant trajectories. However, with such a small sample size, any conclusions warrant caution.

Finally, Hatta and Koike (1991) reported a left-hand preference in frightened mother monkeys when picking up their babies. Fischer et al. (1982; see also Lockard, 1984) found that female gorillas usually hold an infant cradled with the left arm during tripedal locomotion. Manning and Chamberlain (1990) and Manning, Heaton, and Chamberlain (1994) extended these findings to chimpanzees and gorilla infant-mother pairs. (A similar effect failed to reach significance for gibbons, and there was no population bias for orang-utans.) They noted a higher asymmetry in gorillas for cradling male infants, as with humans (and see Saling and Kaplan-Solms, 1989), with similar nonsignificant sex differences in chimpanzees, orang-utans, and gibbons. They speculate that male infants may be more restive, requiring the soothing, left-sided, maternal heartbeat or attention (via the right hemisphere and left hemispace). Of course, as may especially be the case in humans, this posture permits freedom of movement to the normally preferred right limb. Indeed Nishida (1993) invokes a similar explanation when he found a preference for suckling from a left nipple in 34 mother-infant pairs of wild chimpanzees, though again the asymmetry was far stronger for suckling male infants. Hopkins et al. (1993) also found a left-lateral bias in carrying behavior in captive bonobos (*Pan paniscus*), coupled with the opposite bias in leading limb during locomotion, especially in the bipedal posture.

7. NONHUMAN TOOL USE

We are certainly not the only species to use tools (Beck, 1980), though we must first define what we mean. Beaks, claws, and stings can be eliminated if a tool is seen as an object which is not part of the individual's body, which is not attached to a substrate, and which is used somehow to operate upon some other object.

Pepperberg (1989) describes how Australian and Amazonian parrots used empty nut shells, bottle tops, and teaspoons to remove water and seeds from otherwise inaccessible containers. Bluejays shredded newspaper to mop up wet sticky food in order to eat it, and a rook plugged a hole in the floor of its aviary to accumulate water for purposes of bathing and drinking.

Westergaard (1992) reports infant baboons in a captive peer group spontaneously using objects, in play, as containers, drinking utensils, and sponges. They later used paper, browse, and other materials as tools to extract sweet liquids from an apparatus designed to accommodate sponging and probing behavior. Indeed, infant baboons aged between 7 and 11 months spontaneously learned to get food by maneuvering a plastic rod into a distant food container, and were able to use objects as rakes to secure otherwise inaccessible food (Westergaard, 1989).

According to Hauser (1988) a wild vervet monkey (*Cercopithecus aethiops pygerythrus*) learned how to use dried seed pods to soak up exudate from otherwise inaccessible recesses in trees, which she would then consume. This behavior was subsequently copied by others. Macaques are known to use stones to hammer open oyster shells and to crush scorpions (Falk, 1989). Moreover, the highly dexterous New World capuchin monkeys (*Cebus capucinus imitator*) have been observed breaking off and dropping branches on each other, probing holes with twigs, and bashing nuts together so as to break them (Chevalier-Skolnikoff, 1989). Captives have even been seen to use objects as rakes or ladders so as to get to food, and to use sticks to push food out of tubes and to pry lids off boxes.

Wild chimpanzees use twigs when "fishing" for termites, stone hammers to crack nuts, and leaves as sponges to collect water (Goodall, 1968). However, according to McGrew and Marchant (1992) who studied 15 wild animals, roughly equal numbers preferred either hand, although a subsequent reanalysis of these data revealed a weak but significant preference to use the left hand (McGrew and Marchant, 1994). Nishida and Hiraiwa (1982) similarly failed to find any evidence of hand asymmetries at a population level in wild chimpanzees using a probe to "fish" for ants. Charles, Dickson, Joyce, Lewin, and Pain (1991) note that a captive chimpanzee bashed flakes off one stone with another hammer stone, and used them to cut string so as to get into a box containing food. Wild chimpanzees may sequentially employ several tools, (i.e., branches of different sizes for different stages of the task) to obtain honey (Brewer and McGrew, 1990) from a bees' nest. We of course also select a sequence of tools appropriate for each new stage in a task. Chimpanzee mothers in the wild may even *coach* their offspring on how to crack nuts, leaving the offspring, and a "hammer," near an appropriate "anvil" (Boesch, 1991b). They demonstrate appropriate ways of positioning the nut and wielding the hammer whenever the offspring encounters difficulties. However, according to Boesch (1991a), there is no evidence of population biases in handedness when chimpanzees perform these dipping and hammering tasks, even though individuals, especially females, were strongly lateralized in either direction.

Just as there are current attempts to define language, consciousness, and tool use in ways that encompass nonhuman participation, the concept of *teaching* has similarly been addressed (Caro and Hauser, 1992). It is to be distinguished from social learning or imitation, and probably need not depend upon evidence of complex intentionality or attribution of mental states. Caro and Hauser note that teaching is likely to be more efficient than mere observational learning by virtue of its being directed, and define it in a nonhuman context as follows: an individual A is said to teach if it modifies its behavior only in the presence of a naive observer B at some cost or at least without obtaining an immediate benefit for itself. A's behavior therefore encourages or punishes that of B, or provides B with experience, or sets B an example so that B acquires skills or knowledge more rapidly or efficiently than otherwise. In this context, even a mother cat may be said to be teaching her kittens to pursue, capture, kill, and eat prey — and mother chimpanzees to teach offspring to open nuts for food.

While tool use, and even coaching in tool use, is therefore not unique to humans, there is no evidence that in their natural environment any other species, chimpanzees included, make tools for more than one purpose, or to make *new* tools. Indeed all behavior that can be inferred from stone tools and archaeological sites associated with the Oldowan culture of *Homo habilis* (see below) seems to fall within the range of chimpanzee capabilities (Wynn and McGrew, 1989); in fact the oldest known archaeological evidence of *Homo* fails to display anything which could be called uniquely human. This conclusion is endorsed by Westergaard and Suomi (1994) who found that of nine captive capuchin monkeys (*Cebus apella*), three used bone fragments to crack hard-shelled nuts and to cut acetate; one even used bone fragments as both chisels and hammers (striking the former against a surface with the latter), and used a stone to modify bone-fragment tools — perhaps the first report of the use and modification of bone tools by nonhuman primates.

Ingestion of herbs, apparently for medicinal or therapeutic purposes, is a newly reported form of animal behavior which is not unique to humans (Newton and Nishida, 1990; Newton and Wolfe, 1992), and which has close parallels to tool-using behavior. Sick chimpanzees may hold leaves containing pharmacologically active substances between the tongue and buccal surface, a procedure which would avoid inactivation of the substance in the stomach. Monkeys, pigs, bears, and elephants are also known to ingest or topically absorb plant substances apparently to control diarrhea or parasites.

8. HUMAN TOOL USE

The first human stone tools, crude scrapers, choppers, and sharp flakes struck off a core, date to around 2.5 million years ago, the Oldowan industry associated with *H. habilis*. Until *H. erectus* one million years later with the appearance of the Acheulian culture, there was very little change or development. Thereafter, there were steady evolutionary trends culminating 35,000 years ago with the advent of anatomically modern Cro-Magnon *Homo sapiens* in Eurasia and explosive cultural changes. Many have invoked cognitive categorization and language as guiding forces in tool behavior, appealing to common syntactic processes in both domains. Tool making and behavior even now are often far better taught by demonstration and initation.

Piagettian principles may be used to assess spatial thinking (though see the criticisms of Chevalier-Skolnikoff, 1989), and Wynn (1989) adopts them in an attempt to measure the evolution of spatial thought as manifested in stone tools and other artifacts of the archaeological record. He concludes that Oldowan hominids possessed a very limited spatial repertoire, and it was not until Acheulian times, when tools became more standardized and symmetrical, that the makers seemed to have a clear idea of what they were trying to make, and a sense of the aesthetic. By 300,000 years ago, Wynn (1989) argues, perspective had been discovered, together with essentially modern ideas of three-dimensional symmetry, straight edges, regular cross sections viewed from any direction, and parallel lines.

9. DEXTRALITY IN ANCIENT TOOL USE

According to Toth (1985), detailed analysis of prehistoric stone artifacts from Lower Pleistocene sites in Kenya (*H. habilis*) and Acheulian horizons in Spain (*H. erectus*) reveals a mode of manufacture consistent with the operation of holding the core in the left hand and sequentially striking off flakes with the right. Moreover, microwear analysis of flake tools from the Acheulian (200 kya) horizons at Clacton, England, which were used for boring, indicates a clockwise (and therefore for biomechanical reasons probably dextral) direction of rotation during pressure (Keeley, 1977). Similarly, according to Oakley (1972), tools associated with *H. erectus* from Choukoutien (China) appear mostly to have been chipped by dextrals. Cornford (1986) likewise concludes that resharpening or modification of the edge of flint tools was performed predominantly by dextral individuals intermediate between *H. erectus* and Neanderthals at La Cotte de St. Brelade, France. Finally, Bermúdez de Castro, Bromage, and Jalvo (1988) studied the direction of striations on the front teeth of Neanderthals and Anteneanderthals from sites in France and Spain. From experiments they conducted and reports of similar behavior in certain peoples even today, they concluded that predominantly dextral individuals held meat or hide between the teeth, cutting it with a tool held by the right hand.

10. THE EVOLUTION OF PRAXIS

Without hands, we would of course not be tool makers or users. While various species of marsupial and squirrel can hold and manipulate food with varying degrees of efficiency (Megirian, Weller, Martin, and Watson, 1977), as indeed can the parrot, prehensile manipulative grasping is very much a mark of the primates. It cannot, however, have been the sole or maybe even the major factor in the evolution of increasing relative brain size — witness the degree of encephalization (ratio of brain to body size; Jerison, 1973, 1982, 1986) of the cetacea (Martin, 1982), limbless and as far as we know quite unable to use tools. We get our large adult brains through prolonged growth, rather than via an unusual growth rate. In fact, primates generally grow their brains at the same rate as those of other mammals, but grow their bodies more slowly. Humans, moreover, continue their brain growth for up to a year after birth, leading to an effective 21 month gestation, and a brain three times the size of a human-sized ape. Stanley (1992) argues that this postnatal growth period was not possible until our early *Homo* ancestors became terrestrial and bipedal, rather than semi-arboreal like the earlier gracile australopithecines. Thus, one initial driving force may have been major climatic change with resultant loss of forest habitat and increase in grasslands between 2.5 and 1.8 mya. *H. habilis* was the first to demonstrate increased encephalization, and while an upright bipedal posture may have contributed (along with concomitant pelvis adaptations and obstetric consequences therefrom, (Foley and Dunbar, 1989; Harvey and Nee, 1991; Smith, 1990), we can again reject a major role for tool use in further increased encephalization at the human end of the primate lineage, as changes and improvements in lithic industries lagged far behind brain growth (Bradshaw and Rogers, 1993). Nor is a large brain a *sine qua non* for articulate speech; thus *intraspecifically*, people with microcephaly, with head sizes two or more standard deviations below the norm, may have near normal speech and even intelligence (Dorman, 1991). We do of course have enormous "spare capacity," as evident from the fact that individuals who have undergone hemispherectomies during infancy (Goodman and Whitaker, 1985) may later experience surprisingly little overall intellectual deficit. It is in the prefrontal regions that our brain has expanded most, compared to that of other primates (Deacon, 1986a,b; 1989), and we know that these structures also subserve those quintessentially human attributes of forward planning, strategic deployment, social restraint, and attentional set (Benson, 1993; Levin, 1991). Indeed Davidson, Kalin, and Shelton (1992) found asymmetries in these regions in rhesus monkeys when tested under conditions of restraint and stress, with greater right than left sided levels of EEG activation.

We may assume that, as with the great apes, our major foes are members of our own species, and argue the need for the evolution of a special sort of social intelligence, "Machiavellian" intelligence (Whiten and Byrne, 1988), so as to outwit our peers and competitors by predicting their likely responses to our own changes in behavior, alliance relationships, etc. Consciousness is of course a tool for attributing states of mind to others, for putting oneself as it were in another's mind or "empathizing" with them (Gibbons, 1993), and it may be no accident that humans and the great apes seem to be particularly able to attribute intentionality to others (Premack, 1988; Whiten, 1991) and to recognize *themselves* in a mirror (Gallup, 1983). Thus Povinelli, Parks, and Novak (1992) found that pairs of rhesus macaques, unlike chimpanzees and humans, could not reverse roles after being trained to carry out complementary parts of a single task; thus, for example, one member could see where food was hidden, but could not retrieve it, while the other could retrieve food if shown where it was hidden. Apes, however, can reverse roles, and learn by watching others.

If humans and chimpanzees are particularly noteworthy for their capacity of social intelligence, and primates generally are masters of cross-modal integration, of recognition of an object irrespective of the sensory channel by which it is received, and of the ability to construct and use complex spatial maps, where does this leave the evolution of language? *H. habilis*, the first hominid with a substantial allometric increase in brain size, and thought to be the first maker of stone tools which have survived in the archaeological record, perhaps thereby developed a more complex social structure requiring better communication and language. Language therefore as *we* know it may itself ultimately be a byproduct of social intelligence and group complexity (Dunbar, 1993), whatever its other evolutionary antecedents and preadaptations (Wind, 1989). Tobias (1987) notes that the gyral and sulcal impressions left on the inner surface of fossil *habilis* skulls are very similar to our own, and are distinct from those of pongids. A prominent Broca's motor speech area in the posterior part of the inferior frontal convolution of the left hemisphere may foreshadow speech. The well-developed inferior parietal lobule, especially in the regions of Wernicke's receptive speech area and the supramarginal and angular gyri, all tend to confirm these impressions. It is possible that the evolution of language and of tool use occurred hand-in-hand, as it were, in tandem, to their mutual advantage, given the remarkable parallels between speech and praxis. Thus with praxis the left hand may delineate the *frame* into which the right inserts the *contents* (cf. the right-hemisphere-global-holistic, left-hemisphere-serial-analytic dichotomy, Bradshaw and Nettleton, 1981). With language, at a phonological level consonant and vowel elements are inserted into syllabic frames, and at a morphological level words (contents) are inserted into syntactic frames (MacNeilage, Studdert-Kennedy, and Lindblom, 1984). The syntax of language may have its counterpart in the syntax of manual praxis (Frost, 1980), as in making and using tools, and it may be no accident (Kimura, 1982) that the motor areas for language in the left hemisphere are closely adjacent to those that control manual praxis. Indeed, our manual gestures tend to closely follow the rhythms of speech. Note however that the syntax of language involves hierarchical organization and embedding, whereas manual praxis tends to be rather more a matter of sequential chaining. Even sophisticated modern languages are far inferior to simple imitation and observation in the transmission of skills in tool manufacture and use. In fact, the constraints of imitative learning may be another reason why most of us share the same patterns of hand asymmetries — two individuals of mixed handedness are far less efficient in instructing each other in knot tying (Michel and Harkins, 1985). Yet, as we have seen, *H. habilis* was probably already dextral at the dawn of lithic technology, and its tools were almost certainly too simple to require dyadic tutoring.

If we can draw some general conclusions, it is first that tool use, language, intellect, self-awareness, and culture have all interacted to their mutual evolutionary benefit, in the form of an autocatalytic feedback system. As so often in medicine, ecology, evolutionary biology, and social behavior, it is a mistake to seek a single line of causality. We should reject Chomsky's (1980) view of the absolute uniqueness of human speech as an event without evolutionary precedent, and stress the evolutionary continuity of human speech with the neural structures subserving primate call systems (Deacon, 1986a,b), and indeed the general evolutionary continuity of our manual (and other) asymmetries with those now being demonstrated in other vertebrate genera. Secondly, we might conclude that the vertebrate left hemisphere is specialized for sequential, feature-analytic behaviors which may underlie communication, while the right hemisphere's spatial and affective functions may constitute a less coherent set which may in fact be prior, perhaps operating in terms of an attentional vector for directed responses to meaningful or significant stimuli.

REFERENCES

Ádám, G. Y., Szilagyi, N., and Lang, E. (1992). The effect of monocular viewing on hemispheric functions. *Int. J. Psychol.*, 27, 401.

Andrews, P. (1992). Evolution and environment in the Hominoidea. *Nature*, 360, 641.

Annett, M. and Annett, J. (1991). Handedness for eating in gorillas. *Cortex*, 27, 269.

Bard, K. A., Hopkins, W. D., and Fort, C. L. (1990). Lateral bias in infant chimpanzees (*Pan troglodytes*). *J. Comp. Psychol.*, 104, 309.

Bear, D., Schiff, D., Saver, J., Greenberg, M., and Freeman, R. (1986). Quantitative analysis of cerebral asymmetry. *Arch. Neurol.*, 43, 598.

Beck, B. B. (1980). *Animal Tool Behavior: The Use and Manufacture of Tools by Animals*. New York. Garland STPM Press.

Beecher, M. D., Petersen, M. R., Zoloth, S. R., Moody, D. B., and Stebbins, W. C. (1979). Perception of conspecific vocalizations by Japanese macaques: Evidence for selective attention and neural lateralization. *Brain Behav. Evol.*, 16, 443.

Benson, D. F. (1993). Prefrontal abilities. *Behav. Neurol.*, 6, 75.

Benton, A. (1990). Facial recognition. *Cortex*, 26, 491.

Bermúdez de Castro, J. M. B., Bromage, T. G., and Jalvo, Y. F. (1988). Buccal striations on fossil human anterior teeth: Evidence of handedness in the Middle and early Upper Pleistocene. *J. Human Evol.*, 17, 403.

Bishop, P. O., Jeremy, D., and Lance, J. W. (1953). The optic nerve. Properties of a central tract. *J. Physiol.*, 121, 415.

Boesch C. (1991a). Handedness in wild chimpanzees. *Int. J. Primatol.*, 12, 541.

Boesch, C. (1991b). Teaching among wild chimpanzees. *Anim. Behav.*, 41, 530.

Box, H. O. (1977). Observations on spontaneous hand use in the common marmoset (*Callithrix jacchus*). *Primates*, 18, 395.

Bradshaw, J. L. and Nettleton, N. C. (1981). The nature of hemispheric specialization in man. *Behav. Brain Sci.*, 4, 51.

Bradshaw, J. L. and Rogers, L. J. (1993). *The Evolution of Lateral Asymmetries, Language, Tool Use and Intellect*. San Diego; Academic Press.

Brewer, S. M. and McGrew, W. C. (1990). Chimpanzee use of a tool set to get honey. *Folia Primatol.*, 54, 100.

Bryden, M. P. (1988). Correlates of the dichotic right-ear effect. *Cortex*, 24, 313.

Byrne, R. W. and Byrne, J. M. (1991). Hand preferences in the skilled gathering tasks of mountain gorillas (*G. gorilla berengei*). *Cortex*, 27, 521.

Cain, D. P. and Wada, J. A. (1979). An anatomical asymmetry in the baboon brain. *Brain Behav. Evol.*, 16, 222.

Caro, T. M. and Hauser M. D. (1992). Is there teaching in nonhuman animals? *Quart. Rev. Biol.*, 67, 151.

Charles, D., Dickson, D., Joyce, C., Lewin, R., and Pain, S. (1991). Chimp learns stone age use of tools. *New Sci.*, February 23, 11.

Chevalier-Skolnikoff, S. (1989). Spontaneous tool use and sensorimotor intelligence in *Cebus* compared with monkeys and apes. *Behav. Brain Sci.*, 12, 561.

Cheverud, J. M., Falk, D., Hildebolt, C., Moore, A. J., Helmkamp, R.C., and Vannier, J. (1990). Heritability and association of cortical petalias in rhesus macaques (*M. mulatta*). *Brain Behav. Evol.*, 35, 368.

Chomsky, N. (1980). Rules and representations. *Behav. Brain Sci.*, 3, 1.

Cole, J. (1957). Laterality in the use of the hand, foot, and eye in monkeys. *J. Comp. Physiol.*, 50, 296.

Coren, S. and Porac, C. (1976). Size accentuation in the dominant eye. *Nature*, 260, 527.

Cornford, J. M. (1986). Specialised resharpening techniques and evidence of handedness. In P. Calloway and J. Cornford (Eds.), *La Cotte de St. Brelade 1961–1978 Excavation*, Norwich, Geo Books, 337.

Costello, M. and Fragaszy, D. (1988). Prehension in *Cebus* and *Saimiri*: grip type and hand preference. *Am. J. Primatol.*, 15, 235.

Davidson, R. J., Kalin, N. H., and Shelton, S. E. (1992). Lateralized effects of diazepam on frontal brain electrical asymmetries in rhesus monkeys. *Biol. Psych.*, 32, 438.

Deacon, T. W. (1986a). Human brain evolution: 1. Evolution of language circuits. In H. J. Jerison and I. Jerison (Eds.), *Intelligence and Evolutionary Biology*, New York, Springer, 363.

Deacon, T. W. (1986b). Human brain evolution: 11. Embryology and brain allometry, In H.J. Jerison and I. Jerison (Eds.), *Intelligence and Evolutionary Biology*, New York, Springer, 381.

Deacon, T. W. (1989). The neural circuitry underlying primate calls and human language. *Human Evol.*, 4, 367.

Deuel, R. K. and Schaffer, S. P. (1987). Patterns of hand preference in monkeys. *Behav. Brain Sci.*, 10, 270.

Dewson, J. H. (1977). Preliminary evidence of hemispheric asymmetry of auditory function in monkeys. In S. Harnad, R. W. Doty, l. Goldstein, J. Jaynes, and G. Krauthamer (Eds.), *Lateralisation in the Nervous System*, New York, Academic Press, 63.

Dimond, S. J. and Harries, R. (1984). Face touching in monkeys, apes and man: Evolutionary origins and cerebral asymmetry. *Neuropsychologia*, 22, 227.

Domangue, B. B. (1984). Hemisphere dominance, cognitive complexity, and nonverbal sensitivity. *Percept. Motor Skills*, 58, 3.

Dorman, C. (1991). Microcephaly and intelligence. *Dev. Med. Child Neurol.*, 33, 267.

Dunbar, R. I. M. (1993). Co-evolution of neocortex size, group size and language in humans. *Behav. Brain Sci.*, 16, 681.

Ettlinger, G. (1988). Hand preference, ability and hemispheric specialization: In how far are these factors related in the monkey? *Cortex*, 24, 389.

Fagot, J. (1993). Ontogeny of object manipulation and manual lateralization in the Guinea baboon: Preliminary observations. In J. P. Ward and W. D. Hopkins (Eds.), *Primate Laterality: Current Behavioral Evidence of Primate Asymmetries*, New York, Springer, 235.

Fagot, J., Bard, K. A., and Fort, C. L. (1992). Lateralization of the grasping reflex in neonatal chimpanzees. *Folia Primatolog.*, 58, 168.

Fagot, J., Drea, C.M., and Wallen, K. (1991). Evidence for an asymmetrical hand usage in rhesus monkeys in tactually and visually regulated tasks. *J. Comp. Psychol.*, 105, 260.

Fagot, J. and Vauclair, J. (1988a). Handedness and bimanual coordination in the lowland Gorilla. *Brain Behav. Evol.*, 32, 89.

Fagot, J. and Vauclair, J. (1988b). Handedness and manual specialization in the baboon. *Neuropsychologia*, 26, 795.

Fagot, J. and Vauclair, J. (1991). Manual laterality in nonhuman primates: A distribution between handedness and manual specialization. *Psychol. Bull.*, 109, 76.

Fagot, J. and Vauclair, J. (1994). Video-task assessment of stimulus novelty effects on hemispheric lateralization in baboons (*P. papio*). *J. Comp. Psychol.*, 108, 156.

Falk, D. (1989). Primate tool use: But what about their brains? *Behav. Brain Sci.*, 12, 595.

Falk, D., Hildebolt, C., Cheverud, J., Vannier, M., Helmkamp, R. C., and Konigsberg, L. (1990). Cortical asymmetries in frontal lobes of rhesus monkeys (*M. mulatta*). *Brain Res.*, 512, 40.

Falk, D., Pyne, L., Helmkamp, R. C., and DeRousseau, C. J. (1988). Directional asymmetry in the forelimb of *M. mulatta*. *Am. J. Phys. Anthropol.*, 77, 1.

Fischer, R. B., Meunier, G. F., and White, P. J. (1982). Evidence of laterality in the lowland gorilla. *Percept. Motor Skills*, 54, 1093.

Foley, R. A. and Dunbar, R. (1989). Beyond the bones of contention. *New Scientist,* October, 14, 21.

Forsythe, C. and Ward, J. P. (1988). Black lemur (*Lemur macaco*) hand preference in food reaching. *Primates*, 29, 369.

Fragaszy, D. M. and Adams-Curtis, L. E. (1993). An exploration of manual preference and performance in crabeating macaques. In J. P. Ward and W. D. Hopkins (Eds.), *Primate Laterality: Current Behavioral Evidence of Primate Asymmetries*, New York, Springer-Verlag, 75.

Frost, G. T. (1980). Tool behavior and the origins of laterality. *J. Human Evol.*, 9, 447.

Galaburda, A. M. (1984). Anatomical asymmetries. In N. Geschwind and A. M. Galaburda (Eds.), *Cerebral Dominance: The Biological Foundations,* Cambridge, MA, Harvard University Press, 11.

Galaburda, A. M., LeMay, M., Kemper, T. L., and Geschwind, N. (1978). Right-left asymmetries in the brain. *Science*, 199, 852.

Gallup, G. G. (1983). Toward a comparative psychology of mind. In R. L. Mellgren (Ed.), *Animal Cognition and Behavior*, Amsterdam, North-Holland, 473.

Garn, S. M., Mayor, G. H., and Shaw, H. A. (1976). Paradoxical bilateral asymmetry in bone size and bone mass in the hand. *Am. J. Phys. Anthropol.*, 45, 209.

Geschwind, N. and Galaburda, A. M. (1985). Cerebral lateralization: Biological mechanisms, associations and pathology I-III: A hypothesis and program for research. *Arch. Neurol.*, 42, 428, 521, 634.

Geschwind, N. and Levitsky, W. (1968). Human brain: Left-right asymmetry in temporal speech region. *Science*, 161, 186.

Gibbons, A. (1993). Empathy and brain evolution. *Science*, 259, 1250.

Goodall, J. van Lawick. (1968). The behavior of free living chimpanzees in the Gombe Stream Reserve (Tanzania). *Anim. Behav. Monogr.*, 1, 161.

Goodman, R. A. and Whitaker, H. A. (1985). Hemispherectomy: A review (1928-1981) with special reference to the linguistic abilities and disabilities of the residual right hemisphere. In C. T. Best (Ed.), *Hemispheric Function and Collaboration in the Child*, New York, Academic Press, 121.

Hamilton, C. R. and Vermeire, B. A. (1985). Complementary hemispheric superiorities in monkeys. *Soc. Neurosci. Abs.*, 11, 869.

Hamilton, C. R. and Vermeire, B. A. (1991). Functional lateralization in monkeys. In F. L. Kitterle (Ed.), *Cerebral Laterality: Theory and Research. The Toledo Symposium*, Hillsdale, N.J., Erlbaum, 19.

Harris, L. J. and Carlson, D. F. (1992). Hand preference for visually guided reaching in human infants and adults. In J. P. Ward (Ed.), *Current Behavioral Evidence of Primate Asymmetries*, New York, Springer, 285.

Harvey, P. H. and Nee, S. (1991). How to live like a mammal. *Nature*, 350, 23.

Hatta, T. and Koike, M. (1991). Left-hand preference in frightened mother monkeys in taking up their babies. *Neuropsychologia*, 29, 207.

Hauser, M. D. (1988). Invention and social transmission: New data from wild vervet monkeys. In R. Byrne and A. Whiten (Eds.), *Machiavellian Intelligence: Social Expertise and the Evolution of Intellect in Monkeys, Apes and Humans*, Oxford, Oxford University Press, 327.

Hauser, M. D. (1993). Right hemisphere dominance for the production of facial expression in monkeys. *Science*, 261, 475.

Hauser, M. D. and Andersson, K. (1994). Left hemisphere dominance for processing vocalizations in adult, but not infant, rhesus monkeys: Field experiments. *Proc. Natl. Acad. Sci.*, 91, 3946.

Hauser, M., Perry, S., Manson, J. H., Ball, H., Williams, M., Pearson, E., and Berard, J. (1991). It's all in the hands of the beholder: New data on free ranging rhesus monkeys. *Behav. Brain Sci.*, 14, 342.

Heestand, J. (1987). Asymmetric hand preference in four species of captive apes. *Soc. Neurosci. Abs.*, 13, 44.

Heffner, H. E. and Heffner, R. S. (1984). Temporal lobe lesions and perception of species-specific vocalizations by macaques. *Science*, 226, 75.

Heffner, H. E. and Heffner, R. S. (1986). Effect of unilateral and bilateral auditory cortex lesions on the discrimination of vocalizations by Japanese macaques. *J. Neurophysiol.*, 56, 683.

Heilbroner, P. L. and Holloway, R. L. (1988). Anatomical brain asymmetries in New World and Old World monkeys: Stages of temporal lobe development in primate evolution. *Am. J. Phys. Anthropol.*, 76, 39.

Helmkamp, R. C. and Falk, D. (1990). Age and sex-associated variations in the directional asymmetry of rhesus macaque forelimb bones. *Am. J. Phys. Anthropol.*, 83, 211.

Hochberg, F. H. and LeMay, M. (1975). Arteriographic correlates of handedness. *Neurology*, 25, 218.

Hodgkinson, M. A. and Rogers, L. J. (1994). Handedness, mouthedness and eye preference in the common marmoset (*Callithrix jacchus*). *Proc. Int. Primatol. Conf.*, Bali, Indonesia, p. 203.

Holloway, R. L. and de LaCoste-Lareymondie, M. C. (1982). Some preliminary findings on the palaeontology of cerebral dominance. *Am. J. Phys. Anthropol.*, 58, 101.

Hopkins, W. D. (1993). Posture and reaching in chimpanzees (*Pan troglodytes*) and orang-utans (*Pongo pygmaeus*). *J. Comp. Psychol.*, 107, 162.

Hopkins, W. D. and Bard, K. A. (1993). Hemispheric specialization in infant chimpanzees (*Pan troglodytes*): Evidence for a relation with gender and arousal. *Dev. Psychobiol.*, 26, 219.

Hopkins, W. D., Bard, K. A., Jones, A., and Bales, S. L. (1993). Chimpanzee hand preference for throwing and infant cradling: Implications for the origin of human handedness. *Curr. Anthropol.*, 34, 786.

Hopkins, W. D. and Bennett, A. J. (1994). Handedness and approach-avoidance behavior in chimpanzees (*Pan*). *J. Exp. Psychol: Anim. Behav. Proc.*, 20, 413.

Hopkins, W. D., Bennett, A. J., Bales, S. L., Lee, J., and Ward, J. P. (1993). Behavioral laterality in captive bonobos (*Pan paniscus*). *J. Comp. Psychol.*, 107, 403.

Hopkins, W. D. and Morris, R. D. (1989). Laterality for visuo-spatial processing in two language trained chimpanzees (*Pan Troglodytes*). *Behav. Neurosci.*, 103, 227.

Hopkins, W. D. and Morris, R. D. (1993). Handedness in great apes: A review of findings. *Int. J. Primatol.*, 14, 1.

Hopkins, W. D., Morris, R. D., and Savage-Rumbaugh, E. S. (1991). Evidence for asymmetrical hemispheric priming using known and unknown warning stimuli in two language trained chimpanzees (*Pan troglodytes*). *J. Exp. Psychol.: Gen.*, 120, 46.

Hopkins, W. D., Morris, R. D., Savage-Rumbaugh, E. G., and Rumbaugh, D. M. (1992). Hemispheric priming by meaningful and nonmeaningful symbols in language-trained chimpanzees (*Pan troglodytes*): Further evidence of a left hemisphere advantage. *Behav. Neurosci.*, 106, 575.

Hopkins, W. D., Washburn, D. A., Berke, L., and Williams, M. (1992). Behavioral asymmetries of psychomotor performance in rhesus monkeys (*M. mulatta*): A dissociation between hand preference and skill. *J. Comp. Psychol.*, 106, 392.

Hopkins, W. D., Washburn, D., and Rumbaugh, D. (1989). Note on hand use in the manipulation of joysticks by rhesus monkeys (*M. mulatta*) and chimpanzees (*Pan troglodytes*). *J. Comp. Psychol.*, 103, 91.

Hörster, W. and Ettlinger, G. (1985). An association between hand preference and tactile discrimination performance in the rhesus monkey. *Neuropsychologia*, 21, 411.

Ifune, C.K., Vermeire, B.A., and Hamilton, C.R. (1984). Hemispheric differences in split-brain monkeys viewing and responding to videotape recordings. *Behav. Neural Biol.*, 41, 231.

Jerison, H. J. (1973). *Evolution of the Brain and Intelligence*, New York, Academic Press.

Jerison, H. J. (1982). The evolution of biological intelligence. In R. Sternberg (Ed.), *Handbook of Intelligence*, Cambridge, Cambridge University Press, 723.

Jerison, H. J. (1986). Evolutionary biology of intelligence: The nature of the problem. In H. J. Jerison and I. Jerison (Eds.), *Intelligence and Evolutionary Biology*, New York, Springer, 1.

Kaplan, G. and Rogers, L.J. (1994). *Orang-utans in Borneo*. Armidale, University of New England Press.

Kawai, M. (1967). Catching behavior in the Koshima troop: A case of newly acquired behavior. *Primates*, 8, 181.

Keeley, L. H. (1977). The functions of Paleolithic flint tools. *Sci. Am.*, November, 237, 108.

Kertesz, A., Polk, M., Black, S. E., and Howell, J. A. (1990). Sex, handedness and the morphometry of cerebral asymmetries on magnetic resonance imaging. *Brain Res.*, 530, 40.

Kimura, D. (1982). Left hemisphere control of oral and brachial movements and their relation to communication. *Philos. Trans. R. Soc. London B*, 298, 135.

King, J. E. and Landau, V. I. (1993). Manual preference in varieties of reaching in squirrel monkeys. In J. Ward and W. D. Hopkins (Eds.), *Primate Laterality: Current Behavioral Evidence of Primate Asymmetries*, New York, Springer, 107.

King, J. E., Landau, V. I., Scott, A. G, and Berning, A.L. (1987). Hand preference during capture of live fish by squirrel monkeys. *Int. J. Primatol.*, 8, 540.

Kolb, B., Sutherland, R. J., Nonneman, A. J., and Whishaw, I. Q. (1982). Asymmetry in the cerebral hemispheres of the rat, mouse, rabbit and cat: The right hemisphere is larger. *Exp. Neurol.*, 78, 348.

Kruper, D. C., Boyle, B. E., and Patton, R. A. (1966). Eye and hand preference in rhesus monkeys (*M. mulatta*). *Psychon. Sci.*, 5, 277.

Kuhl, P. K. (1988). On handedness in primates and human infants. *Behav. Brain Sci.*, 11, 727.

Lehman, R. A. W. (1980). Distribution and changes in strength of hand preference of cynomolgus monkeys. *Brain Behav. Evol.*, 17, 209.

LeMay, M. (1985). Asymmetries of the brains and skulls of nonhuman primates. In S. D. Glick (Ed.), *Cerebral Lateralization in Nonhuman Species*, New York, Academic Press, 233.

LeMay, M., Billig, S., and Geschwind, N. (1982). Asymmetries of the brains and skulls of nonhuman primates. In E. Armstrong, and D. Falk (Eds.), *Primate Brain Evolution: Methods and Concepts*, New York, Plenum Press, 263.

LeMay, M. and Culebras, A. (1972). Human brain: Morphological differences in the hemispheres demonstrable by carotid arteriography. *N. Engl. J. Med.*, 287, 168.

LeMay, M. and Geschwind, N. (1975). Hemispheric difference in the brains of great apes. *Brain Behav. Evol.*, 11, 48.

Levin, H. S. (Ed.) (1991). *Frontal Lobe Function and Dysfunction*. Oxford, Oxford University Press.

Lockard, J. S. (1984). Handedness in a captive group of lowland gorillas. *Int. J. Primatol.*, 5, 356.

McGrew, W. C. and Marchant, L. F. (1992). Chimpanzees, tools and termites: Hand preference or handedness. *Curr. Anthropol.*, 23, 114.

McGrew, W. C. and Marchant, L. F. (1994). Laterality in tool-use by wild chimpanzees: new data on termite fishing. *Proc. Int. Primatol. Conf.*, Bali, Indonesia, p. 105.

Macho, G. A. (1991). Morphological asymmetries in southern African populations: Further evidence for lateralization. *Int. J. Anthropol.*, 6, 215.

MacNeilage, P. F., Studdert-Kennedy, M. G., and Lindblom, B. (1984). Functional precursors of language and its lateralization. *Am. J. Physiol.: Reg. Integr. Comp. Physiol.*, 15, 246, R 912.

MacNeilage, P. F., Studdert-Kennedy, M. G., and Lindblom, B. (1987). Primate handedness reconsidered. *Behav. Brain Sci.*, 10, 247.

MacNeilage, P. F., Studdert-Kennedy, M. G., and Lindblom, B. (1988). Primate handedness: A foot in the door. *Behav. Brain Sci.*, 11, 737.

MacNeilage, P. F., Studdert-Kennedy, M. G., and Lindblom, B. (1991). Primate handedness: The other theory, the other hand, and the other attitude. *Behav. Brain Sci.*, 14, 344.

Manning, J. T. and Chamberlain, A. T. (1990). The left side cradling preference in great apes. *Anim. Behav.*, 39, 1224.

Manning, J. T., Heaton, R., and Chamberlain, A. T. (1994). Left-side cradling: similarities and differences between apes and humans. *J. Human Evol.*, 26, 77.

Marchant, L. F. and McGrew, W. C. (1994). Laterality in hand-use in daily activities by wild chimpanzees: first exhaustive field study. *Proc. Int. Primatol. Conf.*, Bali, Indonesia, 104.

Marchant, L. F. and Steklis, H. D. (1986). Hand preference in a captive island group of chimpanzees (*Pan troglodytes*). *Am. J. Primatol.*, 10, 301.

Martin, R. D. (1982). Allometric approaches to the evolution of the primate nervous system. In E. Armstrong and D. Falk (Eds.), *Primate Brain Evolution: Methods and Concepts*, New York, Plenum, 39.

Masataka, N. (1989). Population level asymmetry of hand preference in lemurs. *Behaviour*, 110, 1.

Masataka, N. (1990). Handedness of capuchin monkeys. *Folia Primatol.*, 55, 189.

Matoba, M., Masataka, N., and Tanioka, Y. (1991). Cross generational continuity of hand use preference in marmosets. *Behaviour*, 117, 281.

Mattingley, J. B., Bradshaw, J. L., Phillips, J. G., and Bradshaw, J. A. (1993). Reversed perceptual asymmetry for faces in left unilateral neglect. *Brain Cognit.*, 23, 145.

Megirian, D., Weller, L., Martin, G. F., and Watson, C. R. R. (1977). Aspects of laterality in the marsupial *Trichosurus vulpecula* (brush-tailed possum). *Ann. N. Y. Acad. Sci.*, 299, 197.

Mehta, Z. and Newcombe, F. (1991). A role for the left hemisphere in spatial processing. *Cortex*, 27, 153.

Michel, G. F. and Harkins, D. A. (1985). Concordance of handedness between teacher and student facilitates learning manual skills. *J. Human Evol.*, 4, 597.

Morris, R. D. and Hopkins W. D. (1993). Perception of human chimeric faces by chimpanzees: Evidence for a right hemisphere advantage. *Brain Cognit.*, 21, 111.

Morris, R. D., Hopkins, W. D., and Bolser-Gilmore, L. (1993). Assessment of hand preference in two language-trained chimpanzees (*Pan troglodytes*): A multimethod analysis. *J. Clin. Exp. Neuropsychol.*, 15, 487.

Morse, P. A., Molfese, D., Laughlin, N. K., Linnville, S., and Wetzel, F. (1987). Categorical perception for voicing contrasts in normal and lead treated rhesus monkeys: Electrophysiological indices. *Brain Lang.*, 30, 63.

Newton, P. N. and Nishida, T. (1990). Possible buccal administration of herbal drugs by wild chimpanzees, *Pan troglodytes*. *Anim. Behav.*, 39, 798.

Newton, P. and Wolfe N. (1992). Can animals teach us medicine? Over the counter and into the forest. *Brit. Med. J.*, 305, 1517.

Nishida, T. (1993). Left nipple suckling preference in wild chimpanzees. *Ethol. Sociobiol.*, 14, 45.

Nishida, T. and Hiraiwa, M. (1982). Natural history of a tool using behavior by wild chimpanzees in feeding upon wood-boring ants. *J. Human Evol.*, 11, 473.

Oakley, K. P. (1972). Skill as a human possession. In S. L. Washburn and P. Dolhinow (Eds.), *Perspectives on Human Evolution, Vol. 2*, New York, Holt, Rinehart and Winston, 14.

Olson, D. A., Ellis, J. E., and Nadler, R. D. (1990). Hand preferences in captive gorillas, orang-utans and gibbons. *Am. J. Primatol.*, 20, 83.

Pepperberg, I. M. (1989). Tool use in birds: An avian monkey wrench? *Behav. Brain Sci.*, 12, 604.

Peters, M. (1988). Footedness: Asymmetries in foot preference and skill and neuropsychological assesment of foot movement. *Psychol. Bull.*, 103, 179.

Petersen, M. R., Beecher, M. D., Zoloth, S. R., Green, S., Marler, P. R., Moody, D. B., and Stebbins, W. C. (1984). Neural lateralization of vocalizations by Japanese macaques: Communicative significance is more important than acoustic structure. *Behav. Neurosci.*, 98, 779.

Petersen, M., Beecher, M., Zoloth, S., Moody, D., and Stebbins, W. (1978). Neural lateralization of species-specific vocalizations by Japanese macaques (*M. fuscata*). *Science*, 202, 324.

Plato, C. C., Wood, J. L., and Norris, A. H. (1980). Bilateral asymmetry in bone measurements of the hand and lateral hand dominance. *Am. J. Phys. Anthropol.*, 52, 27.

Pohl, P. (1983). Central auditory processing V: Ear advantages for acoustic stimuli in baboons. *Brain Lang.*, 20, 44.

Pohl, P. (1984). Ear advantages for temporal resolution in baboons. *Brain Cognit.*, 3, 438.

Porac, C. and Coren, S. (1981). *Lateral Preferences and Human Behavior*, New York, Springer-Verlag, 192.

Porac, C. and Coren, S. (1982). The relationship between sighting dominance and the fading of a stabilized retinal image. *Percept. Psychophy.*, 32, 571.

Porac, C. and Coren, S. (1986). Sighting dominance and egocentric localization. *Vision Res.*, 26, 1709.

Povinelli, D. J., Parks, K. A., and Novak, M. A. (1992). Role reversal by rhesus monkeys, but no evidence of empathy. *Anim. Behav.*, 43, 269.

Preilowski, B., Reger, M., and Engele, H. C. (1986). Handedness and cerebral asymmetry in nonhuman primates. In D. M. Taub and F. A. King (Eds.), *Current Perspectives in Primate Biology*, New York, Van Nostrand and Reinhold, 270.

Premack, D. (1988). "Does the chimpanzee have a theory of mind?" revisited. In R. Byrne and A. Whiten (Eds.). *Machiavellian Intelligence: Social Expertise and the Evolution of Intellect in Monkeys, Apes and Humans*, Oxford, Oxford University Press, 160.

Rogers, L. J. and Kaplan, G. (1994). Handedness in orang-utans. *Proceedings of the International Orang-utan Conference: The Neglected Ape*. Fullerton, CA.

Rogers, L. J., Ward, J. P., and Stafford, D. (1994). Eye dominance in the Small-Eared Bushbaby, *Otolemur garnetti*. *Neuropsychologia*, 32, 257.

Rubens, A. B., Mahowold, M. W., and Hutton, J. T. (1976). Asymmetry of the lateral sylvian fissures in man. *Neurology*, 26, 620.

Saling, M. M. and Kaplan-Solms, K. L. (1989). On lateral asymmetry in cradling behavior and breast sensitivity. *Curr. Anthropol.*, 30, 210.

Schaller, G. B. (1963). *The Mountain Gorilla: Ecology and Behavior*. Chicago, Chicago University Press.

Schell, L. M., Johnston, F. E., Smith, D. R., and Paolone, A.M. (1985). Direction asymmetry of body dimensions among white adolescents. *Am. J. Phys. Anthropol.*, 67, 317.

Sergent, J., Ohta S., and MacDonald B. (1992). Functional neuroanatomy of face and object processing. *Brain*, 115, 15.

Shafer, D. D. (1993). Patterns of handedness: Comparative study of nursery school children and captive gorillas. In J. P. Ward and W.D. Hopkins (Eds.), *Primate Laterality: Current Behavioral Evidence of Primate Asymmetries*, New York, Springer, 267.

Smith, B. H. (1990). The cost of a large brain. *Behav. Brain Sci.*, 13, 265.

Smith, L. (1970). Eye dominance in a monkey. *Percept. Motor Skills*, 31, 657.

Sohmiya, T. and Sohmiya, K. (1985). Analysis of temporal suppression mechanism in binocular rivalry. *Percept. Motor Skills*, 60, 995.

Stafford, D. K., Milliken, G. W., and Ward, J. P. (1990). Lateral bias in feeding and brachiation in *Hylobates*. *Primates*, 31, 407.

Stanley, S. M. (1992). An ecological theory for the origin of Homo. *Paleobiology*, 18, 237.

Strauss, E. and Goldsmith, S. M. (1987). Lateral preference and performance on non-verbal laterality tests in a normal population. *Cortex*, 23, 495.

Suarez, S. D. and Gallup, G. G. (1986). Face touching in primates: A closer look. *Neuropsychologia*, 24, 597.

Tobias, P. V. (1987). The brain of *H. habilis*: A new level of organization in cerebral evolution. *J. Human Evol.*, 16, 741.

Toth, N. (1985). Archaeological evidence for preferential right handedness in the Lower and Middle Pleistocene, and its possible implications. *J. Human Evol.*, 14, 607.

Vauclair, J. and Fagot, J. (1987). Spontaneous hand usage and handedness in a troop of baboons. *Cortex*, 23, 265.

Vauclair, J. and Fagot, J. (1993). Manual and hemispheric specialization in manipulation of a joystick by baboons (*Papio papio*). *Behav. Neurosci.*, 107, 210.

Ward, J. P., Milliken, G. W., Dodson, D. L., Stafford, D. K., and Wallace, M. (1990). Handedness as a function of sex and age in a large population of lemur. *J. Comp. Psychol.*, 104, 167.

Ward, J. P., Milliken, G. W., and Stafford, D. K. (1993). Patterns of lateralized behavior in prosimians. In J. P. Ward, and W. D. Hopkins (Eds.), *Primate Laterality: Current Behavioral Evidence of Primate Asymmetries*, New York, Springer, 43.

Watanabe, K. and Kawai, M. (1993). Lateralized hand use in the precultural behavior of the koshima monkeys (*M. fuscata*). In J. P. Ward and W.D. Hopkins (Eds.), *Primate Laterality: Current Behavioral Evidence of Primate Asymmetries*, New York, Springer, 183.

Weinberger, D. R., Luchins, D. J., Morihisa, J., and Wyatt, R. J. (1982). Asymmetrical volumes of the right and left frontal and occipital regions of the human brain. *Ann. Neurol.*, 11, 97.

Westergaard, G. C. (1989). Infant baboons spontaneously use an object to obtain distant food. *Percept. Motor Skills*, 68, 558.

Westergaard, G. C. (1991). Hand preference in the use and manufacture of tools by tufted capuchin (*Cebus apella*) and lion-tailed macaques (*Macaca silenus*) monkeys. *J. Comp. Psychol.*, 105, 172.

Westergaard, G. C. (1992). Object manipulation and the use of tools by infant baboons *Papio cynocephalus anubis*). *J. Comp. Psychol.*, 106, 398.

Westergaard, G. C. and Suomi, S. J. (1994). The use and modification of bone tools by capuchin monkeys. *Curr. Anthropol.*, 35, 75.

Whiten, A. (1991). The emergence of mindreading: Steps towards an interdisciplinary enterprise. In A. Whiten (Ed.), *Natural Theories of Mind: Evolution, Development and Simulation of Everyday Mindreading*, Oxford: Blackwell, 195.

Whiten, A. and Byrne, R. W. (1988). The Machiavellian intelligence hypothesis. In R. W. Byrne and A. Whiten (Eds.), *Machiavellian Intelligence*, Oxford, Clarendon Press, 1.

Wind, J. (1989). The evolutionary history of the human speech organs. In J. Wind and E. Pulleyblank (Eds.), *Studies in Language Origins*, Amsterdam, Benjamins, 173.

Witelson, S. F. and Pallie, W. (1973). Left hemisphere specialization for language in the newborn: Neuroanatomical evidence of asymmetry. *Brain*, 96, 641.

Wynn, T. (1989). *The Evolution of Spatial Competence: Illinois Studies in Anthropology, Number 17.* Urbana and Chicago, University of Illinois Press.

Wynn, T. and McGrew, W. C. (1989). An ape's view of the Oldowan. *Man*, 24, 383.

Yeni-Komshian, G. H. and Benson, D. A. (1976). Anatomical study of cerebral asymmetry in the temporal lobe of humans, chimpanzees and rhesus monkeys. *Science*, 192, 387.

Section II

Human Handedness

Chapter 3

The Measurement of Handedness and Its Relation to Neuropsychological Issues

M.P. Bryden, M. Barbara Bulman-Fleming, and Valerie MacDonald

CONTENTS

1. AN INTRODUCTION TO THE PROBLEM

1.1 WHY IS HANDEDNESS INTERESTING?

A major reason for being interested in handedness lies in the assumption that a knowledge of handedness can help us predict something about cerebral organization. It has long been known that the incidence of aphasia following unilateral damage to the left cerebral hemisphere differs in left- and right-handers. In most right-handers, language disturbances frequently occur following left-hemispheric damage, but rarely following right-hemispheric damage. In contrast, the incidence of aphasia following right-hemisphere damage is much higher in left-handers. While the simple assumption that left-handers are the mirror image of right-handers, with their language being lateralized to the right hemisphere, is not tenable, it is clear that the distribution of brain organization differs in the two groups. In general, left-handers are far more likely than right-handers to have a bilateral or right-hemispheric specialization for language (Segalowitz and Bryden, 1983).

0-8493-8999-2/96/$0.00+$.50

However, most left-handers, like most right-handers, have language lateralized to the left hemisphere. This observation has inspired researchers to search for a better predictor of cerebral organization than simple hand preference. Underlying this investigation of the association between handedness and cerebral organization are three major ideas. First, it has often been thought that some lateral preference variable other than the preferred writing hand might show a stronger association with cerebral language lateralization. Writing hand is clearly culturally influenced (Beukelaar and Kroonenberg, 1986), and there are many tales of children who have been literally forced to write with their right hands. Therefore, as the logic goes, it may well be that some other variable associated with handedness but not subject to the same environmental pressures is an even better predictor of cerebral lateralization. Such arguments have led to proposals that eye dominance (Luria, 1970), arm crossing and hand folding patterns (Sakano, 1982), footedness (Searleman, 1980), and the relative proficiency with which pegs can be moved from one place to another (Annett, 1985) are better predictors of cerebral lateralization than is writing hand. They have also led to the belief that improved or more refined measures of handedness will enable a better prediction of functional lateralization.

A second line of reasoning to account for the failure of handedness measures to predict cerebral organization is based on the argument that some individuals are "naturally" left-handed, while others have become so because of minor cerebral insult at or near birth. Rasmussen and Milner (1977) have shown that the incidence of right-hemisphere language representation in left-handers is far higher in those for whom there is some evidence of early brain damage than in those for whom there is no such evidence. Thus, early unilateral brain damage may well lead to a reallocation of cerebral functions to the undamaged hemisphere. A major problem is to determine the prevalence of such reorganization. By one view, only fairly major damage will produce a shift of both handedness and language to the right hemisphere (Satz, 1972). By another view, relatively minor insult may initiate changes in brain organization (Bakan, 1971; Coren, 1992). This latter view has lead to the investigation of birth stress as a determinant of handedness, in an attempt to identify individuals who are "pathological" left-handers (Bakan, 1971; Satz, 1972; McManus, 1983; Satz, Orsini, Saslow, and Henry, 1985). A related argument is that one should distinguish between "familial" left-handers, who are presumably "naturally left-handed," and "nonfamilial" left-handers, who are presumably "really" like right-handers (Hécaen and Sauguet, 1971; McKeever, 1981). Such a view, of course, implies that there is a genetic basis to handedness (McManus and Bryden, 1992). However, it still leaves us with our initial problem: even if we are able to identify certain left-handers as "pathological," we still need to devise and employ appropriate measures of handedness with the nonpathological group.

The third argument is that one should search for an additional variable that, in conjunction with handedness, would predict cerebral organization. Presumably, then, one would look for some behavior that characterized a reasonable number of left-handers (e.g., 20 to 40%), but that was relatively rare in right-handers. Such logic has led to the proposal that handwriting posture predicts whether speech is ipsilateral or contralateral to the writing hand, since a large number of left-handers write with an "inverted" or "hooked" posture, while very few right-handers do (Levy and Nagylaki, 1972; Levy and Reid, 1978). Similarly, Luria (1970) has argued that right-handers who have some characteristics of left-handers are more likely to recover from left-hemisphere aphasias and therefore have a more bilateral language representation. He has termed these people "latent left-handers," and argued that such variables as eye dominance, arm crossing, hand clasping, and the relative size of the fingernails can assist in classifying such individuals. By Luria's arguments, right-handers who are left-eyed or who cross their left arm over their right have signs of being latent left-handers and therefore have some right-hemisphere language involvement. The problem with this concept of latent left-handedness is that a very high percentage of dextrals show at least some of Luria's signs, yet there are relatively few right-handers with bilateral or right-hemisphere language representation (Rasmussen and Milner, 1977). In some ways, the focus is on the wrong place; left-handers are more variable in their language lateralization than are right-handers (Segalowitz and Bryden, 1983), and it is the variability of the left-handers that needs explanation. Nevertheless, it is possible that the variables Luria recommends to predict latent left-handedness may also predict "latent right-handedness" and thereby aid in distinguishing those left-handers with left-hemisphere language from those with right-hemisphere language.

1.2 THE APPROACH OF THIS CHAPTER

This chapter is divided into three major sections. In the initial section, we introduce a number of genetic models that have been proposed to account for the relation between handedness and language lateralization. Rather than being predicated on the assumption that handedness and cerebral lateralization are immutably linked, the models that we shall present are concerned with accounting for both the observed association between language lateralization and handedness and the fact that the two are not perfectly correlated. We have placed this section first because an appreciation of these models is helpful in assessing problems in the measurement of handedness and in relating handedness to cerebral function. In the second section, we shall examine some of the problems in the measurement of handedness. In particular, we shall consider the relative merits of preference inventories and performance measures and attempt to identify some of the major problems in current handedness research. In the third section, we shall examine more closely the relationship between handedness and cerebral organization, as determined from both clinical and experimental studies. In this section, we shall attempt to assess the relevance of various mediating variables, and try to identify the major issues as we see them.

2. MODELS OF HANDEDNESS AND LANGUAGE LATERALIZATION

In developing a model to account for the relation between handedness and cerebral lateralization, one must consider two points. One is that left-handers and right-handers do differ in the incidence of right-hemisphere language representation, and therefore there must be some factor that leads handedness and language functions to be controlled by the same hemisphere. The second is that most people, whether dextral or sinistral, have left-hemisphere language representation, and thus there must be factors that lead to a decoupling of handedness and language. It is therefore not sufficient to postulate that handedness and language both have their origins in motor sequencing (Kimura, 1979) without providing some mechanism by which the two can become separated.

Many of the current genetic theories of handedness and cerebral lateralization have been reviewed by McManus and Bryden (1992). The common feature of most of the successful models (Annett, 1985; McManus, 1985; McManus and Bryden, 1992) is that they postulate one allele (RS+ in the Annett model or D in the McManus models) that leads to both right-handedness and left-hemisphere language, and a second allele (RS– or C) that leads to language and manual praxis being independently and randomly lateralized. Thus, those homozygous for this random factor will include both left-handers and right-handers, with both left- and right-hemisphere speech, in roughly equal proportions. In their present forms, both the Annett (1985) and McManus (McManus and

Bryden, 1992) models are additive in that the heterozygotes are intermediate between the two homozygous genotypes. In addition, McManus and Bryden (1992) have postulated a sex-linked moderator gene to account for the higher incidence of left-handedness in males and the fact that left-handed mothers produce more left-handed offspring than do left-handed fathers.

Yeo and Gangestad (1993) have recently proposed a quite different, yet compelling, model of the origins of handedness variation. Theirs is a polygenic model that posits developmental instability in fetal development leading to handedness phenotypes that differ from the modal norm of moderate right-handedness, namely left-handedness or extreme right-handedness. Essentially, their model denies that handedness per se is under genetic control, rather attributing variations in manifest handedness to variations in heterozygosity.

They cite evidence in support of the idea that left-handers have reduced fitness and propose that the reason left-handedness is still present in the population is that there are advantages to the heterozygous state. Thus, individuals whose genotypes are relatively more homozygous will be less well-buffered from developmental perturbations occurring during critical stages in development and will manifest, in addition to the two nonmodal handedness phenotypes (left- and extreme right-handedness), other physical evidence of developmental instability such as a higher index of fluctuating asymmetry (FA) and more minor physical anomalies (MPA). FA is a measure of the differences in size between paired morphological characters (e.g., tooth size, palm and finger ridge counts, ear lobe and limb bone lengths in humans; Palmer and Strobeck, 1986), irrespective of the direction of the difference. Deviations from the mean difference of zero between bilateral traits is considered an indication of the lack of developmental stability of the organism and generally show significant negative correlations with other measures of genetic heterozygosity (Livshits and Kobyliansky, 1991; Palmer and Strobeck, 1986). MPAs are just that — small variations in morphology of certain physical features such as the ears (malformed, positioned low on the head) or eyes (widely spaced). Yeo and Gangestad (1993) reviewed evidence showing that both left-handers and extreme right-handers have higher indices of MPA and FA than do moderate right-handers (Yeo, Gangestad, and Daniel, 1993) and that left-handed parents produce relatively more *extreme right-handed* as well as left-handed children than do right-handed parents (Gangestad and Yeo, 1994). They also presented some evidence that left- and extreme right-handers are generally more homozygous than are moderate right-handers, a result predicted by their model (Yeo and Gangestad, 1993). Finally, they suggested that environmental agents could mediate handedness variation through genetic differences in human leucocyte antigen (HLA) alleles; possession of certain HLA alleles or haplotypes could predispose one to increased susceptibility to pathogen attack early in development which could be the source of developmental instability.

While these are not the only theories of handedness (see reviews by Hardyck and Petrinovitch, 1977, and Porac and Coren, 1981), they do have the property not only of accounting for the distribution of handedness in families, but also of providing a rationale for why handedness and language lateralization are not immutably linked. Other theories of cerebral asymmetry, such as Kimura's (1979) notion that language is but an oral manifestation of the same motor sequencing system required to control manual gesture or Corballis and Morgan's (1978) idea that there is a left-to-right developmental gradient during fetal growth, seem to encounter difficulty in decoupling handedness from language lateralization. However, rather than evaluating these models at the present time, it seems appropriate to examine the data concerning the relation between handedness and lateralization of cerebral function.

3. THE MEASUREMENT OF HANDEDNESS

3.1 PREFERENCE INVENTORIES

One of the major problems in relating handedness to other variables is that different investigators use different means of assessing handedness. For example, in investigating the relations between handedness and language lateralization, Kimura (1983) and Rasmussen and Milner (1977) have combined "mixed" and "left-handed" people into a single group of "non-right-handers." In contrast, Geffen and Caudrey (1981) distinguished between strong left-handers and people of mixed handedness. While it is easy to see why one might want to combine all non-right-handers together in order to increase the cell sample size, this procedure confounds degree and direction of handedness and makes it very difficult to determine which aspect of handedness is correlated with the observed functional or anatomical asymmetry. Nevertheless, despite years of research, there are no clearly defined conventions for defining handedness or for determining which subgroups to combine. Both performance and preference measures have been used, and the particular tasks or items employed vary greatly from one investigator to another.

Probably the simplest way to assess handedness is to ask the subject (or a close relative or friend) which hand is used to perform various common unimanual activities. Most people are agreed that inquiring about writing hand alone is not sufficient to define handedness; too many people describe situations in which they were encouraged or forced to shift their writing hand. Thus, most questionnaires ask about several activities. The problem is one of selecting the activities and conceptualizing the general properties that one wants the questionnaire to have.

Raczkowski, Kalat, and Nebes (1974) have demonstrated that some common items lack reliability, in the sense that they will not be answered in the same way upon subsequent testing, while others are not valid in the sense that people do not necessarily perform the activities in the way they claim. Items asking about relatively infrequent activities in particular may prove to be invalid. It is common to ask how one holds a needle when threading it, for instance, and those people unaccustomed to sewing may well answer the question in one way, and then do the opposite when actually confronted with the task.

Recent factor analytic studies have shown that many hand preference inventories may be multifactorial (Healey, Liederman, and Geschwind, 1986; Kang and Harris, 1993; Steenhuis and Bryden, 1989a). Geschwind and Galaburda (1987) have suggested that hand preference for fine distal motor movements and arm preference for more gross proximal movements such as those used in hammering or swinging an axe may be controlled by different neural systems, and the Healey et al. (1986) inventory reflects this consideration. However, their data only marginally support the view. Steenhuis and Bryden (1989a) have also used a large number of items to develop a multifactorial preference questionnaire, but were able to find little support for the proximal-distal distinction offered by Geschwind and Galaburda (1987). However, a very large-scale survey carried out through the *National Geographic Magazine* indicates that many people who write with their left hands throw with their right arms, whereas there are relatively few right-handed writers who throw left-handed (Gilbert and Wysocki, 1992). A similar dissociation of writing and throwing in left-handers has been noted by others (Peters and Pang, 1992; Watson and Kimura, 1989). The proximal-distal distinction may therefore be much more critical among left-handed writers than for right-handers.

A further problem is that the criterion against which any handedness questionnaire is evaluated remains unspecified. In effect, the task of constructing a handedness questionnaire is a gigantic bootstrapping operation. One begins with several initial premises: that the majority of people are right-handed; that writing hand is not the sole (or even the best) manifestation of handedness; that there is a legitimate distinction between what people do "naturally" and what they do because of environmental or cultural pressures; and that any good handedness questionnaire must involve items that are both reliable (repeatable) and valid in the sense that people actually behave in the way in which they claim. Beyond this, there seems to be no absolute criterion to determine whether one questionnaire is any better than another, and no *a priori* grounds on which to determine whether one should be looking for one factor or several. The very popular Edinburgh Handedness Inventory (Oldfield, 1971), for example, employs items that differentiate between self-professed left-handers and self-professed right-handers, yet this begs the question by assuming that the criterion for classification is self-professed handedness.

Despite much thought, we have been unable to develop any criterion for validating a handedness measure that will satisfy everyone. To the extent that one believes that handedness assesses some underlying biological variable (Annett, 1985; Bryden, McManus, and Bulman-Fleming, 1994; Geschwind and Galaburda, 1987; McManus and Bryden, 1992), one might expect the best handedness items to be those that show the greatest heritability coefficients. Yet, the search for such effects has been frustrating (Bryden, Singh, and Rogers, 1995). Because we know that handedness is related to cerebral speech organization (Rasmussen and Milner, 1977), a second validation criterion might involve the relation between specific handedness items and brain organization. Again, there appears to be no compelling evidence that any one aspect of hand preference is better related to cerebral organization than another. Finally, one might consider those aspects of handedness that are common across different cultures to be the most important ones (Ida and Bryden, 1996; Payne, 1987; Singh and Bryden, 1994).

A final issue in the construction of handedness questionnaires concerns the gradations of preference asked about in the inventory. Annett (1967), for instance, asks for a dichotomous response (left or right), arguing that further refinements do not add additional valid information. In contrast, the Edinburgh Inventory (Oldfield, 1971) permits scoring in two different ways, which lead to rather different distributions (Schachter, 1993). If one scores the questionnaire as originally proposed, one is asked to mark a "+" in the "left" or "right" column to indicate the preferred hand. If "you would only use the other hand in exceptional circumstances, make a double +;" "mark a + in each of the left and right columns if you would use your two hands equally." Many researchers, without clear explanation, have chosen to employ a 5-point scale, with "always use left or right hand," "usually use left or right hand," and "use both hands equally often" as possible responses, and it is often impossible to determine just how the test was scored. In fact, Briggs and Nebes (1975) have "improved" Annett's questionnaire by using a five-response classification rather than a dichotomous one. The problem with the five-category response continuum is that the distinction between "always" and "usually" is not clearly defined, and people may indicate the weaker "usually" category if they can recall a single instance of using the opposite hand. In a mathematical sense, precision of measurement will be better with a greater number of response catgeories, but this may not be true if the category boundaries mean different things to different people. Furthermore, as Schachter (1993) has clearly pointed out, the specific degree of handedness may depend on the scoring procedure employed.

3.2 PERFORMANCE MEASURES

One alternative to a preference inventory is some form of performance test in which subjects are required to make some simple unimanual movement and are timed at the task. Annett (1985), for example, has regularly employed a peg-moving task in which subjects are asked to move a number of small dowels from one row of holes to another as rapidly as possible. Annett and Kilshaw (1983) presented normative data on this task and reported that the population distribution can be described as two normal distributions, a large one with the mean shifted to the right and a small one with the mean at zero. This breakdown corresponds to the predictions of Annett's (1978; 1985) right-shift model of handedness. In contrast, Tapley and Bryden (1985) reported data on a group test in which subjects were asked to place dots in each of a number of small circles as fast as possible. Their population data also decompose into two normal distributions, but in this case one has a mean shifted to the right and the other a mean shifted to the left. Such a pattern is quite distinct from that predicted by Annett's (1985) model and suggests separate groups of left- and right-handed subjects.

There are several possible reasons for this discrepancy. One is that the Tapley-Bryden task is a group paper-and-pencil task, sharing some properties with handwriting and correlating more highly with writing hand than with other items on a preference inventory (Steenhuis and Bryden, 1989b). In contrast, the Annett task is individually administered and shares little in common with writing; it correlates most strongly with the preferred hand for hammering (Annett, 1985).

In addition to peg-moving and dot-filling, many other performance tests have been proposed. For example, Peters and Durding (1978; 1979) have shown that the rate with which one can tap a key with the index finger is a reliable test and that it correlated with hand preference measures. Borod, Koff, and Caron (1984) have proposed a test in which the task is to place a mark in the center bull's-eye of four concentric circles. This particular task can be administered for speed, when the total time required to hit 32 targets is measured, or for accuracy, when the subject is required to aim for a new target every 1/144th of a minute (every 417 msec.). Borod et al. (1984) have shown that this test differentiates between left- and right-handers, and that both speed and accuracy measures correlate with hand preference and tapping speed.

As with preference inventories, the problem with performance tests is that it is difficult to know what one is trying to measure. Barnsley and Rabinovitch (1970), for instance, found ten distinct factors in an analysis of motor proficiency. Similarly, Van Horn and McManus (1993) found that Annett's (1985) peg-moving task, Tapley and Bryden's (1985) dot-filling task, and Bishop's (1990) square-drawing task loaded on independent factors. These data would suggest that there are a number of dimensions to performance differences between the hands. It is not surprising, therefore, that the Annett peg-moving task is most highly correlated with the hammering item on a preference inventory, while the Tapley-Bryden circle-dotting task is correlated with handwriting preference. In both cases, the most correlated preference item is one that shares common motor components with the performance task.

3.3 AN INTEGRATION OF PREFERENCE AND PERFORMANCE

Performance tasks have two real advantages over preference inventories. First, they involve the observed participation of the subject and not simply his/her claim about the preferred way of performing the activity; in this sense, they provide an intrinsically more valid measure. Second, performance measures can easily provide measurement along a continuum, and most authors would agree that handedness is a continuum, and that it is legitimate to talk about degrees of handedness.

On the other hand, performance measures usually require more equipment than do preference measures, and some of this equipment may be at least modestly expensive. They are normally best administered individually (but cf. Tapley and Bryden, 1985; Borod et al., 1984) and tend to take rather more time than do preference inventories.

Recently, there have been several attempts to develop objective measures of preference (Bishop, Ross, Daniels, and Bright, 1996; Bryden and Edmonds, 1995; Bryden, Singh, Steenhuis, and Clarkson, 1994). In the Bryden and Edmonds task, for instance, subjects were asked to turn one of three knobs, one located to the left, one to the right, and one below a display, to control a cursor on a computer monitor. On each trial, a small light indicated which knob was to be used. Subjects were free to use either hand. Subjects used their preferred hand in a greater region of space than their nonpreferred hand. Within handedness groups, estimates of the region of space in which the preferred hand was used correlated significantly with scores on a hand preference questionnaire. Thus, this technique holds promise for providing an objective measure of the degree of hand preference.

3.4 THE DISTRIBUTION OF HAND PREFERENCE

It is very difficult to compare the actual prevalence of left-handedness in different populations, given that different studies vary in both the specific questions included in their handedness inventories and in their criteria for classifying people as left-handed. However, in a meta-analysis of a large number of surveys of handedness, Seddon and McManus (1993) concluded that the world-wide incidence of left-handedness was approximately 8%. Seddon and McManus (1993) also claimed that there are no significant racial or ethnic differences, although other data suggest that the incidence of left-handedness is lower (about 3 to 5%) in Oriental samples than in Caucasian ones (Porac, Rees, and Buller, 1990; Hatta and Nakatsuka, 1976; Ida and Bryden, 1996; Shimizu and Endo, 1983; Teng, Lee, Yang, and Chang, 1979) At the other extreme, Dawson (1977) reports that the incidence of left-handedness is as high as 15% among Alaskan Inuit.

In many aboriginal societies, the prevalence of left-handedness appears to be extraordinarily low. For example, Bryden, Ardila, and Ardila (1993) have tested over 100 Tucano Indians in South America and failed to find a single left-hander. Likewise, there are reports of very few left-handers among the Katanga in Zaire (0.5%; Verhaegen and Ntumba, 1964), in the Solomon Islands (2.8%; Rhoades and Damon, 1973), and among several other aboriginal African and South American societies (Marchant, McGrew, and Eibl-Eibesfeldt, 1995). Bryden, Singh, and Rogers (1995) have suggested that the relatively low incidence of left-handedness seen in India (about 5%) can be accounted for in a genetic framework by selective marriages and a lower frequency of the allele leading to left-handedness. It remains a matter for further research to determine whether the very low rates of left-handedness seen in some aboriginal societies are the result of particular cultural pressures (Bryden et al., 1993) or of the absence of the allele leading to left-handedness (McManus and Bryden, 1993).

The prevalence of left-handedness is also about 25% higher in males than in females (Seddon and McManus, 1993). This represents an additional problem because there is no evidence that the prevalence of right-hemispheric language is any higher in men than in women, and if anything, the opposite is the case (McGlone, 1980; Kimura and Harshman, 1984). Therefore, the sex difference in handedness implies that there must be differences between men and women in the association between handedness and cerebral organization.

3.5 AGE EFFECTS IN HANDEDNESS

Porac and Coren (1981) and Fennell (1985) indicate that people become more right-handed with age. Not only are young children more ambiguous with respect to handedness than are older children, but adults seem to become more right-handed with increasing age. Thus, for instance, the prevalence of right-handedness is estimated to be 97 to 99% in subjects 55 years old or older (Fleminger, Dalton, and Standage, 1977; Gilbert and Wysocki, 1992; Porac, Coren, and Duncan, 1980). There are several possible explanations for this. First of all, common lore has it that left-handedness is less likely to be discouraged by parents and teachers in recent years, with the result that fewer left-handers are compelled to become right-handed for writing than was the case in the past and this is born out by some research (Hugdahl, Satz, Mitrushina, and Miller, 1993). However, Porac and Coren (1981) found no correlation between the prevalence of left-handedness and the date of the study in a survey of 20th-century studies of handedness.

Coren and Halpern (1991) have suggested that left-handers are at greater risk for early death than are right-handers. They reported that left-handers die, on average, 7 years younger than do right-handers. These data have been questioned by others (e.g., Harris, 1993; Wolf, D'Agostino, and Cobb, 1991), and Coren and Halpern (1991) may have overestimated the magnitude of the effect, but it remains possible that there is a differential mortality for left-handers and right-handers (Coren, 1994; Hugdahl et al., 1993).

Results from a three-generational survey of handedness (Bryden, 1987) suggest a third possibility (Table 3.1). In this study, a simple performance test of handedness (Tapley and Bryden, 1985), and a short hand preference questionnaire (Bryden, 1977) were given to undergraduate students, their parents, and their grandparents. The data support the view that the prevalence of left-handedness is higher among young people than in the elderly. However, they also suggest that the elderly are stronger in their hand preference than are younger people in that they show more extreme scores on the preference questionnaire. Thus, it may not be so much that people are becoming more right-handed as that they are becoming more fixed and determined in their hand preference or more likely to endorse the extreme categories in preference inventories. It may be, then, that not only are right-handers getting more right-handed, but left-handers are becoming more left-handed. By this argument, the apparent increase of right-handedness is due to increasingly stronger preferences in a population that is dominated by right-handers. Therefore, the increase in right-handedness may be viewed as a result of two factors: a strengthening of the degree of preference with age and an increased willingness of society to permit left-handed children to remain left-handed. Note that the same effect is not observed in the performance data and that the older right-handers are actually less strongly right-handed than the younger right-handers.

Table 3.1 Age Effects in Degree and Direction of Handedness

			Preference[a]		Performance[b]	
Age Group	**N**	**%L**	**Left**	**Right**	**Left**	**Right**
Old (64+)	206	1.9	10.7	36.1	–.10	+.17
Middle (35–54)	314	8.6	14.5	35.7	–.20	+.20
Young (20–29)	530	19.8	16.4	34.7	–.19	+.22

[a] Preference score based on 8-item questionnaire, with maximum of 40 (extreme right-handedness) and minimum of 8 (extreme left-handedness).

[b] Performance score based on dot-filling task (Tapley and Bryden, 1985). Positive scores indicate right hand superiority.

3.6 SOME CONCLUSIONS ABOUT THE MEASUREMENT OF HANDEDNESS

In the final analysis, the major issue in the selection of a test for handedness concerns just what aspects of handedness are important to measure. Many hand preference items are reliable, valid in the sense that people actually perform in the way they claim, and distinguish between self-professed left-handers and self-professed right-handers. Likewise, many fairly simple hand proficiency tasks are reliable and distinguish between handedness groups. If, however, handedness is a multidimensional skill, it remains uncertain which dimension is most critical, and for what. If the goal is simply to define objectively those people who will claim to be left- or right-handed, then perhaps the skills that cluster around handwriting are the best, at least in contemporary North American and Western European societies; if, on the other hand, the goal is to predict something about the pattern of cerebral organization, then it is more open to question which aspect of handedness is the most appropriate to measure. Because gross movements of the limbs tend to be controlled bilaterally, and fine movements, especially grasping movements, of the fingers are more likely to be controlled contralaterally, it is tasks related to handwriting and fine motor dexterity that are more likely to be closely related to other lateralized cerebral functions. Nevertheless, there remains much research to be done.

4. HANDEDNESS AND NEUROPSYCHOLOGICAL ISSUES

4.1 HISTORICAL BACKGROUND

The doctrine that control of language functions and control of manual dominance were localized to the same hemisphere became popular shortly after Broca's observation that language was primarily a left-hemisphere function (Benton, 1965). One can find suggestions of a relationship between handedness and the cerebral control of language in the work of Broca, Bastian (1868), and Hughlings Jackson (1958), writing in the 1860s and 1870s. It is true that the infrequent cases of crossed aphasia, in whom damage to the right hemisphere produced aphasia in a right-hander, or damage to the left hemisphere led to aphasia in a left-hander, represented a major problem to the view that there was a direct link between handedness and language lateralization, but this general view has persisted until quite recently (cf. Zangwill, 1960).

During much of this period, any evidence of atypical laterality was viewed as pathological (cf. Geschwind and Galaburda, 1987). For example, Orton (1925; 1937) related reading disability to an inappropriate cerebral dominance, postulating that those individuals with incomplete cerebral lateralization would have difficulty in discriminating mirror-images and would generally have difficulty with perceiving letters in their proper sequence. He felt that poor readers often had poorly developed laterality, mixed hand-eye dominance, or came from families with a high incidence of left-handedness. This general view, suggesting that people with mixed patterns of lateralization are somehow abnormal, was taken to an extreme by Delacato (1966), who recommended retraining one's motor behavior to bring hand and eye dominance into congruence. Orton's views have also been instrumental in focusing attention on measures of lateralization other than handedness, such as eyedness, footedness, and earedness (Porac and Coren, 1981), and on the concept of mixed dominance.

However, the observation of crossed aphasia, particularly in sinistrals, has made it increasingly clear that handedness and language lateralization are not immutably linked. By the 1960s, we not only understood that the majority of left-handers were like right-handers in that they had language represented in the left hemisphere, but also that the right hemisphere had its own unique functions (Benton, 1965; Zangwill, 1960). The problem then became one not only of explaining the association between handedness and language lateralization but also of accounting for the exceptions and dealing with the association between handedness and other cerebral functions. The genetic models described earlier represent one approach to show how handedness and language lateralization can be dissociated.

4.2 CLINICAL STUDIES OF HANDEDNESS AND BRAIN ORGANIZATION

Information concerning the relation of handedness to brain organization has come from two sources: studies of the incidence of aphasia following unilateral brain damage and studies involving the use of sodium amytal to selectively anesthetize the hemispheres prior to surgery. Of course, such studies can tell us only about the lateralization of language functions. Although it is often assumed that "right-hemisphere" functions, such as visuospatial and emotion perceptual processes, are necessarily complementary to left-hemisphere language functions, much evidence suggests that this is not the case (Bryden, Hécaen, and DeAgostini, 1983; Bulman-Fleming and Bryden, 1994; Jäncke, Schlaug, Huang, and Steinmetz, 1994). Thus, it is at least theoretically possible for handedness to bear one predictive relationship to language lateralization and quite another to the lateralization of other functions. Most of the following section focuses on the lateralization of language, but it is wise to remember that the association between handedness and language lateralization may be quite different from the association between handedness and other lateral specializations.

Large-scale surveys of the aphasia literature such as those by Segalowitz and Bryden (1983) and Carter, Satz, and Hohenegger (1984) have provided one means whereby the relation between handedness and language lateralization has been assessed. Both research groups attempted to collect data from as many studies of aphasia following unilateral brain damage as possible, and to use these data to estimate the relative frequency of left, right, and bilateral language representation. One problem with such an approach is that the estimates of the incidence of aphasia will depend on the number of nonaphasic cases included. Most of the studies relating handedness to aphasia have been primarily concerned with the occurrence of aphasia, not with the failure of aphasia to appear. Furthermore, the classification of cases as left-handed is often unclear, with some individuals being categorized as left-handed on the basis of secondary evidence. This is especially true for right-hemisphere aphasias, which conventional wisdom suggests would be more prevalent in left-handers. These considerations, plus rather different criteria for including a particular study in the analysis, resulted in Segalowitz and Bryden (1983) and Carter et al. (1984) having obtained rather different estimates of the relation between handedness and language lateralization (see Table 3.2). In particular, Carter et al. (1984) gave a very high estimate of the proportion of left-handers having bilateral language representation. Furthermore, Kimura (1983) has presented data on the incidence of aphasia in a large series of patients selected solely for unilateral brain damage, and her data do not deviate significantly from those presented in the Rasmussen and Milner (1977) study. Unfortunately, there were very few cases of aphasia following right-hemisphere damage in Kimura's study, and thus any estimate of the incidence of right-hemisphere language representation has a large error of measurement.

Table 3.2 Language Lateralization and Handedness

	Lateralization		
	Left	**Bilateral**	**Right**
Right-handers			
Carter et al. (1984)	99%	0%	1%
Segalowitz-Bryden (1983)	95%	0%	5%
Rasmussen-Milner (1977)	96%	0%	4%
Left-handers			
Carter et al. (1984)	23%	66%	11%
Segalowitz-Bryden (1983)	61%	20%	19%
Rasmussen-Milner (1977)	70%	15%	15%

A second source of evidence about language lateralization has come from individuals given unilateral injections of sodium amytal anesthetic prior to surgery for temporal lobe epilepsy. This technique produces a suppression of speech if the language-dominant hemisphere is affected but not otherwise (Wada and Rasmussen, 1960). Reporting on several hundred patients with this procedure, Rasmussen and Milner (1977) have provided estimates of the association between handedness and language lateralization that are in close agreement with those proposed by Segalowitz and Bryden (1983). More recent amytal data (as reviewed by Beaton, 1996) are more or less consistent with the earlier work. Notwithstanding, concerns have been raised about the validity of the construct of bilateral speech or, perhaps more properly, mixed-speech dominance (Snyder, Novelly and Harris, 1990) and about the lack of uniformity with which the amytal procedure is administered and interpreted (Snyder et al., 1990). The 55 epilepsy programs using the amytal procedure that were surveyed by Snyder and his colleagues made wildly varying estimates of the prevalence of mixed-speech dominance. Therefore, based on these findings and on other concerns, the authors caution against uncritically embracing the amytal procedure as an accurate method for determination of language lateralization in the absence of other corroborating data.

Warrington and Pratt (1973) have estimated the incidence of right-hemisphere language in left-handers by observing the occurrence of dysphasia following unilateral ECT. Among 30 left-handers without signs of organic disease, 70% were left-hemispheric, 23% right-hemispheric, and 7% uncertain. These figures again are in reasonable correspondence with those provided by Rasmussen and Milner (1977) and by Segalowitz and Bryden (1983). Comparable data in right-handers (Pratt and Warrington, 1972) indicated an incidence of right-hemisphere language of about 2%.

There are virtually no comparable studies of the relation of handedness to putative right-hemisphere functions. However, the data of Bryden et al. (1983) do permit a preliminary statement of the relation between handedness and visuospatial function. Although atypical left-hemisphere visuospatial processing is more prevalent in left-handers than in right-handers, the pattern relating handedness to cerebral function is quite different from that obtained for language functions. In right-handers, visuospatial functions are not nearly so dominantly lateralized to the right hemisphere as language functions are to the left hemisphere. In left-handers, the Bryden et al. (1983) data suggest that visuospatial processes are about equally often lateralized to the left, right, or both hemispheres. In comparison, DeRenzi (1982), in his review of visuospatial processes, suggests that the effects of unilateral brain damage are similar in left- and right-handers. Further research is clearly needed before any definitive statements can be made.

One problem with these estimates is that many investigators have divided their groups into "right-handed" and "non-right-handed." While such a division is statistically convenient, the "non-right-hander" group is not only more likely to be left-handed than the "right-hander" group, but it is also less well differentiated with respect to handedness, containing many people who have only weak lateral preferences. As a result, degree of handedness and direction of handedness are confounded, and this may well be an important issue (cf. Bryden, 1987; Collins, 1985).

4.3 HANDEDNESS AND ANATOMICAL ASYMMETRIES

A number of studies have investigated the possible neuroanatomical correlates of manual dominance. The majority of these have focused either on asymmetries in the superior temporal/Sylvian fissure region or on differences in size and shape of the corpus callosum. The question of whether there exists a relation between handedness and cerebral morphological asymmetries is fraught with difficulties, not the least of which are measurement issues.

In assessing cerebral anatomy, researchers use different methods to obtain measurements, measure different regions, and utilize differing methods to analyze data. Because of their proximity to areas thought to subserve language functions, superior temporal regions have been related to individual differences in language lateralization and handedness. But, because of differences in morphology between the two hemispheres, there is no universally accepted algorithm for the measurement of, for example, the length of the Sylvian fissure or the area of the planum temporale (PT). The Sylvian fissure has a longer horizontal component on the left side, and a longer vertical component on the right (Geschwind and Galaburda, 1987; Beaton, 1996), and there are two Heschl gyri more frequently on the right side than on the left, so depending on whether both, if present, are included in the PT area measure, asymmetries may or not be found (see Beaton, 1996, for a discussion of these issues). Recently, there appears to be agreement among researchers on at least some of these measurement issues (but see Habib, Robichon, Lévrier, Khalil, and Salamon, 1995). Also, of course, as far as asymmetries in these brain regions are concerned, even if some anatomical measure were found that was a perfect marker for language lateralization (itself difficult to measure, as mentioned above), there is still a less-than-perfect correlation between language lateralization and any measure of handedness yet developed.

That said, it must be noted that there have been a number of reports of anatomical differences between left- and right-handers (summarized by Geschwind and Galaburda, 1987). In general, these studies demonstrated an asymmetry in right-handers, and a reduction or lack of asymmetry in left-handers. In the last few years, with the advent of sophisticated *in vivo* magnetic resonance imaging (MRI) techniques for neuroanatomical measurement, it has been possible to use larger sample sizes, as well as healthier subjects, than had been possible in the earlier studies.

For example, Jäncke, Steinmetz, and colleagues have published the results of a number of careful studies which used high-resolution MRI techniques and large numbers of healthy subjects (e.g., Jäncke et al., 1994; Steinmetz, Volkmann, Jäncke, and Freund, 1991). In the Jäncke et al. (1994) study, the PT and planum parietale (PP) of each of 106 young adult right-handers and 35 left-handers (by self classification) were measured. The PT results nicely replicated those of the earlier study (Steinmetz et al., 1991), which had a smaller sample size (26 each of self-professed left- and right-handers). Both studies revealed a significant overall leftward asymmetry of the PT with (at least when handedness was defined by hand skill) significantly greater asymmetry in right-handers. In the 1991 study, most of the handedness effect was contributed by left-handers with at least one first-degree left-handed relative. It would be interesting to know if this was also true for the 1994 data, for which familial sinistrality was not reported. The area PP, as defined by Jäncke et al. and which they conjectured may underlie putative right-hemisphere functions such as visuospatial ability and attention, comprises the posterior walls of the right and left posterior ascending Sylvian fissures. The PP showed an overall rightward asymmetry, with a significant sex by handedness interaction: right-handed men and left-handed women exhibited a particularly strong rightward bias (left-handed men, in fact, were slightly leftward biased). Interestingly, however, the PT and PP measures were not correlated within individuals. For the analyses, handedness was determined by several paper-and-pencil tasks. It is not clear from this report whether there was complete correspondence between self classification and the hand dominance tests. In addition, there were 11 people in the original sample who completely lacked a PP on either hemisphere and whose data were not analyzed. One wonders whether left- and right-handers were equally represented in this group and also whether these people had normal visuospatial and attentional functioning.

Habib's group (Habib et al., 1995) used MRI to obtain length measures of both the PT and the parietal operculum in each of 40 normal volunteers who completed the Edinburgh Handedness Inventory. Subjects whose laterality quotient was +80 or higher, when scores ranged from –100 to +100, were classified as right-handed and others as non-right-handed. Significant leftward asymmetries were found for both PT area and the opercular measure, SR (the distance from the end of the Sylvian fissure to the opercular part of the Rolandic, or central, sulcus as measured on the sagittal section where the distance was greatest) but only in right-handers. Four subgroups were formed based on convergent and divergent asymmetries of the two measures and it was found that hand preference distributions differed among these subgroups. The authors speculated that as PT asymmetries may underlie language asymmetries, so parietal opercular asymmetries may be involved in the lateralized control of motor behaviors (Habib et al., 1995). As was the case in the Jäncke et al. (1994) study for PT and PP asymmetries, PT and parietal opercular asymmetry measures within individuals did not correlate significantly. These data offer additional support for the notion of a lack of causal complementarity of lateralized functions (Bryden, 1982; Bryden et al., 1983; Bulman-Fleming and Bryden, 1994).

In another recent study, Foundas and co-workers (Foundas, Leonard, Gilmore, Fennell, and Heilman, 1994) used MRI to measure PT length in six male and six female seizure patients (age range 17 to 55) who had been tested for language lateralization by the Wada technique. PT measurements in this study were based on the methodology established by Steinmetz and colleagues (Steinmetz, Rademacher, Huang, Hefter, Zilles, Thron, and Freund, 1989). The one patient who was a non-right-hander ("determined on the basis of a handedness inventory"; Foundas et al., 1994, p. 1229) exhibited right-hemisphere speech and a longer right planum length, whereas for the 11 right-handers, the opposite (typical) pattern obtained. The sample size was rather small in this study, and as Beaton (1996) points out, it is not clear from this paper whether degree or direction of handedness is the relevant factor.

Thoma, Lewine, Yeo, Provencal, Davis, Orrison, and Hill (1995), investigating asymmetries in the sensorimotor cortex, used magnetic source imaging to measure the distance between cortical points devoted to the thumb and the fifth finger in the two hemispheres. In each of nine cases, the distance was greater on the side contralateral to the dominant hand, as measured by the Waterloo Handedness Questionnaire. In addition, the correlation between the difference in the cortical distance measure and the difference in peg-moving speed in Annett's (1985) peg-moving task across the two hands was 0.81 ($p < 0.01$). The larger the difference between the dominant hemisphere distance and that of the nondominant hemisphere, the larger was the peg-moving time difference between the dominant and nondominant hands. They also found correlations between the total hand-preference scores and both cortical distance and pegboard-difference scores. This admittedly is a small sample but similar results have been obtained by other workers (Purves, White, and Andrews, 1994; White, Lucas, Richards, and Purves, 1994). These results pose interesting questions as to the direction of causality: does a larger cortical area mean that the contralateral hand will be dominant or does the fact one hand is dominant mean that the contralateral hemisphere will be functionally developed to a greater extent than the ipsilateral one (Thoma et al., 1995)?

Measurement issues are no less complicating for conclusions regarding differences in corpus callosum (CC) size between handedness groups. The questions of how best to measure the CC and to analyze the data are still problematic, as is that of sensible subdivisions of the callosum to be measured. With respect to this last point, there may well be differences in connectivity between the hemispheres that are a function of the areas connected. Because there is at least roughly topographic mapping between cortical region and callosal region (De Lacoste, Kirkpatrick, and Ross, 1985; Olavarria and Van Sluyters, 1986), the way the CC is subdivided into measurement units might be crucial for detecting these differences. Also, it must be kept in mind that CC areal differences need not *necessarily* imply differences in connectivity; the diameter and packing density of fibers as well as the proportion of myelinated and unmyelinated axons could differ as a function of handedness, as has been shown to be the case as a function of sex in rats (Juraska and Kopcik, 1988). Conversely, similar CC areas do not necessarily indicate similar numbers of fibers connecting the two hemispheres. These issues notwithstanding, there have been several investigations of CC size as a function of handedness.

Witelson (1985) was the first to suggest callosal differences between consistent right-handers and non-consistent right-handers. She found that the midline area of the callosum in *post-mortem* brains of 15 nonconsistent right-handers was about 11% larger than that of 27 subjects who showed consistent right-hand preference (Witelson, 1985). Her subsequent work indicates that some effects may only be true for males and in certain callosal regions, namely the isthmus, which is just anterior to the splenium (Witelson, 1989). On the other hand (as it were!), handedness effects were not found in a subsequent study (Steinmetz, Jäncke, Kleinschmidt, Schlaug, Volkmann, and Huang, 1992) which used the handedness classification method that Witelson (1989) used, 52 subjects (including consistent left-handers, which the Witelson sample lacked), and high-resolution MRI technology. A larger proportional isthmus area in women, however, was found in the Steinmetz et al. (1992) study, a result that also emerged from the later Witelson (1989) work but that was *not* upheld in a subsequent study reported by Jäncke and Steinmetz (1994).* In another recent article, Habib and co-workers describe a study in which MRI was used to measure callosal size in normal subjects (Habib, Gayraud, Oliva, Regis, Salamon, and Khalil, 1991). This group partially replicated Witelson's work, in that the callosa of nonconsistent right-handers were found to be larger than those of consistent right-handers, but only for males, and most particularly in the *anterior* half. Consistent right-handed females had significantly larger callosa in the area of the posterior mid-body than did nonconsistent right-handed females. Burke and Yeo (1994), in a study involving 96 healthy elderly subjects (mean age 78), have added to the evidence for there being a gender effect in some callosal regions (females > males when total cerebral volume was taken into account). In addition, they found that increasing posterior callosal size was associated with increasing right-handedness for men, but in women, increasing right-handedness was associated with smaller anterior and posterior CC areas, and mid-callosal width. It should be very clear from the above discussion that more research in this area is required before anything like a clear picture emerges.

4.4 HANDEDNESS AND NONINVASIVE TECHNIQUES FOR ASSESSING LATERALIZATION

Given the problems of the clinical literature, it should be no great surprise that behavioral techniques that can be related to functional lateralization have become very popular in the past several years. Much of the impetus for this research comes from the seminal work of Kimura (1961a,b), who showed a relation between language lateralization and the ear advantage obtained with dichotic listening. Although other techniques such as visual hemifield presentation, bimanual stimulation, and lateralized dual-task performance have also been employed to assess cerebral lateralization in normal subjects (see Bryden, 1982, for a review), by far the most thorough studies have employed dichotic

* The issue of sex differences in callosal size is a contentious one and will not be discussed at length here. The interested reader is referred to a recent article by Beaton (1996) and a recent meta-analysis on the topic by Wahlsten and Bishop (1994).

listening tasks, and the present review will focus on such studies. Although several recent studies (Bryden and Bulman-Fleming, 1995; Jäncke, Steinmetz, and Volkmann, 1992) have revealed a disturbing lack of significant within-subjects correlations between the results using various dichotic procedures, carefully conceived dichotic tasks have been shown to reliably predict lateralization of language production as determined by the amytal procedure (e.g., Zatorre, 1989). In a dichotic listening procedure, subjects are presented with two competing auditory messages simultaneously, one arriving at the left ear and the other arriving at the right ear, usually with the aid of earphones. Kimura (1961a) discovered that patients about to undergo surgery for temporal lobe epilepsy who had known right-hemisphere language lateralization were more accurate in identifying numbers presented to the left ear, while patients with left-hemisphere language were better on the right ear. Furthermore, normal right-handed subjects also showed a right-ear advantage (REA).

A review of dichotic listening studies (Bryden, 1988) revealed that left-handers are significantly less likely to show an REA for language tasks than are right-handers. As is so often the case, the data on nonverbal functions are more sparse, and no clear conclusions can be drawn. However, we have recently described a dichotic technique with which simultaneous left- and right-hemisphere functions can be demonstrated. With it, we have been able to demonstrate the superiority of the right hemisphere (left ear) for processing the affective components of words and the well documented left-hemisphere (right car) advantage for processing of the words themselves (Bulman-Fleming and Bryden, 1994, 1996). This method overcomes some of the problems that have made interpretation of dichotic studies difficult and, in addition, may be able to be modified for use in different sensory modalities, and shed some light on the nature of interhemispheric integration of information (Bulman-Fleming and Bryden, 1994). Kim (1994) has recently reviewed those dichotic listening and divided visual field tasks of perceptual asymmetry that have employed both left- and right-handers and has concluded that right-handers have greater asymmetry whereas left-handers have greater variance and that, within left-handers, those with sinistral relatives show less variability than do those without.

Witelson (1983), Strauss, Lapointe, Wada, Gaddes, and Kosaka (1985), and Kertesz and co-workers (Kertesz, Polk, Black, and Howell, 1992) have all reported correlations between dichotic listening performance and anatomical asymmetries. Jäncke and Steinmetz (1993), however, found no correlations between PT asymmetry and laterality indices for any of four dichotic tests given to 52 normal volunteers. It is interesting to note that Strauss et al. (1985) found that dichotic asymmetries were more closely related to posterior asymmetries measured from arteriograms than to amytal-determined speech lateralization. This would suggest some independence of posterior (receptive) and anterior (expressive) language systems. In addition, a study by O'Kusky, Strauss, Kosaka, Wada, Li, Druhan, and Petrie (1988), while not finding differences in callosal size between "handedness" groups (groupings were formed by taking asymmetries in addition to manual ones into account), found a significant correlation suggesting that the larger the REA, the smaller the callosal area. Clarke, Lufkin, and Zaidel (1993) also obtained this result and proposed a model relating CC size to differences in interhemispheric inhibition. Again, it is difficult to compare many of these studies, because of their employing differing methodologies, and much careful research will be required in order to discover the (no doubt complex) interrelations between handedness and lateralization of function.

To summarize, the existing literature would suggest a relation between handedness and speech lateralization. It remains true, nevertheless, that the majority of left-handers are, like right-handers, left-hemispheric for language. As a result, a knowledge of handedness, at least as defined conventionally, adds relatively little to our accuracy in predicting speech lateralization for any specific individual.

4.5 PATHOLOGICAL LEFT-HANDEDNESS

Rather than there being any single aspect of handedness that correlates with cerebral organization, it may be that there are different types of left-handers, and that some of these are anomalous in their cerebral organization. Certainly, Rasmussen, and Milner (1977) have shown that the incidence of right-hemispheric language representation is far higher in left-handers with evidence of early brain abnormalities than it is in more normally-developing left-handers. Their population, however, was composed of people who were about to undergo surgery for the relief of temporal lobe epilepsy. It may not be appropriate to generalize from such a group to a more normal population. Nevertheless, it remains a tenable hypothesis that some left-handers differ in cerebral organization from others for pathological reasons.

Satz and his colleagues (cf. Satz, 1972; Satz, Orsini, Saslow, and Henry, 1985; Orsini and Satz, 1986; Soper and Satz, 1984) have proposed a model that describes how manifest left-handedness (MLH) may develop in more than one way. They suggest that for the majority of left-handers, MLH is determined by genetic and/or environmental factors. For a smaller group of left-handers, MLH reflects neurological trauma and is therefore referred to as pathological left-handedness (PLH). Satz notes that the incidence of MLH is elevated among individuals with early brain injury. He suggests that this group includes natural right-handers for whom an early (i.e., before 6 years of age) left-hemisphere injury causes motor impairment of the contralateral hand and thereby leads to a shift in hand preference. Satz et al. (1985) also suggest that the incidence of familial sinistrality would be similar to that of right-handers since these left-handers would presumably have been right-handed were it not for the early brain injury.

The evidence that major perinatal left-hemisphere damage can produce left-handedness (PLH) is relatively strong (Orsini and Satz, 1986; Rasmussen and Milner 1977). The proportion of left-handers who have become so for pathological reasons remains a matter of some debate. Bakan (Bakan, Dibb, and Reid, 1973) might claim that all left-handedness results from some pathology or birth stress; Coren (1992) suggests that about half of left-handers are PLH, while the genetic models of Annett (1985) and McManus and Bryden (1992) consider PLH to be sufficiently rare that it can be ignored in their formulations. It is difficult, however, to demonstrate more frequent birth stress among left-handers (Searleman, Coren, and Porac, 1989).

4.6 "LATENT" LEFT-HANDEDNESS

Luria (1970) argued that there were many behaviors that suggested a "latent" left-handedness. He suggested that such things as the way in which one crossed one's arms or clasped one's hands might reflect a latent preference for the left hand and provided some evidence to suggest that right-handers with latent left-handedness were more likely to recover from aphasic disturbances following unilateral left hemispheric brain damage than were those with no such signs.

Sakano (1982) showed that both arm crossing and hand clasping were related to handedness. On average, left-handers were more likely than right-handers to fold their arms with the left arm uppermost, and to clasp their hands with the left thumb above the right. In addition, Sakano provided some evidence that these variables were related to cerebral lateralization.

Bryden (1988) investigated arm crossing by comparing people who preferred to fold their arms with the left arm uppermost to those who preferred the right arm uppermost. On a dichotic listening task, there was no difference between the two groups. In this study, only eyedness and familial sinistrality showed any evidence of affecting lateralization. Thus, while arm-crossing and hand-clasping may have some value, there is little evidence at the present time to suggest that they predict hemispheric specialization.

Another variable often considered as possibly interacting with handedness is that of eyedness, usually defined as the dominant eye for sighting. Most people are right-eyed for sighting, and eyedness is correlated with handedness (Bourassa, McManus, and Bryden, 1996). The argument is that parents and teachers do not notice the preferred sighting eye, and therefore do not attempt to modify it. Thus, one might expect eyedness to be a better predictor of cerebral lateralization than handedness.

There is, unfortunately, little evidence on this point. Searleman (1980) reported that eyedness did not correlate significantly with the ear effect in a verbal dichotic listening task, although Bryden (1988) reported that it does.

Yet another possibility is that foot preference, which is presumably less confounded by cultural and environmental factors, is a better predictor of cerebral organization than is handedness. For instance, Searleman (1980) and Strauss (1986) have found that footedness correlates well with the dichotic REA. One should note that most foot questionnaires involve relatively gross movements of the whole leg (e.g., kicking a ball, stamping out a fire) and thus may be more analogous to the gross arm movement factor of handedness (e.g., hammering) than to handwriting preference. It thus remains quite unclear as to whether these findings are a result of hand/foot differences or of proximal/distal differences.

Handwriting posture has also been suggested as a moderator variable. Levy and Reid (1978) classified writing posture as either inverted or noninverted and provided evidence to support this assertion that those who used an inverted writing posture also wrote with the hand ipsilateral to the speech hemisphere. They defined the inverted posture as one in which the hand is held above the line of writing and the pen points toward the bottom of the page. Levy and Reid reported that right-handed noninverters and left-handed inverters were left-hemisphere dominant on their verbal task (nonsense syllable identification) and right-hemisphere dominant on their spatial task (dot localization), whereas left-handed noninverters displayed the opposite pattern of hemispheric dominance for language and spatial functions.

Attempts to replicate the results of Levy and Reid's visual tasks have yielded conflicting results. Smith and Moscovitch (1979) found a similar result with a verbal task, but not with a nonverbal one. Weber (1980, as cited in Weber and Bradshaw, 1981) found no difference between inverters and noninverters in the pattern of lateralization of either language or spatial functions. MacDonald (1985) also failed to support Levy and Reid's predictions using similar tasks and writing posture criteria.

Some support for Levy and Reid's predictions comes from a study reporting that left-handed noninverters showed greater right-hemisphere involvement (measured by EEG alpha-asymmetries) than left-handed inverters while reading and writing (Herron, Galin, Johnstone, and Ornstein, 1979). These results, taken together with those of Smith and Moscovitch (1979), suggest that among left-handers writing posture may be related to the lateralization of visual language processes in the manner predicted by Levy and Reid (1978). The results of Weber (Weber and Bradshaw, 1981) and MacDonald (1985), though, challenge the usefulness of writing posture as a predictor of visual language processes. It seems that writing posture is not the simple indicator of hemispheric specialization as it first appeared to be. It continues to be an intriguing variable, however, because of its relationship to such variables as familial sinistrality (McKeever and VanDeventer, 1980), hand preference (Searleman, Porac and Coren, 1984), and hand performance (Parlow and Kinsbourne, 1981).

5. CONCLUSIONS

We started this chapter by indicating three ways in which an improved measurement of handedness or a refined conceptualization of handedness and laterality would be of relevance to neuropsychology and how it would aid in predicting individual patterns of cerebral organization. These ways included the improved measurement of handedness, the discovery of some variable that would distinguish between true or natural left-handers and pathological left-handers, and the possibility that some additional variable, added to information about handedness, would prove to predict cerebral organization. Although much progress has been made in the past decade, it is not yet possible to provide definitive statements about any of the possibilities.

In recent years, new ideas about the measurement of handedness have emerged. It is now considered at least reasonable to conceptualize handedness as multidimensional (Healey et al., 1986; Steenhuis and Bryden, 1989a). Furthermore, Bryden (1987) has provided evidence to suggest that degree and direction of handedness are separable in humans, much as they are in the mouse (Collins, 1985). Two major issues, however, need to be resolved. One concerns how replicable these various factors are (Peters and Murphy, 1993); the results of any factor analysis are influenced by the items that are entered and their specific wording, and it remains uncertain whether any of the various secondary factors will prove to be reliable. Assuming that they are, then it is important to determine whether scores on any one of these secondary factors provide a better prediction of cerebral organization than a simple indication of hand preference or writing hand. It would be most desirable to have a large series of patients with unilateral brain damage; lacking this, studies associating the various handedness factors with noninvasive performance measures such as those obtained with dichotic and visual half-field procedures are needed.

The data relating individual differences in neuroanatomical features to handedness variation are confusing and conflicting, to some extent because of the varying methodologies that have been used. There may well be differences in certain aspects of brain structure between handedness groups, but it is far from clear at this stage where these differences may occur, their magnitude, or their importance to neuropsychological function. With the incredibly rapid development of sophisticated techniques of *in vivo* brain imaging, this picture will undoubtedly become much more clear over the next decade.

There is little evidence to support the notion that a large percentage of left-handers are so for pathological reasons. While it is certainly true that right-hemisphere language is far more common in those left-handers with evidence of significant early left-hemisphere brain damage (Rasmussen and Milner, 1977), there is little to lead us to believe that left-handedness is generally a consequence of early brain damage (McManus, 1983). As a consequence, attempts to divide left-handers into "natural" and "pathological" subgroups have not proven to be particularly useful (Orsini, Satz, Soper, and Light, 1985). It is clear that truly pathological left-handers should be excluded from large-scale surveys in that they may be distorting the associations between variables, but most handedness research is carried out on undergraduate populations, and significant early brain damage is relatively rare in such groups. However, one might also consider omitting twins from the analyses of large-scale surveys on the grounds that twinning is a disorder of symmetry (Boklage, 1980) or that it is an indicator of birth stress.

The notion that some other variable, either alone or in conjunction with handedness, would prove to generate clear predictions of cerebral organization has been more promising than fruitful. However, there are now two studies showing that footedness is a better predictor of language lateralization than handedness (Searleman, 1980; Strauss, 1986), and some data suggesting the relevance of sighting-eye dominance (Bryden, 1989). It would be advantageous to study these variables in a clinical population. In addition, there are relatively little data on the relation of handedness to the lateralization of putative right-hemisphere functions such as spatial ability or musical ability, and this oversight needs to be corrected.

ACKNOWLEDGMENTS

Preparation of this manuscript was aided by a grant from the Natural Sciences and Engineering Research Council of Canada to the first author. The authors wish to thank Dr. Runa Steenhuis for her insightful comments on early drafts of this chapter and Thomasin Adams-Webber for her assistance in editing first drafts of the typescript for the inevitable gremlins. We are also indebted to Dr. Lutz Jäncke for his helpful suggestions and comments.

REFERENCES

Annett, M. (1967). The binomial distribution of right, mixed and left-handedness. *Q. J. Exp. Psychol.*, 19, 327.

Annett, M. (1978). *A Single Gene Explanation of Right and Left-handedness and Brainedness*. Lanchester Polytechnic, Lanchester, U.K.

Annett, M. (1985). *Left, Right, Hand and Brain: The Right Shift Theory*. Lawrence Erlbaum, Hillsdale, NJ.

Annett, M. and Kilshaw, D. (1983). Right- and left-handed skill II: Estimating the parameters of the distribution of L-R differences in males and females. *Br. J. Psychol.*, 74, 269.

Bakan, P. (1971). Birth order and handedness. *Nature*, 229, 195.

Bakan, P., Dibb, G., and Reed, P. (1973). Handedness and birth stress. *Neuropsychologia*, 11, 363.

Bastian, H.C. (1868). *A Treatise on Aphasia and Other Speech Defects*. London, Lewis.

Barnsley, R.H. and Rabinovitch, M.S. (1970). Handedness: Proficiency vs. stated preference. *Percept. Motor Skills*, 30, 343.

Beaton, A.A. (1996). The relation of planum temporale asymmetry and morphology of the corpus callosum to handedness, gender and dyslexia: A review of the evidence. *Brain Lang*. (in press).

Benton, A.L. (1965). The problem of cerebral dominance. *Can. Psychol.*, 6a, 332.

Beukelaar, L.J. and Kroonenberg, P.M. (1986). Changes over time in the relationshipo between hand preference and writing hand among left-handers. *Neuropsychologia*, 24, 301.

Bishop, D.V.M. (1990). *Handedness and Developmental Disorder*. Oxford, Blackwell Scientific Publications.

Bishop, D.V.M., Ross, V. A., Daniels, M. S., and Bright, P. (1996). The measurement of hand preference: a validation study comparing three groups of right-handers. *Br. J. Psychol.* (in press).

Boklage, C.E. (1980). On the distribution of nonrighthandedness among twins and their families. *Acta Genet. Med. Gemellol.*, 30, 167.

Borod, J.C., Koff, E., and Caron, H.S. (1984). The Target Test: A brief laterality measure of speed and accuracy. *Percept. Motor Skills*, 58, 743.

Bourassa, D.C., McManus, I.C., and Bryden, M.P. (1996). Handedness and eye-dominance: A meta-analysis of their inter-relations. *Laterality*, 1 (in press).

Briggs, G.C. and Nebes, R.D. (1975). Patterns of hand preference in a student population. *Cortex*, 11, 230.

Bryden, M.P. (1977). Measuring handedness with questionnaires. *Neuropsychologia*, 15, 617.

Bryden, M.P. (1982). *Laterality*. Academic Press, New York.

Bryden, M.P. (1987). Handedness and cerebral organization: Data from clinical and normal populations. In D. Ottoson (Ed.), *Duality and Unity of the Brain*. Macmillan, Harmondsworth, U.K., 55.

Bryden, M.P. (1988). Correlates of the dichotic right-ear effect. *Cortex*, 24, 313.

Bryden, M.P. (1989). Handedness, cerebral lateralization, and measures of "latent left-handedness." *Int. J. Neurosci.*, 44, 227.

Bryden, M.P., Ardila, A., and Ardila, O. (1993). Handedness in native Amazonians. *Neuropsychologia*, 31, 301.

Bryden, M.P. and Bulman-Fleming, M.B. (1995). Dichotic tasks: Relating the emotional words test to the fused dichotic words test. *J. Int. Neuropsychol. Soc.*, 1, 177.

Bryden, M.P. and Edmonds, A. (1995). An objective measure of hand preference. *J. Int. Neuropsychol. Soc.*, 1, 322.

Bryden, M.P., Hécaen, H., and DeAgostini, M. (1983). Patterns of cerebral organization. *Brain Lang.*, 20, 249.

Bryden, M.P., McManus, I.C., and Bulman-Fleming, M.B. (1994). Evaluating the empirical support for the Geschwind-Behan-Galaburda model of cerebral lateralization. *Brain Cognit.*, 26, 103.

Bryden, M.P., Singh, M., and Rogers, T.T. (1995). Heritability for Degree and Direction of Human Hand Preference. *Soc. Neurosci. Abstr.* 21, 200.

Bryden, M.P., Singh, M., Steenhuis, R.E., and Clarkson, K.L. (1994). A behavioral measure of hand preference as opposed to hand skill. *Neuropsychologia*, 32, 991.

Bulman-Fleming, M.B. and Bryden, M.P. (1994). Simultaneous verbal and affective laterality effects. *Neuropsychologia*, 32, 787.

Bulman-Fleming, M.B. and Bryden, M.P. (1995). Noncomplementarity of verbal and affective processes. *Brain Cognit.* (in press).

Burke, H.L. and Yeo, R.A. (1994). Systematic variations in callosal morphology: The effects of age, gender, hand preference, and anatomic asymmetry. *Neuropsychology*, 8, 563.

Carter, R.L., Satz, P., and Hohenegger, M. (1984). On the statistical estimation of speech-organization distributions from aphasia data. *Biometrics*, 40, 937.

Clarke, J.M., Lufkin, R.B., and Zaidel, E. (1993). Corpus callosum morphometry and dichotic listening performance: Individual differences in functional interhemispheric inhibition? *Neuropsychologia*, 31, 547.

Collins, R.L. (1985). On the inheritance of direction and degree of asymmetry. In *Cerebral Lateralization in Nonhuman Species*. (Ed. S.D. Glick). Academic Press, Orlando, FL.

Corballis, M.C. and Morgan, M.J. (1978). On the biological basis of human laterality: I. Evidence for a maturational left-right gradient. *Behav. Brain Sci.*, 1, 261.

Coren, S. (1992). *The Left-Hander Syndrome*. Free Press, New York.

Coren, S. (1994). The diminished number of older left-handers: Differential mortality or socio-historical trend? *Int. J. Neurosci.*, 75, 31.

Coren, S. and Halpern, D. F. (1991). Left-handedness: A marker for decreased survival fitness. *Psychol. Bull.*, 109, 90.

Dawson, J.L.M.B. (1977). An anthropological perspective on the evolution and lateralization of the brain. *Ann. N. Y. Acad. Sci.*, 299, 424.

Delacato, C.H. (Ed). (1966). *Neurological Organization and Reading*. Springfield, IL: Charles Thomas.

De Lacoste, M.C., Kirkpatrick, J.B., and Ross, E.D. (1985). Topography of the human corpus callosum. *J. Neuropathol. Exp. Neurol.*, 44, 578.

DeRenzi, E. (1982). *Disorders of Space Exploration and Cognition*. Wiley, Chichester, U.K.

Fennell, E.B. (1985). Handedness in neuropsychological research. In *Experimental Techniques in Human Neuropsychology*. (Ed. H.J. Hannay). Oxford University Press, New York, 15.

Fleminger, J.J., Dalton, R., and Standage, K.F. (1977). Handedness in psychiatric patients. *Br. J. Psych.*, 131, 448.

Foundas, A.L., Leonard, C.M., Gilmore, R., Fennell, E., and Heilman, K.M. (1994). Planum temporale asymmetry and language dominance. *Neuropsychologia*, 32, 1225.

Gangestad, S.W. and Yeo, R. (1994). Parental handedness and relative hand skill: A test of the developmental instability model. *Neuropsychology*, 8, 572.

Geffen, G. and Caudrey, D. (1981). Reliability and validity of the dichotic monitoring test for language laterality. *Neuropsychologia*, 19, 413.

Geschwind, N. and Galaburda, A.M. (1987). *Cerebral Lateralization*. M.I.T. Press, Cambridge, MA.

Gilbert, A. N. and Wysocki, C. J. (1992). Hand preference and age in the United States. *Neuropsychologia*, 30, 601.

Habib, M., Gayraud, D., Oliva, A., Regis, J., Salamon, G., and Khalil, R. (1991). Effects of handedness and sex on the morphology of the corpus callosum: A study with brain magnetic resonance imaging. *Brain Cognit.*, 16, 41.

Habib, M., Robichon, F., Lévrier, O., Khalil, R., and Salamon, G. (1995). Diverging asymmetries of temporo-parietal cortical areas: A reappraisal of Geschwind/Galaburda theory. *Brain Lang.*, 48, 238.

Hardyck, C. and Petrinovitch, L.F. (1977). Left-handedness. *Psychol. Bull.*, 84, 385.

Harris, L.J. (1993). Do left-handers die sooner than right-handers? Commentary on Coren and Halpern's (1991) "Left-handedness: A marker for decreased survival fitness." *Psychol. Bull.*, 114, 203.

Hatta, T. and Nakatsuka, Z. (1976). Note on hand preference of Japanese people. *Percept. Motor Skills*, 42, 530.

Healey, J.M., Liederman, J., and Geschwind, N. (1986). Handedness is not a unidimensional trait. *Cortex*, 22, 33.

Hécaen, H. and Sauguet, J. (1971). Cerebral dominance in left-handed subjects. *Cortex*, 7, 19.

Herron, J., Galin, D., Johnstone, J., and Ornstein, R.E. (1979). Cerebral specialization, writing posture and motor control of writing in lefthanders. *Science*, 205, 1285.

Hugdahl, K., Satz, P., Mitrushina, M., and Miller, E.N. (1993). Left-handedness and old age: Do left-handers die earlier? *Neuropsychologia*, 31, 325.

Ida, Y. and Bryden, M.P. (1996). A comparison of hand preference in Japan and Canada. *Can. J. Exp. Psychol.*, in press.

Jackson, J.H. (1958). *Selected Writings of John Hughlings Jackson*. Taylor (Ed.). New York, Basic Books.

Jäncke, L. and Steinmetz, H. (1993). Auditory lateralization and planum temporale asymmetry. *NeuroReport*, 5, 169.

Jäncke, L. and Steinmetz, H. (1994). Interhemispheric transfer time and corpus callosum size. *NeuroReport*, 5, 2385.

Jäncke, L., Schlaug, G., Huang, Y., and Steinmetz, H. (1994). Asymmetry of the planum parietale. *NeuroReport*, 5, 1161.

Jäncke, L., Steinmetz, H., and Volkmann, J. (1992). Dichotic listening: what does it measure? *Neuropsychologia*, 30, 941.

Juraska, J.M. and Kopcik, J.R. (1988). Sex and environmental influences on the size and ultrastructure of the rat corpus callosum. *Brain Res.*, 450, 1.

Kang, Y. and Harris, L. J. (1993). Is Human HandednessUnifactorial or Multifactorial? A Factor-Analytic Study of Hand Preference in American College Students. Unpublished manuscript, Michigan State University.

Kertesz, A., Polk, M., Black, S.E., and Howell, J. (1992). Anatomical asymmetries and functional laterality. *Brain*, 115, 589.

Kim, H. (1994). Distributions of hemispheric asymmetry in left-handers and right-handers: Data from perceptual asymmetry studies. *Neuropsychology*, 8, 148.

Kimura, D. (1961a). Cerebral dominance and the perception of verbal stimuli. *Can. J. Psychol.*, 15, 166.

Kimura, D. (1961b). Some effects of temporal lobe damage on auditory perception. *Can. J. Psychol.*, 15, 156.

Kimura, D. (1979). Neuromotor mechanisms in the evolution of human communication. In H. D. Steklis and M.D. Raleigh (Eds.), *Neurobiology of Social Communication in Primates*. New York, Academic Press, 197.

Kimura, D. (1983). Speech representation in an unbiased sample of left-handers. *Hum. Neurobiol.*, 2, 147.

Kimura, D. and Harshman, R. (1984). Sex differences in brain organization for verbal and non-verbal functions. In G.J. DeVries, J.P.C. DeBruin, H.B.M. Uylings, and M.A. Corner (Eds.), *Sex Differences in the Brain*. Elsevier, Amsterdam, 423.

Levy, J. and Nagylaki, T. (1972). A model for the genetics of handedness. *Genetics*, 72, 117.

Levy, J. and Reid, M. (1978). Variations in cerebral organization as a function of handedness, hand posture in writing and sex. *J. Exp. Psychol.: Gen.*, 107, 119.

Livshits, G. and Kobylianski, E. (1991). Fluctuating asymmetry as a possible measure of developmental homeostasis in humans: A review. *Hum. Biol.*, 63, 441.

Luria, A.R. (1970). *Traumatic Aphasia*. The Hague, Mouton.

MacDonald, V. (1985). *The Relationship of Writing Posture with Cerebral Organization, Familial Sinistrality, and Strength of Handedness*. Unpublished M.A. thesis, University of Waterloo.

Marchant, L.F., McGrew, W.C., and Eibl-Eibesfeldt, I. (1995). Is human handedness universal? Ethological analyses from three traditional cultures. *Ethology,* 101, 239.

McGlone, J. (1980). Sex differences in human brain organization: A critical survey. *Behav. Brain Sci.*, 3, 215.

McKeever, W.F. (1981). Sex and cerebral organization: Is it really so simple? In A. Ansara, N. Geschwind, A. Galaburda, M. Albert, and N. Gartrell (Eds.), *Sex Differences in Dyslexia*. Orton Dyslexia Society, Towson, MD, 97.

McKeever, W.F. and van Deventer, A.D. (1980). Inverted handwriting position, language laterality, and the Levy-Nagylaki genetic model of handedness and cerebral organization. *Neuropsychologia*, 18, 99.

McManus, I.C. (1983). Pathologic left-handedness: does it exist? *J. Comm. Disorders*, 16, 315.

McManus, I.C. (1985). Handedness, language dominance and aphasia: a genetic model. *Psychol. Med.*, Monograph Supplement 8.

McManus, I.C. and Bryden, M.P. (1992). The genetics of handedness and cerebral lateralization, In I. Rapin, and S.J. Segalowitz (Eds.) *Handbook of Neuropsychology, Vol. 6*. Elsevier, Amsterdam, 115.

McManus, I.C. and Bryden, M.P. (1993). Handedness on Tristan da Cunha: The genetic consequences of social isolation. *Int. J. Psychol.*, 28, 831.

O'Kusky, J., Strauss, E., Kosaka, B., Wada, J., Li, D., Druhan, M., and Petrie, J. (1988). The corpus callosum is larger with right-hemisphere cerebral speech dominance. *Ann. Neurol.*, 24, 379.

Olavarria, J. and Van Sluyters, R.C. (1986). Axons from restricted regions of the cortex pass through restricted portions of the corpus callosum in adult and neonatal rats. *Dev. Brain Res.*, 25, 309.

Oldfield, R.C. (1971). The assessment and analysis of handedness: The Edinburgh Inventory. *Neuropsychologia*, 9, 97.

Orsini, D.L. and Satz, P. (1986) A syndrome of pathological left-handedness: Correlates of early left hemisphere injury. *Arch. Neurol.*, 43, 333.

Orsini, D.L., Satz, P., Soper, H.V., and Light, R.K. (1985). The role of familial sinistrality in cerebral organization. *Neuropsychologia*, 23, 223.

Orton, S.T. (1925). "Word blindness" in school children. *Arch. Neurol. and Psychiatry*, 14, 481.

Orton, S.T. (1937). *Reading, Writing, and Speech Problems in Children*. New York, Norton.

Palmer, A.R. and Strobeck, C. (1986). Fluctuating asymmetry: Measurement, analysis, patterns. *Annu. Rev. Ecol. Sys.*, 17, 391.

Parlow, S. and Kinsbourne, M. (1981). Handwriting posture and manual motor asymmetry in sinistrals. *Neuropsychologia*, 19, 687.

Payne, M.A. (1987). Impact of cultural pressures on self-reports of actual and approved hand use. *Neuropsychologia*, 25, 247.

Peters, M. and Durding, B. (1978). Handedness measured by finger tapping: A continuous variable. *Can. J. Psychol.*, 32, 257.

Peters, M. and Durding, B. (1979). Left-handers and right-handers compared on a motor task. *J. Motor Behav.*, 11, 103.

Peters, M. and Murphy, K. (1993). Factor analysis of pooled hand questionnaire data are of questionable value. *Cortex*, 29, 305.

Peters, M. and Pang, J. (1992). Do "right-armed" left-handers have different laterality of motor control for the proximal and distal musculature? *Cortex*, 28, 391.

Porac, C. and Coren, S. (1981). *Lateral Preferences and Human Behavior*. New York, Springer-Verlag.

Porac, C., Coren, S., and Duncan, P. (1980). Life span trends in laterality. *J. Gerontol.*, 35, 715.

Porac, C., Rees, L., and Buller, T. (1990). Switching hands: A place for left hand use in a right hand world. In S. Coren (Ed.), *Left-handedness: Behavioral Implications and Anomalies*, Amsterdam, North-Holland, 259.

Pratt, R.T.C. and Warrrington, E.K. (1972). The assessment of cerebral dominance with unilateral E.C.T. *Br. J. Psych.*, 121, 327.

Purves, D., White, L.E., and Andrews, T.J. (1994). Manual asymmetry and handedness. *Proc. Natl. Acad. Sci.*, 91, 5030.

Raczkowski, D., Kalat, J.W., and Nebes, R. (1974). Reliability and validity of some handedness questionnaire items. *Neuropsychologia*, 12, 43.

Rasmussen, T. and Milner, B. (1977). The role of early left-brain injury in determining lateralization of cerebral speech functions. *Ann. N. Y. Acad. Sci.*, 299, 355.

Ratcliff, G., Dila, C., Taylor, L., and Milner, B. (1980). The morphological asymmetry of the hemispheres and cerebral dominance for speech: A possible relationship. *Brain Lang.*, 11, 87.

Rhoades, J.G. and Damon, A. (1973). Some genetic traits in Solomon Island populations: II. Hand clasping, arm folding and handedness. *Am. J. Phys. Anthropol.*, 39, 179.

Sakano, N. (1982). *Latent Left-Handedness: Its Relation to Hemispheric and Psychological Functions*. VEB Gustav Fischer Verlag, Jena DDR.

Satz, P. (1972). Pathological left-handedness: An explanatory model. *Cortex*, 8, 121.

Satz, P., Orsini, D.L., Saslow, E. and Henry, R. (1985). The pathological lefthandedness syndrome. *Brain Cognit.*, 4, 27.

Schachter, S.C. (1993). Studies of handedness and anomalous dominance: Problems and progress. In A.M. Galaburda (Ed.), *Dyslexia and Development: Neurobiological Aspects of Extra-ordinary Brains*. Harvard University Press, Cambridge, MA, 269.

Searleman, A. (1980). Subject variables and cerebral organization for language. *Cortex*, 16, 239.

Searleman, A., Coren, S., and Porac, C. (1989). Relationship between birth order, birth stress, and lateral preferences: a critical review. *Psychol. Bull.*, 105, 397.

Searleman, A, Porac, C., and Coren, S. (1984). Lateral preferences and writing hand posture in left-handers: A reply to Levy. *Brain Cognit.*, 3, 451.

Seddon, B. and McManus, I.C. (1993). The incidence of left-handedness: A meta-analysis. Unpublished manuscript, University College, London.

Segalowitz, S.J. and Bryden, M.P. (1983). Individual differences in hemispheric representation of language. In *Language Functions and Brain Organization*. (Ed. S.J. Segalowitz). Academic Press, New York, 341.

Shimizu, A. and Endo, M. (1983). Handedness and familial sinistrality in a Japanese student population. *Cortex*, 19, 265.

Singh, M. and Bryden, M.P. (1994). The factor structure of handedness in India. *Int. J. Neurosci.*, 74, 33.

Smith, L.C. and Moscovitch, M. (1979). Writing posture, hemispheric control of movement and cerebral dominance in individuals with inverted and noninverted hand postures during writing. *Neuropsychologia*, 17, 637.

Snyder, P.J., Novelly, R.A., and Harris, L.J. (1990). Mixed speech dominance in the intracarotid sodium amytal procedure: Validity and criteria issues. *J. Clin. Exp. Neuropsychol.*, 12, 629.

Soper, H.V. and Satz, P. (1984). Pathological left-handedness and ambiguous handedness: A new explanatory model. *Neuropsychologia*, 22, 511.

Steenhuis, R.E. and Bryden, M.P. (1989a). Different dimensions of hand preference that relate to skilled and unskilled activities. *Cortex*, 25, 289.

Steenhuis, R.E. and Bryden, M.P. (1989b). Hand preference and performance: Right-handers, left-handers, and left-handers who are not consistently left-handed. *J. Clin. Exp. Neuropsychol.*, 11, 37.

Steinmetz, H., Jäncke, L., Kleinschmidt, A., Schlaug, G., Volkmann, J., and Huang, Y. (1992). Sex but no hand difference in the isthmus of the corpus callosum. *Neurology*, 42, 749.

Steinmetz, H., Rademacher, J., Huang, Y., Hefter, H., Zilles, K., Thron, A, and Freund, H. (1989). Cerebral asymmetry: MR planimetry of the human planum temporale. *J. Comp. Assist. Tomogr.*, 13, 996.

Steinmetz, H., Volkmann, J., Jäncke, L., and Freund, H-J. (1991). Anatomical left-right asymmetry of language-related temporal cortex is different in left- and right-handers. *Ann. Neurol.*, 29, 315.

Strauss, E. (1986). Hand, foot, eye and ear preferences and performance on a dichotic listening test. *Cortex*, 22, 475.

Strauss, E., Lapointe, J.S., Wada, J.A., Gaddes, W., and Kosaka, B. (1985). Language dominance: Correlation of radiological and functional data. *Neuropsychologia*, 23, 415.

Tapley, S.M. and Bryden, M.P. (1985). A group test for the assessment of performance between the hands. *Neuropsychologia*, 23, 215.

Teng, E.L., Lee. P.-H., Yang, K.S., and Chang, P.C. (1979). Lateral preferences for hand, foot, and eye, and their lack of association with scholastic achievement in 4143 Chinese. *Neuropsychologia*, 17, 41.

Thoma, R.J., Lewine, J.D., Yeo, R., Provencal, S.L., Davis, J.T., Orrison W.W., and Hill, D.E. (1995). Magnetic source imaging ot the neural substrates of handedness. Poster presented at the 1995 annual meeting of the Society for Cognitive Neuroscience, San Francisco, CA.

Van Horn, J.D. and McManus, I.C. (1993). *Task difficulty and hand differences in peg moving, circle marking, and square tracing*. Unpublished manuscript, University College, London.

Verhaegan, P. and Ntumba, A. (1964). Note on the frequency of left-handedness in African children. *J. Educ. Psychol.*, 55, 89.

Wada, J. and Rasmussen, T. (1960). Intracarotid injection of sodium amytal for the lateralization of cerebral speech dominance. *J. Neurosurg.*, 17, 266.

Wahlsten, D. and Bishop, K.M. (1994). Sex differences in the human corpus callosum: Myth or reality? Paper presented at the annual meeting of the Canadian Society for Brain, Behavior and Cognitive Science, Vancouver, BC (June; abstracts vol. 4, p. 61).

Warrington, E.K. and Pratt, R.T.C. (1973). Language laterality in left-handers assessed by unilateral E.C.T. *Neuropsychologia*, 11, 423.

Watson, N.V. and Kimura, D. (1989). Right-hand superiority for throwing but not for intercepting. *Neuropsychologia*, 27, 1399.

Weber, A.M. and Bradshaw, J.L. (1981). Levy and Reid's neurological model in relation to writing hand/posture: An evaluation. *Psychol. Bull.*, 90, 74.

White, L.E., Lucas, G., Richards, A., and Purves, D. (1994). Cerebral asymmetry and handedness. *Nature*, 368, 197.

Witelson, S.F. (1983). Bumps on the brain: Right-left asymmetry as a key to functional lateralization. In S. J. Segalowitz (Ed.), *Language Functions and Brain Organization*. Academic Press, New York, 117.

Witelson, S.F. (1985). The brain connection: The corpus callosum is larger in left-handers. *Science*, 229, 665.

Witelson, S.F. (1989). Hand and sex differences in the isthmus and genu of the human corpus callosum: A post-mortem morphological study. *Brain*, 112, 799.

Wolf, P. A., D'Agostino, R.B., and Cobb, J. (1991). Left-handedness and life expectancy: Letter. *N. Engl. J. Med.*, 325, 1042.

Yeo, R. and Gangestad, S.W. (1993). Developmental origins of variation in human hand preference. *Genetica*, 89, 281.

Yeo, R., Gangestad, S.W., and Daniel, W.F. (1993). Hand preference and developmental stability. *Psychobiology*, 21, 161.

Zangwill, O.L. (1960). *Cerebral Dominance and Its Relation to Psychological Functions*. Edinburgh, Oliver and Boyd.

Zatorre, R.J. (1989). Perceptual asymmetry on the dichotic fused words test and cerebral speech lateralization determined by the carotid sodium amytal test. *Neuropsychologia*, 27, 1207.

Chapter 4

Pathological Causes and Consequences of Left-Handedness

Stanley Coren

CONTENTS

1. INTRODUCTION

There was a recent television documentary about the Marx Brothers comedy team who created a number of hilarious films during the late 1920s through the 1930s. At one point, as a black and white image of a man in curly hair playing a harp appeared, the narrator noted "Even when compared to Groucho and Chico, there was something different, something strange and bizarre, something crazy about Harpo Marx. But then, this might have been expected since he was the only left-hander in the group." While this comment clearly reflects a popular stereotype about "wacky southpaws," there is now a large body of scientific data that suggests that right- and left-handers really do differ on a multiplicity of dimensions which extend well beyond simple hand use patterns. These dimensions are quite varied and include cognitive and personality differences, health status, predispositions toward abnormal psychological states, brain organization, and perhaps even longevity (see Coren, 1993, for a general review). To understand why left- and right-handers may differ psychologically and physically, the initial question which must be asked is "How does an individual come to be right- or left-handed in the first place?"

2. SOCIAL PRESSURE, LEARNING, AND HANDEDNESS

If you had first became interested in handedness in the middle of the 20th century, you would have found that there were only two seriously considered hypotheses used to explain how the majority of people in the population come to be right-handed. One invoked genetic mechanisms and the other social or learning processes.

The suggested nongenetic origin of handedness was based upon the presumption that handedness was learned and enforced by cultural pressures in society. Some theorists

0-8493-8999-2/96/$0.00+$.50

argued that having everyone as right-handed simplified the use and design of tools. Others suggested that the pressures toward a right-handed population came from religious, cultural, or social considerations (Coren, 1993; Harris, 1990). As the anthropologist Robert Hertz, writing at the beginning of the 20th century, noted "One of the signs which distinguish a well-brought up child is that its left hand has become incapable of any independent action" (Hertz, 1973). Ideas of social pressure on handedness are often discussed as a means of explaining why so many left-handers learn to do a variety of things with their right hand (e.g., Harris, 1990).

The social-cultural pressure theory of handedness has never been very convincing. The major reason is that handedness is not easily changed, even when pressures are applied at a young age or are quite harsh (Porac, Coren, and Searleman, 1986). A study by Porac, Rees, and Buller (1990) shows the general pattern of results obtained. They looked at cases where deliberate attempts were made to switch handedness. Much to everyone's surprise, they found that even those respondents who felt that the attempt to switch their hand use was successful still performed more skilled actions with their left hand than their right hand. Thus only hand use for a few "targeted" activities had actually changed. This is similar to the results of Hoosain (1990) who found that apart from the more socially monitored activity of writing, even the so-called "switched" left-handers had hand preference patterns more similar to sinistrals than dextrals.

Perhaps the major reason why the cultural pressure hypothesis as an explanation for handedness has only been used in special instances comes from the logic of the situation, rather than any particular piece of data. Certainly social pressures might account for some additional right-handers in the world (the switched left-handers). What this learned handedness hypothesis cannot do is to account for the relatively constant proportion of around 10% left-handers usually found in population surveys. Certainly no social-cultural theorist would argue that there are people who are actively teaching right-handers to be left-handed. In other words, even if it is possible that learning in response to societal pressure can explain the existence of so many right-handers, we would still have to deal separately with the problem of why left-handers exist in the population. One possibility would be to argue that left-handed children are simply too stupid or stubborn to learn how to use the hand that everyone else learns to favor. Yet it is difficult to imagine that the great scientist Albert Einstein, the diplomat-scientist-writer-inventor Benjamin Franklin, the famous lawyer Clarence Darrow, the painter-inventor Leonardo da Vinci, and the great lexicographer Samuel Johnson were all "too dumb" to learn to be right-handed and hence ended up as left-handers.

3. THE GENETIC BASIS OF RIGHT-HANDEDNESS

The more popular hypothesis to explain handedness was genetic in nature. Whenever the etiology of handedness is considered, the vast majority of researchers assume that whether individuals are right- or left-handed is determined, at least in part, by genetic contributions from their parents (e.g., Annett, 1985; Bryden, 1982; Corballis, 1983; Coren, 1994a; McManus, 1985).

Since we are about to discuss the interaction between genetics and handedness, we ought to be clear about some concepts that tend to be glossed over when neuropsychologists speak about the genetic basis of features and traits. Generally, when we discuss heritability, we are directing our attention to a characteristic that exists in several forms in a population. Our goal is to explain why some individuals show one set of characteristics while others show a different set of characteristics. The textbook example of this would be eye color. There are two dominant varieties of eye color in the population, namely brown and blue. Whether an individual has brown or blue eyes can be shown to depend upon the eye color of his or her parents. The presence of at least one brown-eyed gene results in a brown-eyed phenotype, while to be phenotypically blue-eyed requires the absence of any brown eyed gene. This means that blue- and brown-eye individuals are genetically different. We could have used numerous other examples of genetically determined characteristics that vary from individual to individual. Curly vs. straight hair, skin color, night blindness, strabismus, hemophilia, tendencies toward schizophrenia, degree of intelligence (especially in the extremes, such as mental retardation), some forms of personality disorders, and numerous diseases (such as sickle cell anemia) have all been shown to be genetically determined to the extent that we can predict the child's characteristics based upon a knowledge of the parents' characteristics. Notice that we attempt to predict how individuals will vary within the population (that is to say have different phenotypes), based upon genetic combinations resulting from particular mating pairs (or different genotypes). We will refer to characteristics that operate in this manner as being *genetically variable*.

The reason why it is important to clearly understand the nature of genetically variable characteristics is because there are another set of characteristics that are also genetically determined, but cannot be usefully explored using traditional measures of the similarity between parents and offspring. Human beings, for example, have a series of genetically determined traits which distinguish them from other species. These include the presence of exactly two eyes (no more, no less), the ability to grow hair on the head and underarms (but not on the palms of the hands or the soles the feet), the presence of an opposable thumb, leg insertion into the hips to allow upright walking, and the absence of a visible tail. All of these characteristics are part of the genetic heritage of all humans. It should be obvious that we would learn very little about these characteristics by looking trying to predict the characteristics of the offspring from those of its parents. Since *all* human beings have five fingers on each hand, it makes no sense to ask the question "What happens if we mate a man with six fingers to a woman with four fingers?" simply because the characteristic of having five fingers is a species specific trait, genetically encoded with all of the other characteristics that make the subject human. These invariant, but obviously genetically determined traits, that are found in all members of a species, we will call *genetically fixed* characteristics.

The reason that I am stressing this distinction is that there is some evidence which suggests that right-handedness may be a genetically fixed characteristic within humans. If this were the case, then human beings, throughout their history as the definable biological sub-type *homo sapiens*, should have been right-handed in the same way that they are two-eyed. In Coren and Porac (1977), we studied this issue using artistic productions ranging from early cave drawings through to the present era. We reasoned that artists, even without obvious attention to details, try to produce depictions of the world that reflect the reality that they see. Consider a palaeolithic (old stone age) artist trying to draw a picture representing the hunt he and his comrades have just completed. Suppose that the majority of his fellow cavemen are *not* consistently right-handed as we are today. If, for example, half of the people used their right hand and half the left hand for tool and weapon use, then this palaeolithic artist's sense of aesthetics or representational accuracy should not be affected much by which hand he depicted a spear or other weapon as being held in. However, if most of the people that he observed manipulating tools and weapons did so with their right hands, then he would be more likely to place the implements in the picture in the right hands of his characters. This need not be done at any conscious level, it is simply a reflection of the fact that if the majority of people that he saw were right-handers then the picture would appear to be more "natural" and life-like if he placed most of the tools and implements in the right hand. In our study we looked at over 10,000 artistic depictions spanning over 50 centuries of human history.

In the palaeolithic set of art works, the distribution showed 90% right-handedness. In samples of drawings made in the 1950s (which is 16,950 years after the earliest dated drawing that we used) we found 89% right-handedness. In between these times, except for some minor fluctuations, right-handedness continued at about the same level with only one out of ten drawings showing left-handed tool or weapon use. This finding suggests that the predisposition towards right-handedness is a genetically fixed and relatively invariant feature of the human species.

Other research pushes the heritage of right-handedness back further than the palaeolithic time period that we started with. For example, Semenov (1964) microscopically examined wear patterns on stone tools dated between 8,000 and 35,000 B.C., drawn from sites as widely spaced as Eastern Europe and North Africa. His analysis confirmed the predominance of right-handers during this period. Keeley (1977), gathered even earlier samples of tools from English sites dating from 100,000 to 500,000 years ago. His conclusion was that these tool makers were "consistently" right-handed. Finally, there is even evidence that right-handedness may go back to a human precursor, *Australopithecus africanus*. This early hominid dates from the Pleistocene period which is around 2 million years ago. Dart (1959) examined the killing blows to the skulls of baboons hunted by *Australopithecus* and concluded that these were predominantly made by simians wielding rocks or sticks as weapons, using their right-hands.

Let us add to our examination of artifacts and the fossil record the observation that while other animals (e.g., rats, cats, and monkeys) have been shown to have handedness, the proportion of right- and left-pawed individuals is relatively equal. It appears that the strong bias toward right-sidedness seen in humans is almost unique to hominids (see Annett, 1985 and Warren, 1980 for reviews).

All of the evidence discussed above is consistent with the genetic determination of handedness, at least at the species level. However, the conclusion that we reach is that *right-handedness* is a genetically fixed trait of humans. What then is the origin of left-handedness? Is it also due to genetic factors, or is it some form of mutation, or some failure in the genetic coding to be right-handed? To answer such questions we must consider the evidence that there may be a genetically variable form of handedness that might explain why some people are left-handed while the majority are right-handed.

4. GENETIC VARIABILITY AND LEFT-HANDEDNESS

The most persistent theory used to explain the appearance of left-handedness refers it to genetically variable mechanisms, using the handedness of an individual's parents as predictors. Since the early 1900s, there have been numerous studies that have evaluated handedness patterns as a function of familial relationship in the hopes of demonstrating familial inheritance patterns that contribute to the handedness phenotype. The persistence of the genetically variable model for handedness is, in some respects, a tribute to the resiliency of scientific belief systems in the face of inconclusive and ambiguous data. Generally speaking, despite large samples of subjects, most family studies of handedness (e.g., Ashton, 1982; Coren and Porac, 1980; Porac and Coren, 1979; Porac, Coren, and Searleman, 1983) have concluded that there is no compelling evidence to support the notion that right and left handedness is under simple genetically variable control. A similar negative conclusion was reached by several extensive literature reviews (e.g., Corballis, 1980, 1983; Porac and Coren, 1981), although some other authors of reviews disagree with this conclusion (e.g., Annett, 1985; McManus, 1985).

Perhaps the major reason for the persistence of the belief in genetically variable transmission of handedness comes from the one consistent finding in virtually all family studies thus far. This is an observed maternal effect on handedness. For example, in one study (Coren and Porac, 1980), we measured handedness in 459 families. We noted that if the mother was left-handed, the chance of the offspring being left-handed was approximately doubled (in our data the probability of non-right-handedness went from 17% in matings with no left-handed parents to 31% in matings with a left-handed mother). The father's handedness simply did not seem to make much difference. These results are very similar to the results that many other family studies of handedness have produced. For example, in Coren (1992) I surveyed the existing scientific literature and have found 11 family studies on handedness, published between 1913 and 1982, that had large enough numbers of families to make comparisons meaningful. Basically I learned that, on average, the presence of a left-handed mother raises the likelihood of left-handedness from about 1 out of 10 to 2 out of 10. The father's handedness has virtually no effect. Matings between two left-handed parents only raises the likelihood of sinistrality to about 3.5 out of 10. These increases in the probability of left-handedness when a left-handed mother is present are almost always statistically significant, and this finding seems to have been reliable enough to keep the hope of finding a genetically variable mechanism alive despite the fact that the remaining family correlations do not show the expected patterns based upon Mendelian genetic models.

Unfortunately, the case for a genetically variable contribution to handedness starts to fall apart when we turn to the methodology which should produce the best evidence for familial inheritance factors, namely studies of twins. It is with twin samples that we instead find the most compelling evidence against a simple, strong genetic determinant for handedness. It is generally accepted that the strongest evidence for genetically variable transmission of a characteristic involves comparisons of monozygotic (identical) twins with dizygotic (fraternal) twins. Monozygotic twins, coming from a single fertilized egg, have 100% genetic overlap, while dizygotic twins, coming from two fertilized eggs from the same parents only have an average of 50% genetic material in common (equivalent to any other sibling pair). Thus, if there is a genetically variable component in handedness, at the minimum we should expect that pairs of monozygotic twins would be much more likely to have the same handedness patterns than would pairs of dizygotic twins. In Coren and Halpern (1981), we analyzed data from 13 studies published over the time period 1933 to 1985, each of which looked at the handedness of twin pairs based upon their zygosity. We simply measured the concordance of handedness in each pair (whether both twins had the same handedness). Much to my surprise, we found no difference in the concordance of handedness for monozygotic vs. dizygotic twin pairs (both at about 76% concordance). Furthermore, neither sets of twin findings were significantly different from the percentage of concordance that would be expected on the basis of chance (78%), which would be equivalent to randomly drawing pairs of unrelated individuals from a population where right-and left-handedness was distributed in the proportions reported by Porac and Coren (1981).

Faced with the failure to find the expected genetic patterns normally obtained when characteristics are genetically variable in nature, several researchers have attempted to fit more complex genetic models to the family and twin data. The best known of these are the models by Annett (1985) and McManus (1985), both of which add the notion that in addition to genes for right- and left-handedness, there are also genes (or gene-like mechanisms) that introduce a chance or "wild card" or random element. While providing better fits than simple Mendelian models, both of these models fail by overestimating the number of left-handed offspring when both parents are left-handed. Most importantly, both also fail by predicting differences in the handedness concordance for monozygotic and dizygotic twins. Corballis (1980) summarized these attempts at model fitting by saying: "On the grounds of parsimony, then, adding further assumptions to the genetic model can only strengthen the case against it, and in favor of the much simpler hypothesis that the distribution of handedness among twins is simply a matter of chance." (p. 166).

The conclusion which we then come to seems to be that there may be reasonable evidence that right-handedness is a genetically fixed, species characteristic of humans. When it comes to predicting left-handedness, however, there appears to be little evidence for genetically variable components. Other than the usually observed maternal effects, most of the family data has provided poor support for genetic transmission of left-handedness based upon parental hand use patterns. The twin data, which ought to have provided the strongest evidence for any heritable characteristic, gives no support at all for familial heritability of left-handedness.

5. PATHOLOGICAL DETERMINANTS OF HANDEDNESS

If we accept the above conclusion, then, to explain left-handedness, it appears that we need an additional mechanism. Suppose that we have a species-typical, genetically fixed characteristic which does not appear in an individual, or appears in a modified or atypical form. Thus, consider one characteristic discussed earlier, namely that humans are genetically programmed to have five fingers on each hand. Given this fact, when we encounter an individual who is born with an atypical number of digits, the most natural presumption is that that person must have suffered from some form of pathology that has caused him or her to deviate from the standard pattern. This pathology could be something that directly interfered with normal *in utero* development, such as the introduction of a teratogenic substance, mechanical interference (e.g., accident related injuries), maternal illness, or some aberrance in the interuterine environment. A more passive pathological possibility is that despite a normal genotype, the gene controlling the characteristic is simply not activated. An example of this for a characteristic other than handedness is albinism, where, for reasons not fully understood, during the course of development the gene associated with the normal production of the skin and hair pigment (melanin) does not activate or express itself. Notice, that the failure of an expected species-specific, genetically-fixed characteristic to appear, then serves as prima facie evidence that there was some pathological condition associated with the individual's development.

This same reasoning has been applied to left-handedness. For example, in 1913, Brewster summarized the research of the previous half century and concluded (somewhat colorfully) "A sound and capable stock, like a right-handed one, breeds true generation after generation. Then something slips a cog, and there appears a left-handed child, a black sheep, or an imbecile." (p. 183). By "slips a cog" Brewster clearly meant the intervention of some pathological condition. In contemporary form, research on this hypothesis has generally been operationalized by a search for pre- and perinatal problems that may be associated with an increased incidence of left-handedness.

The research that has been going on in my laboratory over the past 25 years has often focused on the possibility that left-handedness may be a marker for the presence of some form of neuropathological insult. We have been most interested in perinatal stressors, such as delivery complications, whose presence or absence is relatively easy to determine through maternal retrospective report. Such problems can include deviations from normal maturational pattern (such as premature birth or low birth weight), mechanical factors (such as pressure from breech birth position or the use of forceps which may interfere with blood flow to the brain), or exposure to high concentrations of certain hormones during gestation. Generally speaking, results from my lab have been consistent with the findings of other researchers and have shown that the presence of any of these pathological conditions seems to be associated with an increased likelihood of left-handedness (see Bakan, 1990; Coren, 1993; Geschwind and Galaburda, 1987; Habib, Touze, and Galaburda, 1990; or Searleman, Porac, and Coren, 1989 for reviews).

For example, in Searleman, Porac, and Coren (1989) we reviewed the research literature on handedness and birth stress over the time period 1973 to the beginning of 1987 and performed a meta-analysis of these studies. We found that there was a consistent and statistically significant association between handedness and birth stress. Specifically in 30 out of 33 comparisons, we found that birth stress was associated with elevated levels of left-handedness. Since we completed that review, I have continued to monitor research findings in this area, and there has been a steady stream of findings demonstrating that there are a variety of pregnancy and birth related risk factors that increase the likelihood of left-handedness. Some studies showing global confirmation of our conclusions include Ellis and Peckham (1991) who confirmed more recalled birth stress in mothers of left-handers, and van Strien, Bouma, and Bakker (1987) report that the effect size can be quite large, with left-handers in their sample being twice as likely to have been born with a history of birth stress than their right-handed counterparts.

Many studies, too recent to have been included in our meta-analysis, have isolated specific birth stress or birth risk factors that seem to contribute to the probability of left-handedness. For instance, O'Callaghan, Tudehope, Dugdale, Mohay, Burns, and Cook (1987) reported that in their sample of children born with extremely low birth weights (e.g., below 1000 g), 54% were left handed, while among those with close to normal birth weight, only 8% were left-handed. Similarly, Ross, Lipper, and Auld (1987) found that at age 4 years, 80% of their normal-term children showed right-handedness while only 63% of their sample who had been born prematurely did. Elliman, Bryan, Elliman, Walker, and Harvey (1991) confirmed that both prematurity and reduced birth weight were associated with increased rates of left-handedness. Colburne, Kaplan, Crawford, and McLeod (1993) found that difficult delivery and induced labor increased sinistrality. Williams, Buss, and Eskenazi (1992) report that if resuscitation is required at birth, the probability of non-right-handedness went up. In Coren (1990) I found increased left-handedness when mothers were an older age at the time of parturition, with mothers over 40 years of age being 60% more likely to have left-handed children than were mothers who were around 20 years of age.

Exposure to various chemicals that have teratogenic or fetotoxic effects can also result in pathological development and increase the likelihood of sinistrality. For example, Bakan (1991) found more left-handed offspring of mothers who smoked during pregnancy. A particularly interesting example of a teratogenic factor associated with increased probability of left-handedness comes from Schachter (1994). He looked at women who during their period of fetal development, had been exposed to diethylstilbestrol (DES). This exposure occurred because during the period 1945 to 1955 DES was prescribed to prevent miscarriage, prematurity, and still birth in high-risk patients, and as prophylaxis for these problems in normal pregnancies. The use of DES was later stopped when it became apparent that it had toxicological actions, acting as a teratogenic and carcinogenic agent on the Mullerian tissue, with occasional manifest malformations of the genitalia. Schachter found that these DES-exposed children were significantly more likely to be non-right-handed.

If the hypothesis that birth stress can cause left-handedness is correct, then an interesting population in which to study handedness would be twins. The interest in this case is not because of any genetic similarities, but because having two fetuses developing in the same uterus elevates the risk of birth complications. Twinning could be viewed as a birth risk factor simply because twins are more likely to be born with low birth weights; however, it is also true that twin births are more likely to be associated with a number of specific gestational and delivery problems, including prolonged labor, premature delivery, intermittent bleeding, incorrect position at birth, and asphyxial problems (see Akerman and Fischbein, 1991). Thus, if pregnancy complications are related to increased sinistrality, the obvious prediction is that we should find an increased incidence of left-handedness in twins. My laboratory recently looked at a twin sample to explore this possibility (Coren, 1994d). Specifically, we measured the handedness of 298 twins and compared them to 1192 age and sex matched singletons. The rate of left-handedness rose from 9.9% in singletons to 14.5% in the twins, which represents a 56% increase in the relative risk of left-handedness. Similar results have recently been reported by Davis and Annett (1994), who found that twinning resulted in a 63% increase in the probability of left-handedness (from 7.1% in singletons to 11.7% in twins in their sample).

As should be clear from this brief review, there is now a sizeable literature which links left-handedness to pre- and perinatal birth complications. Thus it seems that there is ample empirical support for the hypothesis that many left-handers may owe their sinistrality to some pathological condition that prevented their normal development, and hence may have interfered with the right-handed phenotype expected in most humans. However, if we accept the idea that the very appearance of left-handedness in an individual may signal that there may have also been a history of developmental disruption and/or neuropathology, we also open the door to the possibility that the implications of handedness may extend well beyond manual dexterity and motor proficiency.

6. IMPLICATIONS OF PATHOLOGICAL LEFT-HANDEDNESS

Most theorists who believe that left-handedness may be due to some form of birth stress also presume that any pathological consequences of birth trauma will be rather diffuse. Accordingly, it would be expected that when we examine a sample of birth stressed individuals, the group would show relatively random damage to various organs, brain centers, and pathways. Handedness is vulnerable to such random damage because it has a *diffuse control system* which refers to the fact that the control of handedness is neurologically complex, involving a number of brain sites and neural pathways. If the current data on upper limb coordination are correct, there are at least 23 neural centers or systems that have been mentioned as being important to manual control (e.g., Brodal, 1992; Goodwin and Darian-Smith, 1985; Kuypers, 1985; Lewis, 1989). The hypothesis is that if any one of these vital loci are damaged, handedness may digress from the course which would eventually lead to a right-handed phenotype (see Coren, 1993). However, this idea of relatively random damage due to birth stress also implies that while non-right-handedness may be a marker for birth or gestation related pathology, left-handedness may also indicate the presence of other problems which resulted from the same trauma that disrupted the normal development of right-handedness (see Bakan, 1990; Coren, 1993; Coren and Halpern, 1991; Coren and Searleman, 1990). Put simply, left-handers may be at higher risk for a number of psychological and physical abnormalities than are their dextral counterparts. There appears to be substantial evidence that this prediction is, in fact, true.

Some problems which left-handers show with higher frequency are quite specific. For example, left-handers have more allergies, are more likely to have asthma, and have a higher probability of a number of immune and auto-immune system problems. The first evidence for this relationship came from Geschwind and Behan (1982, 1984). They showed that auto-immune diseases (especially those involving the intestinal tract and the thyroid gland) and atopic diseases (allergies, asthma, eczema, and hay fever) are 2.5

times more frequent in left-handers than in right-handers. Since that time there have been a number of additional confirmations of these findings (see, for instance, Coren, 1994b; Geschwind and Galaburda, 1987; Habib, Touze, and Galaburda, 1990). In a recent meta-analysis, which covered over a decade of research on this topic, Bryden, McManus, and Bulman-Fleming (1994) were able to confirm an overall relationship between left-handedness and immune system dysfunction, with the strongest associations being for allergies, asthma, and ulcerative colitis. Finally, a recent series of studies has looked at the blood chemistry of left- and right-handers and found systematic differences (Chengappa, Ganguli, Yang, Schurin, Cochran, Brar, and Rabin, 1992; Chengappa, Ganguli, Yang, Schurin, Brar, Rosenbleet, and Rabin, 1994). These blood serum differences have to do with the relative concentration of the interleukins, which are molecules secreted by the T-cells, which are, in turn, intimately involved with the functioning of the immune system. The direction of these blood chemistry differences seems to be consistent with the hypothesis that the immune function in left-handers may be less efficient.

Some pathological correlates of handedness seem to affect all systems to some degree. For example, there appears to be some evidence that left-handers mature more slowly than their right-handed counterparts. For example, in Coren, Searleman, and Porac (1986) we tested 713 females and 467 males and assessed their relative rate of physical maturation using the onset of several secondary sexual characteristics, age of menarche, and relative body size as our indicators. In this study we were able to demonstrate that left-handers mature at a slower rate than do right-handers. I later extended these results, reasoning that if left-handedness is associated with delayed maturation, then it is possible that sinistrals would consistently lag behind their dextral counterparts, never catching up on the growth lost during adolescence (Coren, 1989). This led to the conjecture that left-handers might have smaller body sizes, both in terms of height and weight. To test this prediction, I used archival data on the height and weight of the 3707 professional pitchers who had played major league baseball up to and including the year 1975. I found that the left-handers in this group averaged about a half-inch shorter (1.23 cm) and about 3 pounds lighter (1.35 kg) than their right-handed teammates. This result has been replicated on a larger, updated sample by Fudin, Rinninger, and Hirshon (1994). While the first two studies used only male subjects, Tan (1992) was able to show that diminished body size was also characteristic of women who were left-handed.

We have listed a few conditions above that might be more common in left-handers; however, remember that the hypothesis is that the birth or gestational trauma, which is purported to cause left-handedness affects of a diffuse control system and should show a fairly random pattern of pathology. If this is the case, then we might expect a wide variety of abnormal conditions to be more prevalent in non-right-handers (cf. Coren and Searleman, 1990). In fact, the best summary of left- vs. right-hander status on a plethora of physical and psychological dimensions is that if any difference exists between the handedness groups, it is the left-handers who will (virtually always) show poorer levels of function. A review of the literature shows such a multitude of maladies and problems that are more common in left-handers that there is simply not enough space here for me to detail them all here. For example, Coren (1990, 1993) has listed many clinical and psychological problems that are more frequently found in left-handers, according to research reports published in the past 25 years, and Table 4.1 gives a sampling of these findings.

A general idea as to the type of research supporting some of these associations can be seen from the data relating handedness to alcoholism and other potentially addictive substance use. In this literature there are a number of reports demonstrating that non-right-handers are more common in samples of alcoholics (Bakan, 1973; London, 1986, 1990; Nasrallah, Keelor, and McCalley-Whitters, 1983). In some reports the effects are

Table 4.1 A Listing of Conditions that Research Has Shown to be More Common in Left-Handers

aggressive tendencies	Hashimoto's thyroiditis	reduced weight
alcoholism	hayfever	regional ileitis
allergies	homosexuality	schizophrenia or schizotypal thinking
asthma	hypopigmentation	school failure
attempted suicide	immune system dysfunction	shortened life span
autism	infection susceptibility	smoking
brain damage	juvenile onset diabetes	sleep difficulty
celiac disease	language problems	slow maturation
chromosomal damage	learning disabilities	strabismus
clinical depression	manic-depressive psychosis	stuttering
criminality	mental retardation	suicidal tendencies
Crohn's disease	migraine headaches	sudden heart attack
deafness	myasthenia gravis	death
drug abuse	neural tube defects	transsexuality
dyslexia	neuroticism	ulcerative colitis
emotional problems	personality differences	urticaria
epilepsy	poor verbal ability	vegetarianism
eczema	reduced height	
excessive smoking		

quite large. Thus, in a sample of naval personnel who were alcohol abusers, Chyatte and Smith (1981) found that 30% were left-handed, while in another study of alcoholic men and women Smith and Chyatte (1983) found the incidence of left-handedness to be 39%. In addition to the increased incidence of left-handedness among alcoholics, it appears that treatment outcomes vary as a function of handedness. Two studies have shown that left-handers show less improvement in detoxification programs. Thus, Smith and Chyatte (1983) found that the relapse rate for left-handed alcoholics was nearly three times higher than for right-handed alcoholics. Similarly, London (1985) found that only 29% of left-handers improved after a year of hospitalization for alcoholism, as compared to 56% of right-handers in the same treatment program. Along similar lines, there is evidence that left-handers are more likely to be heavy smokers (Harburg, 1981; Harburg, Feldstein, and Papsdorf, 1978). This tendency toward greater dependency upon alcohol or tobacco may have to do with the fact that left-handers show larger changes in cortical activity in response to a variety of psychoactive drugs (Irwin, 1985).

My own laboratory has recently produced data which agrees with the pattern of findings above. As part of a project exploring the health status and handedness, individuals living in a large Canadian urban center were surveyed on some issues associated with substance use. The subsample tested involved 1009 subjects, ranging in age from 18 to 67 years (mean 31.2). When asked whether they had ever smoked regularly, it was found that 32.5% of left-handers had, as opposed to 22.5% of right-handers, $X^2(1) = 5.81, p<0.05$. When asked if they had ever sought professional help about problems with alcohol, three times as many left-handers had done so (3.3% sinistrals vs. 1.0% dextrals, $X^2(1) = 4.36$, $p<0.05$). Finally, when asked if they had ever sought help for problems associated with the use of drugs, left-handers were seven times more likely to have done so (4.1% left-handers vs. 0.6% right-handers, $X^2(1) = 13.72, p<0.001$). These data clearly confirm the findings that left-handers seem to be more likely to engage in substance use and perhaps to have substance abuse problems.

Notice that the long list of problems which are more common in left-handers presented earlier includes some problems which can be quite serious in nature. It is likely that the raised incidence some of these conditions may, in part, explain why some studies find that left-handers have shorter life spans (e.g., Aggleton, Kentridge, and Neave, 1993; Coren, 1993, 1994c; Coren and Halpern, 1991; Halpern and Coren, 1988, 1991; Rogerson, 1993).

7. HOW MANY PATHOLOGICAL LEFT-HANDERS?

Given the number of problems apparently associated with pathological left-handedness, an important question springs to mind. Are all left-handers pathological? If not, what proportion of the population of sinistrals are pathological? The suggestion that all left-handers may be pathological is not new (see Bakan, 1990) although it does sound somewhat extreme. When Coren and Searleman (1990) attempted to mathematically model the distribution of pathological left-handedness in the population they concluded that *at least half* of all left-handers were pathological, suggesting that the other half might be "natural" left-handers, where the term "natural" could be interpreted as the result of genetically variable factors or passive nonexpression of the right-handedness gene. The data we have reviewed above, however, made it clear that while the evidence for the genetically variable mechanism needed for "natural" left-handedness is, at best, equivocal, there is a good deal of evidence supporting a pathological processes as the cause of left-handedness.

The preceding paragraph looks as if it is leading to the suggestion that the majority of left-handedness is pathological in origin. However, before such an idea can be seriously entertained, we would first have to resolve some questions raised by a highly reliable finding that appears difficult to interpret in any manner other than as support for a genetically variable contribution to handedness. This is the aforementioned finding that the proportion of left-handers in a family with a left-handed mother is approximately twice that found in families where the mother is right-handed. Several extensive reviews and analyses have shown this maternal effect to be reliable (e.g., Annett, 1985; Bryden, 1982; Corballis, 1983; Coren and Porac, 1980; Porac and Coren, 1981; McManus, 1985). This result is sufficiently strong and predictable that it has led researchers to ignore the fact that the contribution of the father to offspring handedness is usually negligible, that the correlations between other family members are small and unreliable, and that the pattern of association observed is usually not consistent with standard genetic interpretations. Based predominantly on this maternal effect, researchers seem to be unwilling to completely abandon the theory that nonpathological, genetically variable factors can account for the appearance of left-handedness in offspring. If this maternal effect can be shown to be due to nongenetically variable mechanisms, we will be left with a literature which suggests that most, if not all left-handedness could be due to pathological causes.

An alternate to a familial inheritance explanation of the maternal effect on handedness is possible. Such an explanation can actually be fashioned around the concept of birth stress related pathology. As a starting point, let us merely assume that the pathological left-handedness theory is correct to the extent that trauma, associated with gestation or the birth process itself, can cause some disruption in the normal developmental course shifting individuals away from the usually expected right-handedness. Clearly, the data we have reviewed here suggest that this is a sound starting point. Staying within this framework, it would make sense to suggest that a large proportion of our sinistral mothers actually arrived at their own left-handedness as the sequelae of some form of birth trauma. All that we need now do is to note that according to the hypothesis, this same set of traumas may have also affected other physiological systems within the individual which may make these left-handed women a bit less healthy overall, and provide them with reduced reserves to deal with trying physical conditions. In other words, it is the left-handed women who, when they become pregnant, are most likely to develop complications during gestation or delivery because of their pre-existing pathologies. If this reasoning is correct, then the manner in which the left-handed mother passes on her sinistrality to her offspring is not by shared genetic material, but rather by the fact that her own difficult birth has produced internal conditions which make it more likely that she will engender a difficult birth for her own offspring. It is the raised probability of birth stress that raises the probability of having left-handed children.

This pathological explanation of the usually observed mother-offspring association in handedness is directly testable. It predicts that if we look at the birth history of a set of randomly selected individuals, the children of left-handed mothers should be more likely to have suffered from pre- or perinatal complications, which in turn could explain their increased probability of being left-handed themselves. This is the prediction that was recently tested in my laboratory.

The sample which I tested consisted of 1398 probands (853 females, 545 males) with a mean age of 20.1 years, living in an urban setting. The handedness of mother and father of each proband was obtained. In addition, the proband's medical history was checked to assess whether the subjects had experienced any of a set of nine birth risk factors. The conditions considered were prolonged labor, breech position during delivery, breathing difficulties at birth, RH incompatibility, low birth weight, premature birth, multiple birth (one of twins or triplets), instrument delivery, or delivery by Caesarian section.

If our prediction is correct, then left-handed mothers should be more likely to have birth and pregnancy complications when giving birth to their own children than right-handed mothers. To check this, I first simply counted the number of birth risk factors reported for each proband and then contrasted the mean birth risk number of birth risks observed for the children of right- and left-handed mothers. The probands with left-handed mothers had a significantly higher average birth risk than the children of right-handed mothers (1.32 for sinistral mothers vs. 0.73, $t(1396) = 4.73$, $p<0.001$). This globally confirms the expectation that left-handed mothers are more likely to conceive children with birth risks than their right-handed counterparts.

It is interesting, however, to look at the results according to each of the nine birth stressors. Table 4.2 presents this more detailed analysis in which each entry represents the percentage of the sample of offspring who have been exposed to each of the birth risk factors, separating the groups based upon whether the mother was left- or right-handed. Notice that left-handed mothers are more likely to have offspring who have birth complications, for seven of the nine risk factors listed. Thus, looking at specific birth stressors confirms that the children of left-handed mothers are at higher risk.

The hypothesis we have considered makes predictions based only on maternal handedness, since it is the left-handed mother's physical problems (due to her own presumed birth stress history) which will impact the birth of the child. Accordingly, we should expect very little in the way of paternal effects. This is clearly the case for the global analysis based upon the simple mean stress count. Now we find that the offspring of left-handed fathers have a mean of 0.91 which not significantly different from the 0.77 mean of the right-handed fathers, with $t(1396) = 1.21$, n.s. Looking at the breakdown by specific birth stressors in Table 4.2, reinforces the minimal association between father's handedness and birth risk for the offspring. The table shows that only one of the nine stressors (Rh incompatibility) reaches conventional levels of statistical significance.

The importance of this study is that it provides an explanation of the maternal effect on handedness without resorting to genetically variable mechanisms. We had hypothesized that the elevated incidence of left-handed offspring observed when the mother is

Table 4.2 The Relationship Between Birth Stress in Offspring as a Function of the Handedness of Their Mother and Father. Data Tabled Indicate the Percentage of Offspring Who Were Subject to the Each Tabled Birth Stressor as a Function of the Left- or Right-Handedness of Their Parents

	Handedness of Family Member			
	Mother		Father	
Birth Stressor	**Left**	**Right**	**Left**	**Right**
Prolonged Labor	29.6%**	18.7	24.6	19.0
Breech Birth	12.2***	3.0	3.6	3.8
Breathing Difficulty	6.1	4.0	7.2	3.9
Rh Incompatibility	11.4***	3.8	8.9**	3.9
Instrument Delivery	16.7**	7.9	13.0	8.2
Caesarean Section	16.5*	9.7	6.5	10.7
Multiple Birth	6.1**	1.7	2.2	2.1
Premature Birth	14.9	12.1	13.0	12.2
Low Birth Weight	19.1*	12.5	11.6	13.2

Note: Significance *** p<0.001; ** p<0.01; * p<0.05.

left-handed was due to a pathological factor. Specifically, left-handed mothers, who themselves may have become sinistrals through a history of birth risk factors, seem to have more difficulty when delivering their own children. Thus the same trauma or pathology which shifted the mother's handedness away from the dextral norm, may have also produced other problems which will be reflected in the mother's physical soundness. These physical problems may later impact on the mother's ability to conceive and bear children easily and safely. We need only add to this the often confirmed observation that birth stressed individuals are more likely to be left-handed to explain the presence of greater sinistrality in offspring of left-handed mothers. Hence, the last remaining datum, which seemed to support familial transmission of handedness based upon the handedness genotypes of the parents, seems to actually support a birth stress, rather than a genetically variable explanation.

8. THE STATUS OF LEFT-HANDERS

We began this investigation by looking for the origin of left-handedness. While a reasonable case can be made that the predisposition for humans to be right-handed is genetically determined, it operates as a species-typical, genetically-fixed trait. This means that it is the appearance of left-handedness that must be explained. The bulk of the evidence seems to favor birth related pathology as a cause for deviation from the expected right-handedness in any given individual. Our search for genetically variable factors, where the genetic material obtained from parents determines the offspring's handedness, was not successful. In fact, as the new data presented here shows, even the one familial relationship which seemed most promising (namely maternal sinistrality predicting offspring sinistrality) now appears to be a case of indirect transmission of a characteristic, through a chain of birth risk factors, rather than through genetic processes. To the extent that this is true, then the actual proportion of pathological left-handers may be considerably higher than we formerly might have guessed. In fact, the proportion of pathological left-handers may be on the increase, as advances in medical technology allows a higher number of birth stressed neonates to survive.

The conclusion that the majority of left-handers may have arrived at their sinistrality through pathological mechanisms has far-reaching implications. This is because of the evidence that the same pattern of trauma that caused the left-handedness in the individual also has other consequences. In this review we have seen that the relatively random processes associated with birth stress related pathology causes left-handers to be more likely to start life with damage to various neurological and organ systems. The end result is that the pathological left-hander is at higher risk for all of the problems listed in Table 4.1, including immune system difficulties, developmental problems, and neural and psychological difficulties of many types. If, as this discussion suggests, the great majority of sinistrals are probably pathological left-handers, then it also means that the simple presence of left-handedness may be a sign that the individual is at higher than average risk for psychological and physical problems.

ACKNOWLEDGMENTS

The research from my laboratory which is reported here was supported in part by grants from the Medical Research Council of Canada, the British Columbia Health Care Research Fund, and the Natural Sciences and Engineering Research Council of Canada. I would like to acknowledge the assistance of David Wong and the various members of the Human Neuropsychology and Perception Laboratory of the University of British Columbia who assisted in the collection of these data.

REFERENCES

Aggleton, J.P., Kentridge, R.W., and Neave, N.J. (1993). Evidence for longevity differences between left- and right-handed men: An archival study of cricketers. *J. Epidemiol. Comm. Health*, 47, 206.

Akerman A. and Fischbein S. (1991). Twins: Are they at risk? A longitudinal study of twins and nontwins from birth to 18 years of age. *Acta Gen. Med. Gemellol.*, 40, 29.

Annett, M. (1985). *Left, Right, Hand and Brain: The Right Shift Theory.* London, Erlbaum.

Ashton, G.C. (1982). Handedness: an alternative hypothesis. *Behav. Gen.*, 12, 125.

Bakan, P. (1973). Left-handedness and alcoholism. *Percept. Motor Skills,* 36, 514.

Bakan, P. (1990). Nonright-handedness and the continuum of reproductive casualty. In Coren, S. (Ed.), *Left-Handedness: Behavioral Implications and Anomalies. Advances in Psychology, No. 67*, Amsterdam, North-Holland, 33.

Brewster, E.T. (1913). The ways of the left hand. *McClure's Magazine,* 168.

Brodal A. (1992). *The Central Nervous System: Structure and Function.* New York, Oxford University Press.

Bryden, M.P. (1982). *Laterality: Functional Asymmetry in the Intact Brain.* New York, Academic Press.

Bryden, M.P., MacManus, I.C., and Bulman-Fleming, M.B. (1994). Evaluating the empirical support for the Geschwind-Behan-Galaburda model of cerebral lateralization. *Brain Cognit.,* 26, 103.

Chyatte, C. and Smith, V. (1981). Brain asymmetry predicts suicide among nave alcohol abusers. *Mil. Med.,* 146, 227.

Chengappa, K.N.R. Ganguli, R., Yang, Z.W., Schurin, G., Brar, J.S., Rosenbleet, J.A., and Rabin, B.S. (1994). Differences in serum interleukin-6 (IL-6) between healthy dextral and non-dextral subjects. *Neurosci. Res.,* 20, 185.

Chengappa, K.N.R., Ganguli, R., Yang, Z.W., Schurin, G., Cochran, J., Brar, J.S., and Rabin, R. (1992). Non-right-sidedness: An association with lower IL-2 production. *Life Sci.,* 51, 1843.

Corballis, M.C. (1980). Is left-handedness genetically determined? In J. Herron (Ed.), *Neuropsychology of Left-handedness.* New York, Academic Press.

Colburne, K.A., Kaplan, B.J., Crawford, S.G., and McLeod, D.R. (1993). Hand asymmetry: Its relationship to nonrighthandedness. *J. Clin. Exp. Neuropsychol.,* 15, 67.

Corballis, M. (1983). *Human Laterality.* New York, Academic Press.

Coren, S. (1989). Southpaws—somewhat scrawnier. *J. Am. Med. Assoc.,* 262, 2682.

Coren, S. (Ed.) (1990). *Left-Handedness: Behavioral Implications and Anomalies. Advances in Psychology, No. 67.* Amsterdam, North-Holland.

Coren, S. (1993). *The Left-Hander Syndrome: The Causes and Consequences of Left-Handedness.* New York, Vintage Books.

Coren, S. (1994a). Are fingerprints a genetic marker for handedness? *Behav. Gen.,* 24, 141.

Coren, S. (1994b). Handedness and allergic response. *Int. J. Neurosci.,* 76, 231.

Coren, S. (1994c). The diminished number of older left-handers: Differential mortality or social-historical trend? *Int. J. Neurosci.,* 75, 1.

Coren, S. (1994d). Twinning is associated with an increased risk of left-handedness and inverted writing hand posture. *Early Human Development,* 40, 23–27.

Coren, S. and Halpern, D.F. (1991). Left-handedness: A marker for decreased survival fitness. *Psychol. Bull.,* 109, 90.

Coren, S. and Porac, C. (1980). Family patterns in four dimensions of lateral preference. *Behav. Gen.,* 10, 333.

Coren, S. and Searleman A. (1990). Birth stress and left-handedness: The rare trait marker model. In S. Coren (Ed.), *Left-Handedness: Behavioral Implications and Anomalies. Advances in Psychology, No. 67,* Amsterdam, North-Holland, 3.

Coren, S., Searleman, A., and Porac, C. (1986) Rate of physical maturation and handedness. *Dev. Neuropsychol.,* 2, 17.

Dart, R.A. (1949). The predatory implemental technique of *Australopithecus. Am. J. Phys. Anthropol.,* 7, 1.

Davis, A. and Annett, M. (1994). Handedness as a function of twinning, age, and sex. *Cortex,* 30, 105.

Elliman, A.M., Bryan, E.M., Elliman, A.D., Walker, J., and Harvey, D.R. (1991). Coordination of low birthweight seven-year-olds. *Acta Ped. Scand.,* 80, 316.

Ellis, L. and Peckham, W. (1991). Prenatal stress and handedness among offspring. *Pre. Peri. Natal Psychol. J.,* 6, 135.

Fudin, R., Renninger, L., and Hirschon, J. (1994). Analysis of data from Reischler's (1979) The Baseball Encyclopedia: Right-handed pitchers are taller and heavier than left-handed pitchers. *Percept. Motor Skills,* 78, 1043.

Geschwind, N. and Behan, P. (1982). Left-handedness: Associations with immune disease, migraine, and developmental learning disorders. *Proc. Nat. Acad. Sci.,* 79, 5097.

Geschwind, N. and Behan, P. (1984). Laterality, hormones and immunity. In N. Geschwind, and A.M. Galaburda (Eds.), *Cerebral Dominance: The Biological Foundations,* Cambridge MA, Harvard University Press.

Geschwind, N. and Galaburda, A. M. (1987). *Cerebral Lateralization: Biological Mechanisms, Associations, and Pathology.* Cambridge, MA, The MIT Press.

Goodwin A.W. and Darian-Smith, I. (1985). *Hand Function and the Neocortex.* New York, Springer-Verlag.

Habib, M., Touze, F., and Galaburda, A.M. (1990). Intrauterine factors in sinistrality: A review. In S. Coren (Ed.), *Left-Handedness: Behavioral Implications and Anomalies. Advances in Psychology, No. 67,* Amsterdam, North-Holland, 99.

Halpern, D.F. and Coren, S. (1988). Do right-handers live longer? *Nature,* 333, 213.

Halpern, D.F. and Coren, S. (1991). Hand preference and life span. *N. Engl. J. Med.,* 324, 998.

Harburg, E. (1981). Handedness and drinking-smoking types. *Percept. Motor Skills,* 52, 279.

Harburg, E., Feldstein, A., and Papsdorf, J. (1978). Handedness and smoking. *Percept. Motor Skills,* 47, 1171.

Harris, L.J. (1990). Cultural influences on handedness: Historical and contemporary theory and evidence. In S. Coren (Ed.), *Left-Handedness: Behavioral Implications and Anomalies. Advances in Psychology, No. 67,* Amsterdam, North-Holland, 195.

Hertz, R. (1973). A study in religious polarity. In R. Needham (Ed.), *Right and Left,* Chicago, University of Chicago press, 3.

Hoosain, R. (1990). Left handedness and handedness switch among the Chinese. *Cortex,* 26, 451.

Irwin, P. (1985). Greater brain response of left-handers to drugs. *Neuropsychologia,* 23, 61.

Keeley, L.H. (1977). The functions of palaeolithic flint tools. *Sci. Am.,* 237 (November), 108.

Kuypers, H.G.J.M. (1985). The anatomical and functional organization of the motor system. In M. Swash and C. Kennard (Eds.), *Scientific Basis of Clinical Neurology,* Edinburgh, Churchill Livingstone, 3.

Lewis, O.J. (1989). *Functional Morphology of the Evolving Hand and Foot.* New York, Oxford University Press.

London, W.P. (1985). Treatment outcome of left-handed vs. right-handed alcoholic men. *Alcohol: Clin. Exp. Res.*, 9, 503.

London, W.P. (1986). Handedness and alcoholism. *Alcohol: Clin. Exp. Res.*, 10, 357.

London, W.P. (1990). Left-handedness and alcoholism. In Coren, S. (Ed.) *Left-Handedness: Behavioral Implications and Anomalies. Advances in Psychology, No. 67,* Amsterdam, North-Holland, 457.

McManus, I.C. (1985). Handedness, language dominance and aphasia: A genetic model. *Psychol. Med. Monograph, Supplement 8*. Cambridge, Cambridge University Press.

Nasrallah, N.A., Keelor, K., and McCalley-Whitter, M. (1983). Laterality shift in alcoholic males. *Biol. Psych.,* 18, 1056.

O'Callaghan, M.J., Tudehope, D.I., Dugdale, A.E., Mohay, H., Burns, Y., and Cook, F. (1987). Handedness in children with birthweights below 1000g. *The Lancet*, May 16, 1155.

Porac, C. and Coren, S. (1979). Individual and family patterns in four dimensions of lateral preference. *Neuropsychologia,* 17, 543.

Porac, C. and Coren, S. (1981). *Lateral Preferences and Human Behavior.* New York, Springer-Verlag.

Porac, C., Coren, S., and Searleman, A. (1983). Inverted vs. straight handwriting posture: A family study. *Behav. Gen.,* 13, 311.

Porac, C., Coren, S., and Searleman, A. (1986) Environmental factors in hand preference: Evidence from attempts to switch the preferred hand. *Behav. Gen.* 16, 251.

Porac, C., Rees, L., and Buller, T. (1990). Switching hands: A place for left hand use in a right hand world. In S. Coren (Ed.), *Left-Handedness: Behavioral Implications and Anomalies. Advances in Psychology, No. 67,* Amsterdam, North-Holland, 259.

Rogerson, P.A. (1993). On the relationship between handedness and longevity. *Soc. Biol.,* 40, 283.

Ross, G., Lipper, E.G., and Auld, P.A.M. (1987). Hand preference of four-year-old children: Its relationship to premature birth and neurodevelopmental outcome. *Dev. Med. Child Neurol.*, 29, 615.

Schachter, S.C. (1994). Handedness in women with intrauterine exposure to diethylstilbestrol. *Neuropsychologia,* 32, 619.

Searleman, A., Porac, C., Coren, S. (1989). The relationship between birth order, birth stress handedness and lateral preference: A critical review. *Psychol. Bull.,* 105, 397.

Semenov, S.A. (1964). *Prehistoric Technology.* London, Cory, McAdams and MacKay.

Smith, V. and Chyatte, C. (1983). Left-handed vs. right-handed alcoholics: An examination of relapse patterns. *J. Stud. Alcohol.*, 44, 553.

Strien, J.W. van, Bouma, A., and Bakker, D.J. (1987). Birth stress, autoimmune diseases, and handedness. *J. Clin. Exp. Neuropsychol.*, 9, 775.

Tan, U. (1992). The relation of body height to handedness in male and female right- and left-handed subjects. *Int. J. Neurosci.*, 63, 217.

Warren, J.M. (1980). Handedness and laterality in humans and other animals. *Physiol. Psychol.,* 8, 351.

Williams, C.S., Buss, K.A., and Eskenazi, B. (1992). Infant resuscitation is associated with an increased risk of left-handedness. *Am. J. Epidemiol.,* 136, 277.

Chapter 5

Hand Preference and Performance in Lefthanders

Michael Peters

CONTENTS

1. INTRODUCTION

The phenotype of handedness in Western industrialized cultures reveals that the large majority of the population can be characterized as having strong and directionally consistent hand preferences. For activities which matter in terms of consequences, the right hand is chosen. It is only for incidental and inconsequential activities, such as picking up objects when these are not hard to pick up, where hand preferences deviate

0-8493-8999-2/96/$0.00+$.50

from the strong right preference pattern. Things are not as easy with reference to lefthanders. I shall allow myself the luxury of defining as lefthanders those who write with the left hand. In doing so I will have to confine much of this chapter to individuals from Western industrialized countries in which there is no large scale pressure against left-handed writing. A basic assumption is that no individual is forced against his/her will to write with the left rather than the right hand while the converse will be the case, albeit to a very minor degree, even in the above-mentioned countries. As a minimal prevalence figure of lefthandedness, I will adopt the proportion of lefthanded writers reported in the survey of more than a million respondents by Gilbert and Wisocki (1992). According to that study, some 10.6% of females and 13.1% of males aged 20 to 30 years write with the left hand.

In many ways, lefthanders represent the most intriguing aspect of handedness in humans because such a polymorphism in phenotype is not easily explained. If one assumes that the majority of humans is righthanded for a reason, then the question of why some individuals do not fit the mold has several possible answers.

1.1 GENETIC MODELS

These models do not make precise predictions about hand performance, but they do consider handedness as part of the normal process of the determination of lateralization of function. McManus' (1991) model of lateralization of function in lefthanders makes no differential prediction of the overall level of motor competence of lefthanders, especially for those lefthanders who have a double dose of the "chance" gene. However, because these are expected to show what he terms "fluctuating asymmetry," they will commit to a clear hand preference which may be either for the left or the right hand. Annett's 1985 and more current models differ in that lefthanders are expected to have smaller between hand differences than righthanders. As pointed out elsewhere (Peters, 1990a), neither model makes predictions that are easily falsified and this is a major problem.

1.2 BALANCED POLYMORPHISM

Annett has introduced an evolutionary element to her handedness theory which suggests why exactly there should be lefthanders: Annett and co-workers (Annett and Manning, 1989) noted that marked right hand superiority, i.e., very strong righthandedness, goes together with weak performance on a variety of tests that are not themselves related to handedness. In short, the suggestion is that lefthandedness is nature's way of avoiding being too righthanded. Lefthanders appear on the scene, therefore, because of some sort of balanced polymorphism. If one accepts this speculation, one would assume that being righthanded is, in general, good, but not being too righthanded. From a conceptual point of view, the question of how to evaluate the performance aspect of "being too righthanded" is of some interest. Annett's method selects individuals for whom the difference between right-hand and left-hand performance is particularly large. There are two aspects that need to be looked at. The first concerns the task. Annett and co-workers mostly use the peg-moving task. Evaluation of the performance of individuals in our lab who were tested on a number of motor tasks shows that the peg-moving task is, in fact, a very good motor task if handedness is to be described. Nevertheless, one would like to know whether an individual who is classed as very strongly righthanded on the basis of the peg-moving task would also be classified in such a way with another task.

The second aspect that needs investigation is the way in which large right-left hand differences can arise. If a subject has average performance in the right hand but a large between-hand difference favoring the right, this can only mean an unusually depressed left-hand performance. Alternatively, a subject can have average performance in the left hand and if this is the case, large between hand differences can only derive from a very high right-hand performance. Annett's data show that righthanders with large between-hand differences have average right-hand performance but strongly depressed left-hand performance. This raises the possibility that her method of identifying strongly dextral individuals amounts to a weak neurological screening for soft neurological signs. One would expect a reverse pattern of strongly depressed right-hand performance if one were to select out of a large number of lefthanders those individuals who showed large between-hand performance differences favoring the left hand.

1.3 PATHOLOGY

This brings us to handedness models which make outright reference to pathology in the genesis of handedness (see also Chapter 4). A strong version of the "pathology" model was most clearly made by Bakan, Dibb, and Reed (1973); with a claim that difficulties during birth selectively damaged the population of cells which is presumed to be active in executing hand movement for the right hand. Here, there is a very clear expectation that the right hand of lefthanders would show a deficit in performance. A somewhat weakened version of this position was provided by Bishop's (1984) suggestion that in the general population of lefthanders there is a subgroup who became lefthanders because the control system for the right hand was in some mild way damaged during early development — or did not develop properly. For this group, one would expect some deficit in some aspects in performance compared to average righthanders. However, to the extent that only a very small proportion of lefthanders are, according to Bishop, affected in this way, testing would have to involve larger numbers in order to identify this group. A much stronger claim for pathological lefthandedness is made in the much-publicized paper by Coren and Halpern (1991). Coren and Halpern suggest that lefthanders do not have the same life expectancy as righthanders, and they attempt to relate this basic contention to diverse sources difficulties faced by lefthanders.

Coren and Halpern (1991) introduce a variety of reasons as to why lefthanders should die earlier, which are not accepted by everybody (Harris, 1993). It does make sense, though, to speculate that lefthanders are exposed to dangers because of their unconventional hand use. Aggleton, Kentridge, and Neave (1993), when exploring life expectancies of left-handed cricket players with a data base that even exceeded that available for baseball players, found that lefthanders, on average, died earlier than righthanders. Interestingly, though, when analyzing causes of death, Aggleton et al. found that there was no significant difference between the two groups in terms of death due to disease. Instead, the differences were derived from different mortality rates incurred during war. There are two other domains in which lefthanders might be exposed to greater risk than righthanders because of their atypical preference pattern. First, there are car accidents, where Coren and Halpern (1991) and Coren (1989) claim greater risks for lefthanders. The other category involves work accidents. Garonzik (1989) makes the perfectly reasonable argument that because individuals do not tend to do as well with their nonpreferred as with their preferred hand, the design of machine controls should take hand preference patterns into account. The fact is that machine control design makes no such concessions. While it would make good sense that lefthanders are exposed to a higher accident risk because of designs favoring righthanders, the evidence is not as convincing as one might think. Dellatolas et al. (1993) looked at the association between temporary hand use shifts due to earlier accidents and handedness and came to the conclusion that while weak righthanders were at a somewhat higher risk for accidents, lefthanders did not have an elevated risk. Porac (1993) looked at a sample of individuals who had unilateral accidental hand injury and compared their preference patterns to that of a comparable control group without hand injury. Her conclusion was that individuals with inconsistent hand preference were more likely to injure the hand than individuals with consistent hand preference, left or right. Porac suggests that injury risk is higher for the preferred hand than for the nonpreferred hand and explains the differences between the consistently handed and the mixed-handed groups in this way.

What does stand out in this discussion is that there is very little direct experimental evidence on the actual performance patterns of lefthanders as related to pathology. However, it is still of some use to look at some available data on the performance of lefthanders in order to see whether there is any evidence, as pathology models suggest, of depressed performance. At the outset, we have to say that the range of motor tasks used in exploring handedness is embarrassingly narrow, and that studies in which sufficient numbers of subjects were tested with adequate measures are rare. There is some interesting older Russian work on this topic, which does examine performance in the context of meaningful industrial tasks (Bragina and Dobrochtowa, 1984). Unfortunately, very little detail on method is available in this work.

2. PERFORMANCE

When we talk about handedness, we have in mind a range of activities which individuals could perform with either the right or left hand, but for which they typically choose one hand to the exclusion of the other. Such choices are subject to a number of influences. Early in life, preferences for one hand or the other do not carry any major baggage of neuromotor specialization which would make it impossible to choose one hand rather than the other. Instead, choices are made on the basis of relatively weak predispositions which then interact with increasing competence which in turn interacts with neuromotor control mechanisms. Because most skilled motor activities require very large amounts of practice, commitment to one hand should not normally waver. These are the inherent elements of hand choice, determined largely from within the individual. As an added complication in what hand is chosen for what activity, there is the cultural element because highly skilled motor activities are culturally transmitted and taught. As any righthanded parent who has obligingly tried to teach his/her lefthanded child how to tie a shoe-lace knows, it is useful for the teacher and the pupil to share hand preference. This adds pressure towards hand choice conformity and in many cases the lefthander will have no choice as to role differentiation. Thus, the piano — built by righthanders, laid out for righthanders, and with music written largely by righthanders — simply has to be played the righthanded way. When we look at hand performance, then, these cultural dictates present a major confounding factor. While the natural righthander finds things just as they should be, the lefthander, willingly or not, will acquire considerable expertise with the nonpreferred right hand simply because there is no way to avoid it.

We may therefore expect, *a priori,* that the nonpreferred hand of the lefthander will tend to be somewhat better than that of the righthander, simply because of a difference in motor experience.

The nature of the motor tasks themselves will also have an influence on the performance of the preferred and nonpreferred hand. If we take a motor task which contains highly practiced elements, such as the circle-filling task described by Tapley and Bryden (1985), we can expect a marked separation of the performances of the preferred and the nonpreferred hands. The circle-filling task contains many motor elements critical in handwriting and can therefore be said to be differentially practiced. Similar comments can be made about tasks like throwing at a target. Throwing is also a very strongly lateralized task in which differential practice of the two hands gives a very strong edge to the hand which is normally used. With tasks like these, the performance differential between the preferred and nonpreferred hand will tell us only that the individual in question has practiced almost exclusively with one hand.

Other tasks are less specifically practiced. For instance, the quite commonly used peg placing tasks require subjects to insert pins into a small target hole and to do this rapidly and repeatedly. While the preferred hand will have more experience in picking up small objects and manipulating them, there will be few individuals who have practiced this task specifically. Similarly, in the finger tapping task which has for years been a staple component of neuropsychological test batteries, there is no specific practice for rapid repetitive finger tapping. Indeed, even typists and pianists will not have practiced this specific movement because in both cases there are few occasions where a single finger will by itself tap rapidly (rapidly repeating single notes on keyboard instruments will tend to be produced by oscillation around the wrist joint).

If we use these two activities as representatives of specifically practiced (throwing) and not specifically practiced (tapping) tasks, we can make some predictions about the magnitude of the effect size of between hand differences. Effect size is defined here as the proportion of variance accounted for by the variable "Hand." For example, if the two hands do not contribute to the inter-interindividual differences in performance on some motor task, the effect size of "Hand" will be close to zero. If hand performance differences are very large, as they would be in, for example, writing speed, then the "Hand" effect size would be very large. Proceeding under the assumption that righthanders are strongly lateralized to the right hand, we can predict that both specifically practiced and non-specifically practiced activities will show a strong "Hand" effect, but that the former will show a distinctly larger effect size because of the differential practice effect. For lefthanders, we can also predict that the hand effect for throwing will be considerably larger than for tapping. However, we will have to differentiate our predictions because of a need to subgroup lefthanders (Kang, 1995; Peters and Murphy, 1992; Peters and Servos, 1989). In North America, there are lefthanders who use the left hand consistently for many activities, and these we call *consistent lefthanders (CL)*. There are also lefthanders who prefer to use the left hand for fine motor activities and the right hand for activities that require strength and ballistic movements. Such lefthanders we call *inconsistent lefthanders (IL)*.

In terms of the relative prevalence figures for these subgroups, the data base provided by Gilbert and Wisocki (1992) provides the best figures at this point. Among males aged 20 to 30, 4.4% write with the left hand and throw with the right hand, and 8.7% write with the left hand and throw with the left hand. Among females aged 20 to 30 years, 4.1% write with the left hand and throw with the right hand, and 6.5% write with the left hand and throw with the left hand. Thus, a sizable proportion of lefthanded writers choose to throw with the left hand, and as pointed out by Peters and Murphy (1992), they do so of their own free will: it is unlikely that they are allowed to write with the left, but forced to throw with the right. The converse is not true because individuals who throw with the left but write with the right might well be natural lefthanders who succumbed to social pressures against writing with the left hand.

2.1 BETWEEN-HAND DIFFERENCES FOR LEFTHANDERS

We assume that the overall magnitude of effect sizes for both of these groups will be smaller than the magnitude of hand effect sizes observed for righthanders. Lacking other information, there is no *a priori* reason to postulate strong differences between these groups but one can adopt a working hypothesis which proposes that ILs do not have strong inherent lateral biases and that, therefore, their effect sizes should be smaller than those for CLs.

For our data base, throwing data were used from the Peters (1990b) throwing data; in that study, no effect sizes were provided. The tapping data comes from our laboratory, and is comprised of data from large numbers of subjects who have been tested over the years. The order of effect sizes for throwing was RHs = .720 > CLs = .436 > ILs = .409. For tapping the order was RHs = .564 > CLs = .385 > ILs = .210. According to Cohen (1969), effect sizes <.25 = small; .25 – .50 = medium; > .50 = large.

It can be seen that while RH's have a larger effect for throwing than for tapping, the effect size of "hand" for tapping is still in the range considered as large by Cohen's criteria. Cl's have a large "hand" effect for throwing (though still markedly lower than the one for righthanders) and a medium effect for tapping. Finally, ILs have a medium effect for throwing and a small effect for tapping. It should be noted here that because of the dissociation of the hand chosen for fine motor activities and strength and ballistic activities, the effect sizes for ILs are based on better left-hand performance in tapping and better right-hand performance in throwing.

These data suggest that while practice has a clear effect on preferred hand performance, this effect is different for righthanders and lefthanders. If one were to ask which task would provide a maximal between/hand separation, throwing would be the task of choice. Here, preference and experience reinforce each other to yield a strong hand effect. Nevertheless, it can be seen that even in this case, the tendency of lefthanders to be less lateralized can be discerned. This is quite significant because if practice were a completely overriding factor, one would suspect that the effect sizes for this task would look similar across the three handedness groups.

2.2 COMPARISON OF THE OVERALL PERFORMANCE LEVELS OF THE TWO HANDS

In addition to the question about the magnitude of between-hand differences, there is also the question of overall performance levels of the two hands. Lefthanders do have greater opportunity (often against their will) to acquire skills with the nonpreferred right hand. For this reason, one would expect that lefthanders excel over righthanders in the dexterity of the nonpreferred hand. This is a somewhat trivial prediction, which nevertheless flies in the face of those pathological theories which attribute lefthandedness to damage in the right hand motor control system. Of greater interest is the question of whether the preferred hand of the two groups differs. To address this question, we can present data from a very recently completed and as yet unpublished study, in which righthanded and lefthanded subjects performed a series of motor tasks.

All subjects performed the Annett peg placing task, the finger tapping task, the O'Connors peg placing task (placing pegs with tweezers), the O'Connors peg placing task (placing pegs with fingers), and the Grooved Pegboard task. The preferred hand was defined as the hand chosen for writing. There were no significant differences when the preferred hands of the three groups were compared. When the performances of the nonpreferred hands were compared, there was an overall significant difference between the groups: while the nonpreferred hand of RHs and CLs did not differ significantly, ILs showed significantly better performance than these two groups. Thus, on these unimanual tasks, the preferred hands of lefthanders and righthanders do not differ, and the nonpreferred hand of inconsistent lefthanders is clearly superior to that of the other groups. Because this superiority emerges most clearly with regard to the tapping task (where practice history is least of a factor), we assume that this group shows a genuinely smaller degree of lateral differentiation than the other groups.

These findings do not provide any indication whatsoever of motor problems in either the preferred or nonpreferred hands of lefthanders, a conclusion that is also supported by other work with similar populations (Levander, Levander, and Schalling, 1989).

In contrast, several studies on bimanual tapping (Peters, 1985, 1987) suggest that righthanders performed better overall with their preferred hand combination (right fast/left slow) than lefthanders. In addition, while righthanders performed significantly better with their preferred combination than with their nonpreferred combination (left fast/right slow), lefthanders showed no clear superiority of one combination over the other, with performance levels that were intermediate between the preferred and nonpreferred hand performances of the righthanders. In tasks such as these, it is not the actual motor execution per se which matters, but the way in which the two hands integrate their activity. This finding points to the possibility that the coordination of motor cortices which are involved in bimanual activities may operate slightly differently in lefthanders than in righthanders.

Against these observations, there is the recent work by Treffner and Turvey (in press) which represents a more sophisticated (both in terms of methodology and conceptual development) approach than the one taken by Peters. Treffner and Turvey investigate an experimental situation where subjects have to move a pendulum with each hand, either in or out of phase. Their design allows for a general index of the variability of the bimanual coordination pattern and they find that in their experimental condition righthanders show a more variable performance than consistent lefthanders and these, in turn, show a more variable performance than inconsistent lefthanders. Treffner and Turvey find meaningful differences between the performances of consistent and inconsistent lefthanders and thus validate this subgrouping with a categorically different task (their task, unlike the tapping tasks described above, does not involve independent movement of the fingers).

In the context of Treffner and Turvey's (1995) observations of variability of performance on bimanual tasks, there are also some interesting data on the variability of unimanual tapping. Over the years, we have accumulated a considerable amount of tapping data in our laboratory. While we collected only tapping rate for the majority of studies, the variability of tapping was collected for a number of studies. We did not generally pay specific attention to the variability of tapping but in a study on finger and arm tapping we did (Peters and Pang, 1992). In that study, as in others, we found that consistent lefthanders in particular and inconsistent lefthanders to a lesser extent tapped faster with the preferred hand than the nonpreferred hand. However, while righthanders showed significantly less variability of intertap interval in the preferred than the nonpreferred hand, neither the consistent nor the inconsistent lefthanders showed any differences in variability between the hands.

This observation cannot be explained in terms of the smaller overall between-hand differences in tapping for the lefthanders; the consistent lefthanders in particular tapped clearly faster with the preferred hand. This trend was confirmed when we looked back at the data of other studies: the variability of intertap intervals for the preferred hand of lefthanders does not differ from that of the nonpreferred hand, and its magnitude is more closely approximated by the variability intertap intervals in the nonpreferred hand of righthanders than in the preferred hand.

2.3 PERFORMANCE DIFFERENCES BETWEEN RIGHT- AND LEFTHANDERS ON A DECISION MAKING TASK

A completely different line of research reveals additional differences between right- and lefthanders. Laeng and Peters (1995) have examined the speed with which righthanders and lefthanders make judgments about spatial coordinates and categories. It turns out that the overall reaction time of lefthanders is appreciably slower when making judgments of this kind than the corresponding reaction time of righthanders. The overall effect is appreciable; handedness accounts for some 32% of the variation in reaction time. We do not know at this point why it is that lefthanders (and especially so consistent lefthanders) have a markedly slower reaction time than righthanders. This may have something to do with the fact that reaction time was signalled by hand movement and thus the delay relative to righthanders may have been introduced in this way. However, it is also possible that the delay may be due to higher level decision processes and if so, this would be the first meaningful indication of differences between handedness groups which are not due to some simple hand movement factors. A preliminary interpretation is that the differences observed here are not due to a simple hand control factor because the mean reaction time for righthanders is 900 msec on this task while it is 941 for inconsistent lefthanders and 1094 for consistent lefthanders. These differences are too large to be explained in any simple way by referring to interhemispheric transmission delays for hand movements.

2.4 SUMMARY

The lack of convincing overall performance differences on the unimanual motor tasks when speed of performance is the measure comes as some surprise. Why surprise? The reasoning is as follows: in righthanders, control of praxis for the preferred hand and motor speech are both located in the left hemisphere and speculations have been advanced of why the common location makes sense in evolutionary and functional terms (Kimura, 1993; Peters, 1990b). If lefthanders had motor speech control on the right side of the brain, the situation would be simple. But they do not. The majority of lefthanders have speech motor control in the left hemisphere, just as righthanders do. This raises the question of where control of the preferred hand is located in lefthanders. There is some indication that lefthanders use the right hemisphere to organize hand movements, as indicated in the observation of apraxia in lefthanders after *right* hemisphere lesions (Faglioni and Basso, 1984; Kimura, 1993). However, there is also evidence that the left hemisphere plays a significant role in some movements (Gur, 1984). This arrangement may be of some advantage in the sense that it allows for flexibility in motor control. However, under some conditions, the involvement of two control systems may be of some slight disadvantage. The lack of a clear lateral advantage in the bimanual coordinated tapping task could be an expression of such a disadvantage. However, it has to be pointed out that in the task used by Treffner and Turvey (1995), similar asymmetries were observed for lefthanders and righthanders. This discrepancy suggests that differences in tasks and/or method may be of importance in the determination of whether or not lateral asymmetries are observed.

Because we have more data on the variability of unimanual tapping, we are more confident that in this case there is a lack of asymmetry in lefthanders. Perhaps this is an indication of a slight disadvantage, revealed in a subtle measure. The term "slight" disadvantage is emphasized here because of the extraordinary flexibility of the human motor system which allows mastery when there is determination. If the motor arrangements in lefthanders exact a small but tangible price for greater flexibility, this price would not be visible in most normal activities, but there is a possibility that the disadvantage would show itself most clearly at the very highest and demanding levels of motor performance, of the distal musculature. To us, such extreme levels of performance are most clearly expressed by virtuosity in musical performance. The question could therefore be posed: can one find, at the very top level of instrumental performance, a proportionate representation of lefthanders? We know from earlier work by Oldfield (1969) that lefthanded musicians are proportionately represented among musicians playing in orchestras, but no information is available at the virtuoso level.

The overall level of motor performance also relates to hypotheses about causes of lefthandedness. Do the performance differences mentioned here relate to the pathological model of lefthandedness? At the most reduced level, one would expect that the right hand of lefthanders should show some clear disadvantage relative to the left hand of righthanders. In the former case, the pathological model predicts that significant damage to the motor control system for this hand caused a switch in the first place. The issue becomes complicated by the question of what to expect from the normal nonpreferred hand. Is it, in principle, capable of performance on par with that of the preferred hand, given sufficient practice? There is no direct experimental evidence on this question, but a most interesting paper by Hiscock et al. (1989) provides some ideas.

Hiscock et al. took an approach parallel to the one taken by investigators who asked the question: if one hemisphere is lost very early in life due to hemispherectomy, will it matter which one is removed in terms of language development? Hiscock et al. compared the level of motor performance in 30 children with right hemiplegia (left hemisphere) with that of 27 children with left hemiplegia (right hemisphere). If the two hemispheres were completely equipotential with regard to motor development, there should not be any appreciable differences between the two groups. However, Hiscock et al. showed that right hemiplegics showed poorer motor performance. This forces the conclusion that the system has some prespecifications which cannot be overcome by selective experience, and just as early damage to the left hemisphere is ultimately more detrimental to language and speech than damage to the right hemisphere, damage to the left hemisphere is more detrimental to the development of motor control than damage to the right hemisphere. This quite fascinating possibility has to be tempered by a caution that relates to the effect of having to reorganize speech and language for the right hemisphere; in children with an intact left hemisphere, no such reorganization has to take place. Thus, it is possible that the conclusion of a "preferred hand" specialization in the left hemisphere is in error because language and speech requirements in the right hemisphere might crowd out or relegate to secondary importance the motor control mechanisms for the hand. However, there is some neuroanatomical evidence which suggests that the region of the motor cortex which deals with the upper extremity is larger in left than in the right hemisphere (White et al., 1994). The observed asymmetry is by no means as pronounced as preference and performance distribution patterns would lead one to expect, but the finding does raise the possibility that the differences favoring the left hemisphere in the Hiscock et al. study have a structural basis. What remains to be determined is the pattern of asymmetry in lefthanders. Would it be reversed, or would it parallel that seen in the planum temporale of lefthanders where lefthanders show a larger planum temporale on both sides rather than a reversed pattern to that seen in righthanders?

Any answer to these questions presupposes a better understanding of another issue that emerged in our discussion: the subclassification of lefthanders. In the following section, some empirical data on hand preferences of lefthanders are presented which indicate the need for subgrouping.

3. LATERAL PREFERENCES OF LEFTHANDERS

This section will consider hand preference patterns of subgroups of lefthanders, and the intent is to relate such preference patterns to everyday concerns of design and usage. Some limited reference will be made to the implications of such preference patterns for models of handedness. The sample on which these data are based is based mostly on citizens of the U.S. who responded to a request for participation in a study on lefthandedness, which was printed in the magazine "Lefthander International." The sample, therefore, is unlike the typical large scale sample which most commonly is comprised of university students and some description of the composition of the sample and how information was collected will be useful.

3.1 METHOD

3.1.1 The Questionnaire

The handedness questionnaire contained 18 items and was printed in the magazine "Lefthander International," and respondents mailed it to the author of this study. In all, 686 usable questionnaires were filled out and returned by lefthanders.

3.1.2 Respondents

These ranged in age from 9 to 81 years, with an average age for males of 35.4 years (n = 270) and 34.3 years for females (n = 416). In order to simplify comparisons where age was involved, two age classes were established: 41 years of age and older and below 41 years of age. The cutoff age was established with reference to Gilbert and Wisocki's (1992) large North-American data set. Their data show that in terms of the prevalence of lefthanded writing, the age cohort beginning in the late 1940s/early 1950s shows contemporary prevalence figures while in older cohorts there is a pronounced decrease in the prevalence of individuals writing with the left hand.

3.2 RESULTS

In the following, the results which are of applied relevance will be presented and discussed. Numbers of respondents in the contingency tables vary according to the number of respondents who answered a particular question.

3.2.1 Difficulties With "Right-Handed" Implements

It is reasonable to suggest that lefthanded writers who prefer the left hand for most activities are less flexible when it comes to using "right-handed" implements than lefthanded writers who prefer the right hand for many activities. If so, the need to accommodate lefthanders covers fewer individuals than would be indicated by the prevalence of lefthanded writers in the population. This possibility was examined directly by evaluating the number of individuals who report having difficulties with righthanded implements relative to hand preference patterns. The responses to 17 preference items (write, draw, hammer, throw, brush teeth, cut bread, comb hair, hold tennis racquet, hold needle when sewing, open jar, pick up penny, hold razor, golf, bat, pick up something heavy, use tweezers to pick up a small object, use eraser) were summed for each individual. With the five point scale, the minimum number of 17 points would be achieved by an individual who chose "left only = 1" for each of the preference items. The maximum number of points would be 85, for an individual who chose "right only = 5" for each item. Four groups of roughly similar size were established, with preference scores as follows: Group 1, 17 to 26; Group 2, 27 to 35; Group 3, 27 to 35; Group 4, 35 and more. For each group, the number of individuals who reported having difficulties with right-handed implements was tabulated, and the result subjected to a chi-square test. Table 5.1 shows the results.

Table 5.1 Difficulties with Righthanded Implements and Degree of Lefthandedness

	Yes	No	N
Group 1	74	72	146
Group 2	85	69	154
Group 3	89	83	172
Group 4	97	59	156
			628

Note: chi-square (df 3) = 5.1, n.s.

There was no significant trend. If anything, lefthanders who prefer the right hand for a number of activities were more likely to report having difficulties with righthanded implements; this can be verified by comparing only the extreme groups, 1 and 4. The results question the assumption that lefthanders with mixed preference choices are more flexible than lefthanders with consistent left hand choices when using righthanded implements.

In all, 54.9% of the respondents reported that they had trouble with tools or activities that were designed for the righthanders. Some 170 items or activities were listed. Considering that some implements are available in "left-handed" form, it may come as an initial surprise that "scissors" and "can openers" are listed as the most common items of complaint. However, even if an individual has a lefthanded version of these implements, such implements are not available in all environments (i.e., office, workplace). The nature of the questionnaire did not allow a judgment as to whether respondents merely suffered inconvenience or felt endangered. Certainly, the 32 respondents who complained about circular saws address not only an inconvenience but a definite hazard. The problems with some items are obvious, such as the pouring spout for ladles, but others are obscure as far as righthanders are concerned. For instance, the 32 respondents who listed "measuring cups" likely react to the fact that the units inside some cups are meant to be read when the handle is held by the right hand. Wristwatches, also indicated, are designed for righthanders, to be held in the left while the right hand adjusts time and date. The great majority of artifacts indicated by the sample as creating difficulties have an inherent laterality, ranging from the direction of thread on bolts to the layout of hand calculators and computer keyboards.

The fact that a sizable minority of lefthanders in the present survey did not indicate difficulties does not suggest that these do, in fact, have no trouble with righthanded implements or procedures. This point will be taken up in the final section of the paper.

3.2.2 Writing Posture

When writing with a posture that is the mirror image of that used by righthanders, lefthanders have to push the pen across the page instead of pulling it. It is not unlikely that part of the reason for a low prevalence of lefthanded writing in the past was dictated by pen nibs that would get caught more easily by impurities in the paper, and the problem of avoiding smudging when the hand passed over wet ink. These technical problems have largely disappeared with the advent of the ballpoint pen and high grade paper. Nevertheless, many lefthanders adopt a writing posture that is not simply the mirror image of the preferred writing posture for righthanders and in which the pen can actually be pulled across the page. This unusual writing posture was called the "hooked" or "inverted" posture by Levy and Reid (1976) who pointed out that in this posture, the pen is held above the line of writing, and part of the hand is held above the line of writing. Levy and Reid's (1976) suggestion that lefthanders with the inverted posture guide their hand with ipsilateral as opposed to the usual contralateral hemisphere is no longer accepted by the majority of researchers (Bishop, 1990). The current understanding is that the inverted writing posture represents a functional adaptation to the demands of writing from the left to the right (Meulenbroek and Van Galen, 1989; Peters, 1986). This view contrasts sharply with the influential opinions expressed by Blau (1946) and Clark (1957) who felt that the inverted posture should be discouraged, an opinion that is still proclaimed in contemporary instruction manuals for handwriting (Peters, 1986).

In the present questionnaire, lefthanders were given illustrations of the inverted and noninverted writing posture and were asked to indicate which posture they used. In addition, they were given the option "parallel to the line of writing" because a sizable proportion of lefthanders cannot be classified in terms of either the inverted or noninverted posture. Because the writing posture was a function of age and sex, the contingency tables take these factors into account. It should be noted that the writing posture also influences the tilt of the writing paper. The clear majority of inverted writers tilts the writing page to the left (65%) while the remaining 35% tilt to the right. Noninverters prefer a right tilt (76.7%) with a minority of 23.3% tilting to the left. A similar pattern, and the fact that the inverted writers are more flexible in terms of the tilt of the writing page, was previously observed for a smaller sample (Peters, 1983).

It can be seen that older individuals are much more likely to write with the non-inverted posture than younger individuals (Table 5.2). This can be interpreted in terms of the degree of tolerance in the educational system for "devious" writing postures. There also is a strong effect of sex. Far more males than females write with the inverted posture (Table 5.3). This is consistent with earlier observations (Levy, 1984). An important aspect to note is that lefthanders can readily adopt either the inverted or noninverted posture and the relative advantages of the inverted posture. In some countries (Weber and Bradshaw, 1981), the inverted posture is quite strongly discouraged.

Table 5.2 Writing Posture and Age

Posture	< 41	> 41	N
Inverted	133	72	205
Noninverted	144	120	264
Parallel	72	31	103
	349	223	572

Note: Chi-square = 9.35; $p < .009$

Table 5.3 Writing Posture and Sex

Posture	Males	Females	N
Inverted	119	86	205
Noninverted	66	198	264
Parallel	43	60	103
	228	344	572

Note: Chi-square = 51.5; $p < .00001$

3.2.3 Pressures to Change Hand Preference

More females than males report that they have been subjected to some pressure by individuals who wished them to change hand choice (Table 5.4). This difference also relates to the higher prevalence of the noninverted writing posture in females. The latter finding suggests that the direct and indirect pressures to conform to an accepted writing posture have differential effects on males and females. Finally, there is a legitimate argument to be made that the lower lefthandedness prevalence in females may not be the result of some complex genetic factors that lead to differential expression of lateral biases in females (McManus, 1991), but rather that fewer females become manifest lefthanders because they are more responsive to direct and indirect social pressures.

In all, some 36.5% of individuals reported having experienced pressures against handedness. Table 5.5 shows pressure relative to age. Two aspects are noteworthy. First, there remain significant pressures against lefthandedness in the current generation. Second, and especially in the older generation, the self-selected nature of the sample may give a very biased impression in terms of the pressures against left-handedness. Thus,

Table 5.4 Pressure to Change Hand Preference as a Function of Sex

Sex	Pressure	No Pressure	N
Males	71	162	233
Females	147	216	363
	218	378	596

Note: Chi-square = 6.14; $p < .013$

especially among the older individuals in this sample, the defining feature is successful resistance to such pressures. Those who did not resist or who did not have some support in their efforts to write with the left hand would of course not be represented in this sample. A cautious interpretation of the present situation is that significant pressures still exist and at the same time there also is likely more support for individuals who wish to be lefthanded. In addition, the existing pressures, especially in the education system, are no longer coercive in character (i.e., left hand tied behind back, slaps on the left hand when used for writing), but indirect.

Table 5.5 Pressure to Change Hand Preference and Age

Age	Pressure	No Pressure	N
<41	121	238	359
>41	97	140	237
	218	378	596

Note: Chi-square = 2.96; $p <.085$

3.2.4 Subgroups of Lefthanders

When considering performance, lefthanders who write with the left and throw with the right were considered a subgroup, and in this section, some of the preference patterns of this subgroup are contrasted with those of lefthanders who write and throw with the left.

In previous work (Peters, 1990b) with smaller samples of lefthanders, it was found that lefthanders who throw with the right also have physical asymmetries favoring the right. In this sample, individuals were asked about ring finger size (Table 5.6), arm strength (Table 5.7), and leg strength (Table 5.8). It can be seen that the majority of lefthanders who throw with the right state that they have a larger right ring finger, while the left ring finger is stated to be larger for lefthanded throwers.

Table 5.6 Ring Finger Size

Hand	Left Larger	Right Larger	Equal	Can't Tell	N
Left	179	95	7	57	338
Right	43	74	32	25	174
	222	169	39	82	512

Note: Chi-square (df 3) = 27.1; $p < .00001$

As in previous work, the majority of lefthanded throwers was found to be stronger in the left arm, while for the righthanded throwers the opposite holds. Also, in the case of the righthanded throwers a relatively larger proportion (16.4%) indicate equal arm strength while the comparable proportion for lefthanded throwers is 5.9%. It can be seen that individuals do not always prefer the stronger limb for throwing. This dissociation between strength and skill is especially marked for righthanded throwers.

Table 5.7 Arm Strength

Arm	Left Stronger	Right Stronger	Equal	Can't Tell	N
Left	350	29	26	30	435
Right	49	80	30	23	182
	399	109	56	53	617

Note: Chi-square (df 3) = 178.4; $p < .00001$

In the case of the legs, there is a similar dissociation between strength and skill, at least for some activities (Tables 5.8 and 5.9). For instance, righthanders prefer the right leg for kicking but the left leg is often preferred as the support leg and the leg that is used for pushing off, (e.g., in the high jump, Peters, 1988). Annett and Turner (1974) have noted that lefthanders with strong left hand preferences prefer the left leg for kicking and preferences for smaller samples of lefthanders (Peters, 1988) suggest that kicking preference follows throwing preference in lefthanders. This is confirmed by the data in Table 5.9. It can be seen that the asymmetries in terms of kicking preference are more clearly expressed than the asymmetries in leg strength; individuals who throw with the right do not necessarily have a stronger right leg but they do prefer the right leg for kicking.

Table 5.8 Leg Strength

Leg	Left Stronger	Right Stronger	Equal	Can't Tell	N
Left	229	52	64	88	433
Right	43	51	40	50	184
	272	103	104	138	617

Note: Chi-square (df 3) = 51.0; $p < .00001$

Table 5.9 Kicking Preference

Leg	AL	ML	ES	MR	AR	N
Left	285	35	32	22	44	418
Right	19	14	22	50	71	176
	304	49	54	72	115	594

Note: Chi-square (df 4) = 194.5; $p < .00001$; AL = always left; ML = mainly left; ES = either side; MR = mainly right; AR = always right

A different test of leg preference is provided by examining which leg swings over when mounting a bicycle. Righthanders prefer to stand on the left and swing over with the right foot, regardless of whether they mount a bicycle or a horse. Table 5.10 shows that in this case lefthanders behave more like righthanders in that the majority of ILs and CLs prefer the right leg to mount. However, it is quite clear that the difference between those who prefer the right and the left leg is quite small for CLs, while the very clear majority of ILs prefer the right leg.

Table 5.10 Leg Used to Mount Bike

Leg	AL	ML	ES	MR	AR	N
Left	123	21	49	77	144	414
Right	25	8	22	40	82	177
	148	29	71	117	226	591

Note: Chi-square (df 4) = 17.5; $p < .002$

In the following tables, the preference patterns for a variety of manual activities are described, and it can be shown that the differences between the CLs and the ILs depend on whether the activity involves fine manual movements, arm movements involving strength, or movements that fall into an intermediate group. We begin with an activity that requires precision of visually guided placement and fine force adjustment in the hand: use of a pair of tweezers.

Both left and right throwing lefthanders show a clear preference for using tweezers in the left hand (Table 5.11). However, the right throwing lefthanders show a greater number of individuals who do not opt for the "left only" choice. In Table 5.12, the distribution for "holding toothbrush" is shown. This is a fine manipulative movement, done by a single hand. Here, the largest component of fine adjustment is accomplished by wrist movements. It can be seen that there is a very similar pattern to that seen in the use of tweezers.

Table 5.11 Using Tweezers

Hand	AL	ML	ES	MR	AR	N
Left	369	37	15	6	4	431
Right	105	21	34	13	8	181
	474	58	49	19	12	612

Note: Chi-square (df 4) = 72.7; $p < .00001$

Table 5.12 Brushing Teeth

Hand	AL	ML	ES	MR	AR	N
Left	380	16	27	3	13	439
Right	128	13	18	9	14	182
	508	29	45	12	27	621

Note: Chi-square (df 4) = 72.7; $p < .00001$

There follow two activities that still yield a clear left hand preference for both groups, but slightly less so than the previous tasks for the ILs. In the case of sewing, a substantial minority of ILs choose "either hand" or even the right hand as preference choices (Table 5.13).

This is even more pronounced in the case of cutting bread, where there is a hint of a bimodal distribution, still favoring the left, but with a relatively larger number of ILs choosing the right hand (Table 5.14). In this case it has to be noted that the scalloping of bread knife edges favors the righthander if there is a laterality to the edge. This will play a role in the preference patterns.

When hammering is considered (Table 5.15), the number of IL individuals who opt for "left only" decreases notably, with the majority indicating that they can use either

Table 5.13 Hand Holding Needle When Sewing

Hand	AL	ML	ES	MR	AR	N
Left	375	15	11	0	6	407
Right	94	21	24	8	22	169
	469	36	35	8	28	576

Note: Chi-square (df 4) = 112.1; $p < .00001$

Table 5.14 Hand Holding Knife While Cutting Bread

Hand	AL	ML	ES	MR	AR	N
Left	385	16	19	7	11	438
Right	94	14	18	21	34	181
	479	30	37	28	45	619

Note: Chi-square (df 4) = 107.5; $p < .00001$

Table 5.15 Hand Holding a Hammer

Hand	AL	ML	ES	MR	AR	N
Left	374	43	17	1	2	437
Right	46	30	49	23	28	176
	420	73	66	24	30	613

Note: Chi-square (df 4) = 251.1; $p < .00001$

hand. Here, it is likely that some balance between the strength and the fine manual skill element of the task is reached.

The shift towards right hand preference is carried even further when the hand preference for a tennis racquet is considered. Now, a clear majority of ILs prefer the right hand. An appreciable number expresses a preference for the left hand, and 20% indicate that they can use either hand. This last figure contrasts with 5% for CLs (Table 5.16).

Table 5.16 Hand Holding Tennis Racquet

Hand	AL	ML	ES	MR	AR	N
Left	348	21	18	2	9	398
Right	44	8	33	19	61	165
	392	29	51	21	70	563

Note: Chi-square (df 4) = 243.7; $p < .00001$

When whole arm movement is used, as in the swinging of a golf club (Table 5.17), ILs show a very clear preference for the right side. Perhaps not unexpectedly, the figures on golfing show a relatively small proportion of individuals reporting "either" hand. When the design of the tool dictates handedness, as is the case with golf clubs, less flexibility can be expected because the individual has to specialize. Indeed, there is a legitimate question as to whether individuals indicating an "either hand" choice would be equally skilled with either hand combination. In addition, there is a rather large proportion of CLs who prefer to play golf righthanded. This proportion is larger than

Table 5.17 Righthanded or Lefthanded Golf

Golf	AL	ML	ES	MR	AR	N
Left	166	8	12	7	91	284
Right	25	2	6	10	86	129
	191	10	18	17	177	413

Note: Chi-square (df 4) = 60.7; $p < .00001$

the proportion indicating a stronger right arm and it can be speculated that the availability of left-handed golf clubs is a factor.

In the case of batting with a baseball bat, there is considerably more flexibility, because the tool itself is directionally neutral. In addition, there is a advantage in being able to bat from either side. However, it is rare that individuals hit equally well from either side. As in the case of golf, a clear majority of ILs prefer the right, and a clear majority of the CLs prefer the left. In baseball, there are some advantages for lefthanded batters because they are, potentially, a step closer to first base.

Table 5.18 Righthanded or Lefthanded Baseball Batting

Batting	AL	ML	ES	MR	AR	N
Left	266	13	36	16	73	404
Right	23	2	32	22	99	178
	289	15	68	38	172	582

Note: Chi-square (df 4) = 152.8; $p < .00001$

3.3 SUMMARY

3.3.1 Subgroups and the Manufacture of Tools

The survey reveals that there is very significant variation in the hand preference patterns of lefthanders. Academic research on handedness tends to emphasize that lefthanders are more variable than righthanders whenever comparisons are made (e.g., Bryden, 1982). However, it is shown here that part of that variability is due to subgroups with significantly different preference patterns. The simplest way of subgrouping seems to be along the lines of throwing preference. Lefthanded writers who throw with the left hand (CL) seem to be quite consistent in preference patterns that tend to favor the left hand. Lefthanded writers who favor the right hand for throwing (IL) show more complex preference patterns. They favor the left hand for fine manual activities, and the right hand for strength and ballistic activities. Tasks that require a combination of manual skill and strength, such as hammering, yield intermediate preference patterns for ILs. In some cases, it is difficult to determine exactly what the preference patterns are. For instance, in the case of golf, preference may be influenced by availability of lefthanded clubs. Nevertheless, it is clear that ILs very clearly prefer righthanded golf, and must do so because of preference rather than availability factors because CLs clearly prefer the left hand.

3.3.2 Tools for Fine Manual Activities

The data provided here show that in designing tools that require fine manual skills, the proportion of the population that would use lefthanded implements closely approximates the proportion that prefers the left hand for writing. For instance, some 86% of lefthanded writers prefer to "mostly" or "always" use the left hand when picking up objects with tweezers and would, by implication, prefer the left hand for fine surgical or mechanical instruments that have a handedness element.

3.3.3 Sports Equipment and Heavy Tools

In contrast, only 48% of lefthanded writers "mostly" or "always" prefer lefthanded golf clubs. As has been pointed out, this figure is somewhat influenced by availability of lefthanded equipment early in life but it is also clear that a manufacturer would do well to produce a proportion of lefthanded equipment that would be significantly below the proportion for lefthanded writers. This applies generally where ballistic movements and arm strength matter; a significant proportion of lefthanders (Table 5.7) was shown to have a stronger right arm.

3.3.4 Adaptation

While 54.9% of lefthanders indicated that they had difficulties with specific righthanded implements, it would be wrong to conclude that the remaining 45.1% experience no such difficulties. Instead, it is appropriate to assume that lefthanders simply learn to live with righthanded implements because there is no choice. For example, in schools and universities, the writing platform is often attached to the chair on which the student sits. If the writing platform is on the right, lefthanders are not able to write without significant rotation of the torso. In addition, they will have difficulties finding support for the writing arm. This is not an insignificant problem when students are required to write for an hour or more. Very few classrooms have sufficient numbers of lefthanded desks. If classrooms have any lefthanded desks at all, their number is not determined by the expected proportion of lefthanded writers but by the number of seats that delimit the left side of a row of chairs. This number can only be sufficient if the number of chairs on the left edge of a row approximates 10% of the total number of chairs. With fixed seating, this ratio can rarely be achieved unless rows of chairs are more commonly interrupted by aisles than they normally are. The case of writing posture is also a good support for the claim that the absence of complaints often indicates resignation and adaptation rather than successful adjustment: all lefthanded writers are seriously hampered by righthanded writing desks but few complaints were expressed in this survey (only five individuals).

3.3.5 Bimanual Coordination

Most skilled activities require the collaboration of the two hands. In cases where simple tools are used, such as hammering in a nail, handedness is of little consequence because there is no inherent lateral bias. However, in the case of more complex machines, vehicles, and musical instruments, it is usually not possible to accommodate both righthanders and lefthanders. For instance, keyboard instruments are designed for the use of righthanders, and the music is composed to meet the preferred hand roles of the righthander. Similarly, the foot pedals of a car are laid out for rightfooted preference (Peters, 1988) regardless of whether the steering wheel is on the left or the right side of the car. In these cases and in the case of very complex operating controls, such as those found in airplanes, no adjustment is possible for lefthanders, because the layout of the controls does not permit choices in hand use. Righthanders have fixed preferences in terms of assigning hand roles in bimanual collaborative actions and arrangements of controls which do not adhere to these preferences lead to inferior performance (Peters, 1985). Because bimanual controls do not favor lefthanders, there is some question as to whether this creates difficulties. Preliminary data indicate that fortunately, lefthanders appear to be somewhat more flexible than righthanders in assigning hand roles to the two hands (Peters, 1987). However, it remains to be seen whether this statement can be generalized to the operation of controls. Ideally, experiments in which the two hands are required to perform concurrent activities that differ from each other (e.g., Korteling, 1993), and especially if principles of man/machine interactions are modeled (Andre and Wickens,

1992), should investigate the effect of varying hand roles assignments across the preferred and nonpreferred hand.

3.3.6 Situations Where Handedness Becomes Important Because of Interactions Between Individuals

So far, handedness was only considered relative to individual activities. However, there are many situations where individuals collaborate and where differing handedness presents a problem. For instance, in infantry formations of antiquity, the shield was held with the left hand and the sword with the right. Uniform hand use ensured overlapping protection and it would not have been possible for an individual to adopt opposite hand roles in the line-up. This still applies in army drills today. Another example would be the teaching of fine manual skills in music and crafts. Here, the righthanded instructor will be challenged in dealing with a lefthanded student. This is no different for the palaeolithic teacher of stone axe manufacture than for the contemporary righthanded parent who wishes to teach a lefthanded child how to tie shoelaces.

Previous discussions of handedness tend to emphasize the element of social deviance in accounting for pressures against lefthandedness, and religious strictures are invoked. However, in a species in which the manufacture and use of artifacts is a defining characteristic and where interactions often presuppose similar hand preferences, there are powerful pragmatic reasons for favoring a uniform hand preference. It may well be that religious invocations against left hand use serve a practical reason, even though they tend to generalize negative attitudes to situations where lefthandedness causes no problems.

3.3.7 Accidents

When lefthanders indicate that they have difficulties with certain implements and tools, the degree to which these difficulties can result in a hazard varies. For instance, a wristwatch designed for righthanders is a nuisance for a lefthander but when a lefthander complains about a circular saw, this complaint refers to a situation in which the lefthander is at risk of injury. This is the case for numerous tools and industrial work station arrangements. Notwithstanding the negative reports by Dellatolas et al. (1993) and Porac (1993) we do take note that under some circumstances, lefthanders who have to live in a world designed by righthanders face concrete danger which does result in disproportionate fatalities (Aggleton, Kentridge, and Neave, 1993).

4. CONCLUSION

This chapter looked at some isolated performance and preference aspects in lefthanders. In the case of performances, reference had to be made to righthanders, in order to have some yardstick by which to measure the behavior of lefthanders. Using this yardstick, we note that for this population of healthy university students there is remarkably little evidence of any major difference between the two groups in terms of overall performance levels. Preferred hand performance levels on a number of selected motor tasks are strictly comparable for lefthanders and righthanders. In terms of nonpreferred hand performance, a meaningful subgrouping of lefthanders could be made: consistent lefthanders behaved much like a mirror image of righthanders while inconsistent lefthanders showed superior nonpreferred hand performance. Indeed, considering that preferred hand performance of the inconsistent lefthanders was on par with that of the other groups, one could say that when both hands are considered, the inconsistent lefthanders perform in a superior way overall. Having said this, there were some indications that when more subtle indicators of performance are looked at, such as in the coordination of bimanual tapping (Treffner and Turvey, 1995) and in the regularity of intertap intervals (which is a measure of very fine distal motor control), there is some indication that lefthanders (both groups) shows different characteristics than righthanders. Ultimately, this might be due to the more flexible and therefore slightly more cumbersome interhemispheric arrangements in lefthanders which might also be involved in the one instance of nonmanual performance differences cited. In that case, both groups of lefthanders show slower reaction times than righthanders in making decisions about coordinate and categorical characteristics of spatial stimuli than righthanders. Of greatest interest in this particular finding is the fact that consistent lefthanders and righthanders form extremes on the performance spectrum, with inconsistent lefthanders being intermediate in their performance. This suggests to us that the distinction between consistent and inconsistent lefthanders is not merely a matter of manual motor control and reaches deeper into interhemispheric communication arrangements. As always in the case of claims in lateralization research, it goes without saying that independent replication of this finding is needed before further speculations are offered.

The preference profiles underline the distinction between subgroups of lefthanders. It is clear that there is considerable variability between lefthanded individuals but even within this variability the usefulness of a distinction between consistent and inconsistent lefthanders emerges. On an applied level, the preference frequencies across lefthanded subgroups allow some estimates as to what proportion of tools, instruments, or procedures have to take into account the preferences of lefthanders, if options for accommodation are available. On a theoretical level, the preference frequencies spell trouble because they indicate that a huge range of idiosyncratic preference patterns can be encountered. Here, a convergence emerges between performance and preference data interpretation: is it the predominance of inherent biases interacting with environmental chance events or is it the predominant environmental influence interacting with weak inherent biases which determines the final pattern of behavior?

ACKNOWLEDGMENT

This work was supported by the Natural Sciences and Engineering Research Council of Canada, Grant No. A 7054.

REFERENCES

Aggleton, J. P., Kentridge, R. W., and Neave, N. J. (1993). *Longevity and Handedness: a Comparison of the Life-Spans of Left and Right-Handed Cricketers*. Paper presented at the meeting of the Experimental Psychology Society, London.

Andre, A. D. and Wickens, C. D. (1992). Compatibility and consistency in display-control systems: implications for aircraft decision aid design. *Hum. Fact.*, 34, 639.

Annett, M. (1985). *Left, Right, Hand and Brain: the Right Shift Theory*. Hillsdale, N. J., Erlbaum.

Annett, M. and Manning, M. (1989). The disadvantages of dextrality for intelligence. *Br. J. Psychol.*, 80, 213.

Annett, M. and Turner, A. (1974). Laterality and the growth of intellectual abilities. *Br. J. Educ. Psychol.*, 44, 37.

Bakan, P., Dibb, G., and Reed, P. (1973). Handedness and birth stress. *Neuropsychologia*, 11, 363.

Bishop, D. V. M. (1990). *Handedness and Developmental Disorder*. Hove, U.K., Lawrence Erlbaum.

Bishop, D. V. M. (1984). Using nonpreferred hand skill to investigate pathological left-handedness in an unselected population. *Dev. Med. Child Neurol.*, 26, 214.

Blau, A. (1946). *The Master Hand*. New York: American Orthopsychiatric Association.

Bragina, N. N. and Dobrochtowa, A. T. (1984). *Funktionelle Asymmetrie des Menschen*. Leipzig, Georg Thieme.

Bryden, M. P. (1982). *Laterality*. New York, Academic Press.

Clark, M. M. (1957). *Left-handedness*. London, University of London Press.

Cohen, J. (1969). *Statistical Power Analysis for the Behavioral Sciences*. New York, Academic Press.

Coren, S. (1989). Left-handedness and accident-related injury risk. *Am. J. Pub. Health*, 79, 1.

Coren, S. (1990). *The Left-Hander Syndrome: The Causes and Consequences of Left-Handedness*. New York, Free Press.

Coren, S. and Halpern, D. F. (1991). Left-handedness: a marker for decreased survival fitness? *Psychol. Bull.*, 109, 90.

Dellatolas, G., Moreau, T., Jallon, P., and Lelouch, J. (1993). Upper limb injuries and handedness plasticity. *Br. J. Psychol.*, 84, 201.

Faglioni, P. and Basso, A. (1984). Historical perspectives on neuroanatomical correlates. In E. Roy (Ed.), *Neuropsychological Studies of Apraxia and Related Disorders*, Amsterdam, North-Holland, 3.

Gilbert, A. N. and Wisocki, C. J. (1992). Hand preference and age in the United States. *Neuropsychologia*, 30, 601.

Garonzik, R. (1989). Hand dominance and implications for left-handed operation of controls. *Ergonomics*, 32, 1185.

Gur, R. (1984). Hemispheric control of the writing hand: The effect of callosotomy in a left-hander, *Neurology*, 34, 904.

Harris, L. H. (1993). Do left-handers die sooner than right-handers? Commentary on Coren and Halpern's (1991) "left-handedness: a marker for decreased survival fitness." *Psychol. Bull.*, 114, 203.

Hiscock, M., Hiscock, M., Benjamins, D., and Hillman, S. (1989). Motor asymmetries in hemiplegic children: Implications for the normal and pathological development of handedness. *Dev. Neuropsychol.*, 5, 169.

Kang, Y. and Harris, L. (1993, May). *Social-Cultural Influences on Handedness: a Cross-Cultural Study of Koreans and Americans*. Paper presented at the TENNET (Theoretical and Experimental Neuropsychology) meeting, Montreal, Quebec, Canada.

Kimura, D. (1993). *Neuromotor Mechanisms in Human Communication*. Oxford, Oxford University Press.

Korteling, J. E. (1993). Effects of age and task similarity on dual-task performance. *Hum. Fact.*, 35, 99.

Laeng, B. and Peters, M. (1995). Cerebral lateralization for the processing of spatial coordinates and categories in left-and right-handers. *Neuropsychologia*, 33, 421.

Levander, M. and Schalling, D. (1988). Hand preference in a population of Swedish college students. *Cortex*, 24, 149.

Levander, M., Levander, S. E., and Schalling, D. (1989). Hand preference and sex as determinants of neuropsychological skill, solving strategy and side preference. *Intelligence*, 13, 93.

Levy, J. and Reid, M. (1978). Variations in cerebral organization as a function of handedness, hand posture in writing, and sex. *J. Exp. Psychol.: Gen.*, 107, 109.

Levy, J. (1984). A review, analysis, and some new data on hand posture distribution in left-handers. *Brain Cognit.*, 3, 105.

Murphy, K. and Peters, M. (1994). Right-handers and left-handers show differences and important similarities in task integration when performing manual and vocal tasks concurrently. *Neuropsychologia*, 32, 663.

McManus, I. C. (1991). The inheritance of left-handedness. In J. Marsh (Ed.) *Biological Asymmetry and Handedness (CIBA Symposium 162)*, London, Wiley, 251.

Meulenbroek, R. G. J. and Van Galen, G. P. (1989). Variations in cursive handwriting performance as a function of handedness, hand posture and gender. *J. Hum. Move. Stud.*, 16, 239.

Oldfield, R. C. (1969). Handedness in musicians. *Br. J. Psychol.*, 60, 91.

Peters, M. (1990a). Phenotype in Normal Lefthanders: An understanding of phenotype is the basis for understanding mechanism and inheritance of handedness. In S. Coren (Ed.), *Left-Handedness: Behavioral Implications and Anomalies, Advances in Psychology Series*, Amsterdam, Elsevier, 167.

Peters, M. (1990b). Subclassification of lefthanders poses problems for theories of handedness. *Neuropsychologia*, 28, 279.

Peters, M. (1988). Footedness: Asymmetries in foot preference and skill and neuropsychological assessment of foot movement. *Psychol. Bull.*, 103, 179.

Peters, M. (1987). A nontrivial motor performance difference between right-handers and left-handers: Attention as intervening variable in the expression of handedness. *Can. J. Psychol.*, 41, 91.

Peters, M. (1986). Incidence of lefthanded writers and the inverted writing position in a sample of 2194 German elementary school children. *Neuropsychologia*, 24, 429.

Peters, M. (1985). Constraints in the coordination of bimanual movements and their expression in skilled and unskilled subjects. *Q. J. Exp. Psychol.*. 37A, 171.

Peters, M. (1983). Inverted and noninverted lefthanders compared on the basis of motor performance and measures related to the act of writing. *Aust. J. Psychol.*, 35, 405.

Peters, M. and Durding, B. (1979). Left-handers and right-handers compared on a motor task. *J. Motor Behav.*, 11, 103.

Peters, M. and Murphy, K. (1992). Cluster analysis reveals at least three, and possibly five distinct handedness groups. *Neuropsychologia*, 30, 373.

Peters, M. and Pang, J. (1992), Do "right-armed" lefthanders have different lateralization of motor control for the proximal and distal musculature? *Cortex*, 22, 391.

Peters, M. and Servos, P. (1989). Performance of subgroups of lefthanders, and righthanders. *Can. J. Psychol.*, 43, 341.

Porac, C. (1993). Hand preference and the incidence of accidental unilateral hand injury. *Neuropsychologia*, 31, 355.

Tapley, S. M. and Bryden, M. P. (1985). A group test for the assessment of performance between the hands. *Neuropsychologia*, 23, 215.

Treffner, P. J. and Turvey, M. T. (1995). Handedness and the asymmetric dynamics of bimanual rhythmic coordination. *J. Exp. Psychol.: Hum. Percept. Perform.*

White, L. E., Lucas, G., Richards, A., and Purves, D. (1994). Cerebral asymmetry and handedness, *Nature*, 368, 197.

Weber, A. M. and Bradshaw, J. L. (1981). Levy and Reid's neuropsychological model in relation to writing hand posture: an evaluation. *Psychol. Bull.*, 90, 74.

Section III

Manual Performance Asymmetries

Chapter 6

Hand Preference and Performance in Skilled and Unskilled Activities

Runa E. Steenhuis

Contents

1. INTRODUCTION

The notion that manual skill is an important factor accounting for and even driving manual preference is not new. Bradshaw and Rogers (1993) state "Humans typically show a right-hand superiority in tasks which entail high accuracy demands with fine corrective movements, frequently, but perhaps not necessarily, under visual control" (p. 197). Many investigators concerned with handedness assume that the preferred hand is more skilled than the nonpreferred hand. According to Ward, Milliken, and Stafford (1993), for example, "There is broadly held an implicit assumption that the right population bias in human handedness arises from the greater inherent capacity of the right hand for fine manipulation, particularly of tools and weapons" (p. 65). Others examine the skill differences in relation to hand preference (e.g., Annett, 1985; Flowers, 1975; Peters and Servos, 1989; Todor and Cisneros, 1985; Vasconcelos, 1993).

My interest in the relation between preference and skill comes from principal components analyses of hand preference questionnaires where the data suggested that in both right- and left-handers, skill may be an important dimension differentiating activities for

0-8493-8999-2/96/$0.00+$.50

which people report strong preferences from those for which they report weak preferences (Steenhuis and Bryden, 1987, 1988, 1989; Steenhuis, Bryden, Schwartz, and Lawson, 1990).

This chapter first reviews data examining the relation between manual skill and manual preference. There is incidental historical data (primarily, from artifacts including tools and artwork) used to infer handedness. In some instances, these data suggest that skill relates to hand preference. In addition, a number of early investigators who recorded hand preferences and examined the capability of the hands to perform a variety of manual tasks speculated that skill was a meaningful dimension. Skill has also been identified as important in eliciting manual preferences in primates. Next, the chapter considers definitions of manual skill and how those definitions might relate to the literature concerning manual performance and preference. Finally, the results of a project examining how several performance tasks relate to hand preference factors representing skilled and less skilled activities is presented.

2. BACKGROUND

2.1 HISTORICAL DATA IN HUMANS

Information allowing inferences about handedness in early humans comes from anthropological artifacts (e.g., tools, artwork, skulls, and teeth). A number of investigators have linked the emergence of hand preferences to tool use (see Bradshaw and Rogers, 1993 and Chapter 2 for a review). According to Bradshaw and Rogers, controversy surrounds analyses of early art which tried to infer hand preference from the direction figures faced or from which hand was shown in outline. Nevertheless, there is ample evidence of manual preferences from art depicting persons engaged in activities involving hand use. For instance, the work of Coren and Porac (1977) recorded right-handedness of 93% over a large number of early works of art. Spennemann (1984) differentiated skilled (e.g., writing and using tools) and unskilled (e.g., holding an object) activities from scenes of daily life drawn over 1000 years ago in Java. There was about 9% left-handedness for skilled unimanual activities and 38% for unskilled actions. Incidental evidence about handedness also comes from written material. Fabbro (1994) documented more biblical references to right than left which he felt reflected, in part, an association of the right hand with superior strength and precision.

Many early investigators considered skill important in handedness. For some it manifests in investigations of the differences in skill between the preferred and nonpreferred hands. Woodworth (1899), for instance, summarized the abilities of the right and left hands (presumably, in right handers) in the following way: (1) the right hand could be controlled more quickly but the left hand could make movements with the same accuracy slowly; (2) the right hand made more uniform movements; and (3) the right hand was better than the left when vision was absent. Durost (1934) observed that handedness became more pronounced as the tests involved finer and finer coordinations. For example, he viewed the differences in capability between the hands as trivial for grip strength but speculated that a task like throwing a ball at a target required such skill and precision that it would be unusual to find a person who could do it equally well with both hands. Some considered skill as they examined the relation between manual preference and performance. For example, Koch (1933) stated that "strength of preference may be conceived more broadly as the expression of many influences, relative skill being only one, though probably the major class" (p. 140–141). Blau (1946) considered laterality as the tendency to use one hand for skilled unimanual acts.

2.2 NONHUMAN PRIMATE STUDIES

Examining hand preferences in nonhuman primates has been as controversial as the human equivalent. A number of variables have been raised as affecting outcome. According to Harris (1993), the level of task difficulty, the amount of manipulation required, distance to the object, possibility of shifting posture, and the location of the object in space may account for differences in findings. Bradshaw and Rogers (1993), in their review of the primate literature, concluded that a failure to demonstrate lateral preferences sometimes related to the choice of task. They blame a focus "on simple rather than the probably more lateralized complex tasks, on spontaneous and unskilled rather than induced or skilled responses" (p. 196) for the negative results of some studies. In his review of the literature, however, Lehman (1993) reported mixed results for task complexity as a variable in demonstrating hand preferences in primates. Despite these difficulties, the consensus appears to be that hand preferences exist at the individual level (for reviews see Bradshaw and Rogers, 1993; Lehman, 1993; and Chapter 2) in many primates.

A number of authors have suggested that the type of activity most likely to demonstrate preferences (usually, at the individual level) are those involving the manipulation of objects or tools (e.g., Marchant and McGrew, 1994; Shafer, 1993). In their examination of gorillas, Shafer reported that the only type of activity lateralized in all animals involved manipulating small objects. Marchant and McGrew observed wild chimpanzees in a natural setting and reported no laterality for activities such as eating or grooming but using a tool to fish for termites showed moderate specialization. Others have also reported that some tasks show preferences but others do not. Byrne and Byrne (1991) recorded manual activities in 44 mountain gorillas. Although there was no population hand preference, there were individual preferences for several multistep feeding tasks. In contrast, preferences were not established for picking a variety of leaves and vines. In sum, though more work is necessary to finally resolve the issue, it is not possible to ignore the level of skill required to execute a task as a possible factor in eliciting manual preferences in primates.

2.3 RECENT STUDIES IN HUMANS

2.3.1 Hand Preference is Multidimensional

There have been a number of reports of hand preference as multidimensional. Two main proposals regarding these dimensions are those of Healey and her colleagues (Healey, Liederman, and Geschwind, 1986; Liederman and Healey, 1986) and Steenhuis and Bryden (Steenhuis and Bryden, 1987, 1988, 1989; Steenhuis et al., 1990). Healey et al. proposed that the main dimensions were related to the musculature used in executing movements. Preferences for movements involving proximal (shoulder and arm) muscles differed from preferences for movements of the distal (hand and fingers) muscles. A distinction between movements of the proximal and distal musculature makes sense from a neuroanatomical point of view, with separate innervation serving them (see Lawrence and Kuypers, 1968a, 1968b). Nevertheless, Steenhuis and colleagues found no evidence of factors related to distal and proximal musculature in their analyses of the Waterloo Handedness Questionnaire (WHQ). In their 1989 work, they specifically included items expected to distinguish a proximal (for example, the shoulder used to open a swinging door or the hand used to throw a basketball) from a distal dimension (for example, hand used for writing or to snap your fingers), but failed to show that distinction. Rather, hand preference items differed primarily in the level of skill required to execute the movement. Both the skill-related factors and items loading on them showed good reliability (Steenhuis et al., 1990) and have been demonstrated in diverse samples. Table 6.1 shows the results of principal components analyses in several adult samples (Obrzut, Dalby, Boliek, and Cannon, 1992; Steenhuis and Bryden, 1989) and one in children (Bryden, MacRae, and Steenhuis, 1991) in North America. It also shows the results from a sample obtained in India (Singh and Bryden, 1994). Though the actual items varied somewhat on different versions of the questionnaire, the basic results remained the same. The level of skill differentiated the items loading on the two factors first reported by Steenhuis and Bryden (1989). It should be noted that Obrzut and colleagues (1992) found a different factor structure in a group of learning disabled students at the same time as replicating Steenhuis and Bryden's findings in their control sample.

Table 6.1 Examples of Factor Loadings of Items Characterized as Relating to Skilled and Unskilled Activities

	Sample 1[1]	Sample 2[2]	Sample 3[3]	Sample 4[4]
		Skilled activities		
Writing	.88	.88	.89	.81
Toothbrush	.85	.84	.74	.67
Erase	.72	.85	.84	—
Throw ball	.87	.66	.71	.72
Sew	.82	.72	.72	—
Hammer	—	—	—	.78
		Less skilled activities		
Pick up small object	.70	—	.68	.78
Pick up paper	—	.64	.66	—
Pick up penny	.68	.60	.61	—
Pick up ball	.65	.62	.61	—
Pet dog or cat	.61	.63	.59	—
Carry a suitcase/briefcase	*	*	.54	.68

[1] Steenhuis and Bryden (1989) — sample 2.
[2] Obrzut et al. (1992) — control subjects.
[3] Bryden, MacRae, and Steenhuis (1991).
[4] Singh and Bryden (1994) — sample 1.
* In these samples similar items loaded onto a separate factor.

Early work supporting the presence of a single hand preference factor used questionnaire items mainly from the skill factor (McFarland and Anderson, 1980; Porac, Coren, Steiger, and Duncan, 1980; Roszkowski, Snelbecker, and Sacks, 1981) or recommended retaining only "Factor 1" items to achieve homogeneity and a single hand preference factor (Bryden, 1977).

Peters and Servos (1989) criticized the principal components approach, stating that the findings are a consequence of variability in the left handers alone, especially those left-handers with preference for the right-hand for some actions (their "inconsistent left-handers"). This criticism may well apply to the work of Healey and Liederman (1986), who selected a high proportion of non-right handers (38%). However, Steenhuis and colleagues used representative samples. Thus, left-handers comprised only a small proportion (10 to 12%) of the entire sample.

The most convincing evidence of the two factors, however, comes from the data itself. Figures 6.1 and 6.2 show the same basic pattern of results in both right- and left-handers. That is, for Factor 1 items, both handedness groups express strong preferences. Most responses fall in the "Always use" category. For left-handers, some always use their right hand. For Factor 2 items, both right- and left-handers shift toward reporting less strong preferences with increases in the "Usually Use" and "Either" categories.

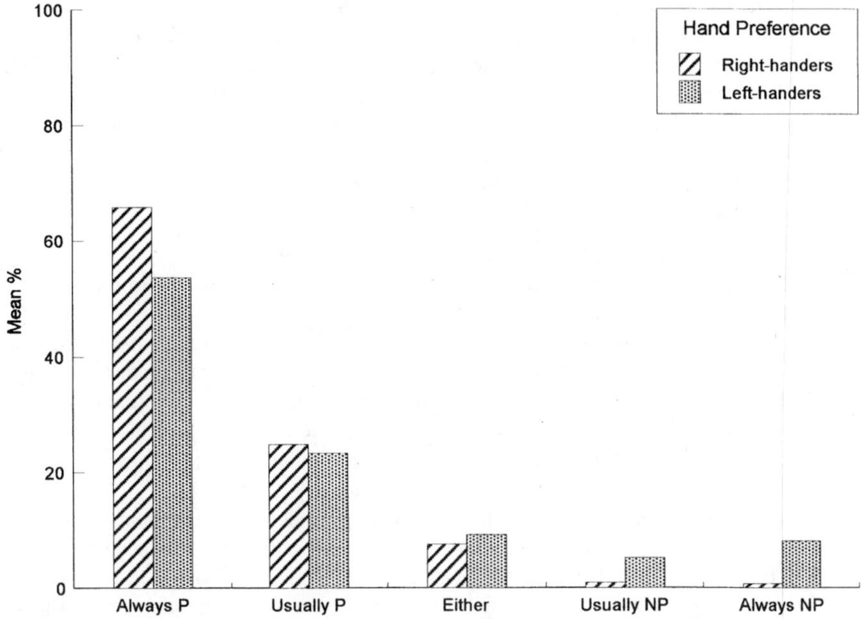

Figure 6.1 Mean percentage of persons reporting hand use (Always, Usually, and Either) in right- and left-handers for Factor 1. These data were adapted from Steenhuis and Bryden (1989).

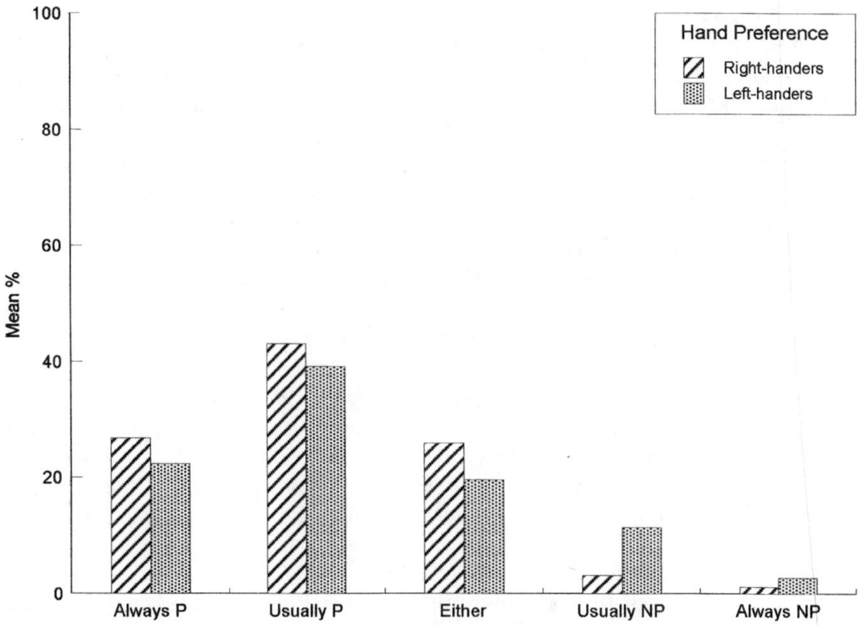

Figure 6.2 Mean percentage of persons reporting hand use (Always, Usually, and Either) in right- and left-handers for Factor 2. These data were adapted from Steenhuis and Bryden (1989).

2.3.2 The Relation Between Skill and Preference

A number of investigators have examined the relation between preference as expressed by hand use or questionnaire responses compared to skill on a proficiency measure. Generally, the preferred hand is the more proficient hand. Nevertheless, there are moderating influences. First, as in the primate work, the characteristics of the performance tasks vary and may account for differences in findings (Annett, 1992; Borod, Caron, and Koff, 1984). Further, classification and subclassification of subjects influences outcome (see for example, Annett, 1985; Peters and Servos, 1989).

2.3.2.1 The Method Used to Measure Handedness

Though infrequently examined, there is good correspondence between hand preference reported on questionnaires and observed hand use (Dean, 1978; Raczkowski, Kalat, and Nebes, 1974; Sherman, Kulhavy, and Bretzing, 1976). Raczkowski et al. observed hand use in 47 college students (selected to include a large number of left-handers) 1 month after they filled out a preference questionnaire. They found high concordances, better than 90% for most items. Items with a high concordance are those typical of Steenhuis and Bryden's skilled factor. There was a lower concordance for items involving less skilled activities.

The relation between hand preference and hand proficiency is less clear. Some data suggest that the distributions of hand preference and hand performance differ. For instance, Borod et al. (1984) collected data on preference and performance in right- and left-handers. They reported that the distribution of scores for preference was J-shaped while performance was normally distributed. On the other hand, Provins, Milner, and Kerr (1982) showed that responses on a 75-item preference questionnaire showed a less skewed distribution than typically found with preference questionnaires. At the same time in that study, a performance measure involving handwriting showed a bimodal distribution of difference scores. Tan (1993) described a 32-item version of the Waterloo Hand Preference Questionnaire as normally distributed. Annett (1992) examined "five tests of manual skill"; several had a bimodal distribution (filling in dots and punching holes) while moving pegs and marking squares were unimodal. Thus, it is possible to demonstrate both bimodal and unimodal distributions of responses for both preference and performance data. Tasks and measures producing bimodal or J-shaped distributions provide clear support for distinct handedness groups (e.g., left-handers and right-handers) whereas those producing unimodal distributions suggest that a continuum or perhaps, a series of groups (e.g., strong, weak, and mixed) might best describe handedness.

As just indicated, some performance tasks show large differences between the hands and some do not. For example, Provins and Magliaro (1989) found, as they expected, a greater discrepancy in proficiency for handwriting than for grip strength. Further, the difference between the hands for handwriting speed is highly reliable whereas grip strength is not (Provins and Cunliffe, 1972). Grip strength has been consistently reported as weakly lateralized (Borod et al., 1984; Provins et al., 1982; Steenhuis and Bryden, in preparation). Often in left-handers, group data imply that the two hands have equal strength. Peters (1990a, 1990b) contends that the substantial number of left-handers who have a stronger right hand account for this finding (also supported by Steenhuis and Bryden, in preparation). Annett (1992) suggests that factors, such as practice (using a pen is highly practiced) or the need to hit a target (as in punching holes) might influence the size of performance differences between the hands.

Intuitively, grip strength represents a different aspect of manual behavior compared to tasks requiring the precise, speeded manipulation of a pen or pencil. Performance data do not correlate highly (Borod et al., 1984; Eling, 1983), supporting the notion that motor behavior is not unitary. A number of aspects of motor performance have been postulated.

On a range of hand and foot laterality tasks, Borod and colleagues identified two main factors: strength and a combination of speed/accurary. Within the motor learning domain, a number of classification systems have developed (see Magill, 1993 for a review). They include those based on the precision of the movement (e.g., fine and gross), the movement end point (e.g., discrete and continuous), and the role of environment (e.g., the need for adaptation to changing conditions and the role of feedback). Given an array of possible tasks and various dimensions of manual performance and preference, it should not be surprising that determining the relation between preference and performance has been challenging.

Additionally, whether one considers all subjects together or separate, handedness groups influences the outcome. For example, Tapley and Bryden (1985) reported a correlation of .75 between dot-filling performance and hand preference in their whole sample. Preference and performance measures correlated only modestly when handedness groups were considered separately. The correlations fell to .17 in right-handers and .20 in left-handers. For dot-filling, therefore, the large correlation in the whole group stemmed from the direction of hand preference. Similarly, Bryden, Singh, Steenhuis, and Clarkson (1994) reported moderate to good correlations between several performance measures and individual preference items in a group containing both right- and left-handers. There were modest correlations between self-professed hand preference and preferences on the two hand preference factors (skilled and less skilled) and several performance tasks in a combined group. This was also true using the absolute value of the performance differences (degree of handedness) between the preferred and nonpreferred hands. However, the pattern of correlations depended on the preference measure and separating left- and right-handers resulted in fewer significant correlations in the left-handers than the right-handers.

Rather than examine differences between the hands, Tan (1992) looked at the relation between hand preference questionnaire scores and performance of each hand in left-handers. She found that the questionnaire score related to the performance of the right hand but not the left hand, using dot-filling and peg-moving tasks. Another approach linking preference and performance has been adopted by Bryden and colleagues who developed modified peg-moving and dot-filling tasks as behavioral measures of hand preference (Bryden et al., 1994). The modification of these tasks produced a situation where subjects had the opportunity to begin the task with one hand but could switch to using the other hand if they wished. For one task, subjects filled in a long strip of dots (about 1 m in length). On a second task, they moved pegs along an elongated pegboard. In each case, the arrangement of the apparatus encouraged subjects to switch to using the other hand before they filled the entire row of dots or moved all the pegs. As they progressed, the task became increasingly difficult to complete with the hand with which they began. These tasks provided information about which hand right- and left-handers persisted in using (or "preferred" to use) on two common performance tasks. Generally, subjects persisted in using their preferred hand longer than their nonpreferred hand on both the dot-filling and peg-moving tasks. Bryden et al. showed the strongest correlations between the long form of the pegboard and the questionnaire preference score (higher than the correlations between the questionnaire score and the traditional peg-moving and dot-filling, and the modified dot-filling task).

2.3.2.2 The Classification of Handedness

How subjects are divided into handedness groups or subgroups can influence the outcome of studies looking at preference and performance. Annett and co-workers (Annett, 1976, 1985, 1992; Kilshaw and Annett, 1983) have placed subjects into different handedness categories (usually, eight classes) and then plotted their peg-moving times (a difference score in seconds between the left and right hands). A linear-looking relationship usually appears across all of the handedness classes in their mean peg-moving times. Nevertheless, if one looks at the right- and left-handers separately, a linear relationship is much less apparent. As noted above with the correlational studies, most of the linearity comes from including right- and left-handers together.

Provins and Cunliffe (1972) matched ten right-handers and ten left-handers for the degree of their preferences on a 31-item questionnaire. In this selected group, they found good agreement between reported preference and manual proficiency on a variety of tasks. While it is possible to match some left-handers to right-handers, matching excludes many left-handers who have no equivalent right-handed counterpart. Some place such left-handers into separate groups. Peters and colleagues (Peters, 1990a, 1990b; Peters and Servos, 1989) recognize a subgroup of left-handers who they have called "inconsistent." These left-handers distinguish themselves by having left hand preferences for activities involving fine dexterity and right hand preferences for activities involving the arm. These individuals are felt to express a variant of left-handedness, not to have a pathological condition.

As outlined above, basic handedness classification can impact how one characterizes associations between manual preference and performance. Other work suggests that pathological conditions might also influence the relationship between preference and performance. For instance, McManus, Murray, Doyle, and Baron-Cohen (1992) examined peg-moving performance in normal, learning disabled, and autistic children. They found that the direction of skill and preference differed in a substantial proportion of children with autism (~50%). There were few discrepancies in the other two groups.

In sum, though the limited data available suggests subjects generally use the hand that they report using, the relationship between preference and the proficiency aspects of manual performance is not straightforward. The data suggests that some types of tasks, especially those involving writing, are more likely to show reliable manual asymmetries that relate to preference. Inclusion of both handedness groups together, looking at the performance of each hand separately, choosing different handedness classifications, or examining groups with pathological conditions will influence the outcome of analyses of preference and performance data. The most popular means of examining the relation between preference and performance has been a correlational approach or some variant of it. This has had limited success, though Bishop (1989) developed a model that supports a common substrate for preference and performance despite the imperfect correlations. An alternate avenue taken by Bryden and colleagues (Bryden et al., 1994) includes a preference dimension in the performance tasks. The usefulness of this approach has not yet been fully evaluated.

2.3.3 Manual Skill

Preference and proficiency data suggest that the skill level of a task may be an important dimension influencing manifest handedness. Thus, consideration needs to be given to defining manual skill. Finding reference to manual skill in relation to human handedness is easy (e.g., Annett, 1992; Annett and Kilshaw, 1983; Kilshaw and Annett, 1983; McManus et al., 1992; Shimrat, 1973). There are also references to skill as an important dimension relating to human footedness (Peters, 1988) and manual preferences in non-human primates (e.g., Byrne and Byrne, 1991; Hopkins, Washburn, Berke, and Williams, 1992). Nevertheless, finding a definition of manual skill in the handedness literature is difficult.

Investigators in other areas, especially those interested in motor learning, have defined and classified motor skills (see Adams, 1987 and Magill, 1993 for reviews). Magill (1993) differentiates the term skill as it relates to *"an action or a task that has a goal and that requires voluntary body and/or limb movement to achieve the goal*" (p. 7) from skill as it relates to the quality of performance (the relative ability of one person compared to other people or compared to a standard). Magill points out several characteristics he sees as important in defining motor skills. These are that motor skills have a goal, require voluntary action (e.g., are not reflexes), need body or limb movement, and success at the task requires learning. Adams, based on historical use of the term, proposed three defining characteristics in his review of human motor skills: (1) skilled activities included a wide range of behaviors, mostly complex; (2) motor skills are learned; and (3) motor behavior is necessary to carry out the skill. Do such definitions apply to measuring handedness?

Though not explicitly stated, there is little doubt that handedness researchers examine a variety of behaviors and tasks requiring voluntary limb action to achieve a goal — the first type of skill referred to by Magill (1993). Sometimes, there is indirect examination of those tasks, using questionnaires (e.g., typical items include writing, using a toothbrush, opening a jar, and the like). At other times, the examination is direct, with performance tasks and observations of hand use. While most handedness researchers are not concerned about the ability or proficiency of individual subjects or their performance compared to a standard, many are concerned about the relative ability or proficiency of the two hands. From the motor control perspective, the precise nature of the differences between the preferred and nonpreferred hands (usually, in right-handers) has been the subject of much interest, investigation, and debate (see Chapter 7 for a review). Thus, both uses of the term "skill" occur in the handedness literature, that is, "skills" as tasks and "skill" denoting the quality of performance. It is less obvious whether these motor behaviors are complex and learned, fulfilling the other aspects of the skill definitions.

2.3.3.1 Variety and Complexity

Certainly, handedness investigators have evaluated a wide variety of manual behaviors, though each may focus on only one or two. The array of possible behaviors is very large and some investigators have included a substantial number. Examples are the 51-item (Beukelaar and Kroonenberg, 1983), 60-item (Steenhuis and Bryden, 1989) and 75-item (Provins et al., 1982) hand preference questionnaires.

Many of the terms applied to handedness imply complexity. Superior manipulation (Bradshaw and Rogers, 1993), dexterity (Flowers, 1975), sequencing (Watson and Kimura, 1989), movement accuracy (Todor and Cisneros, 1985), and movement speed (Todor and Cisneros, 1985) have all been used to describe the advantage that the preferred hand has over the nonpreferred hand. As Elliott and Chua (see Chapter 7) conclude, the advantage of the right hand in right-handers is in more precise control of motor output. One can speculate that precision is more critical with complex movements. Complexity should involve meeting multiple demands such as changing the speed or direction of the movement or coordinating different muscle groups. Many commonly used performance tasks appear complex, for example, dot-filling (Tapley and Bryden, 1985; Tan, 1992; Vasconcelos, 1993), peg-moving (Annett, 1976, 1985; Steenhuis and Bryden, in preparation; Tan, 1992), speeded writing (Borod et al., 1984; Peters and Servos, 1989; Provins and Magliaro, 1989), and throwing at targets (Peters, 1990a; Steenhuis and Bryden, in preparation; Watson and Kimura, 1989). Nevertheless, some tasks only require repetition of a single movement (e.g., rhythmic finger-tapping; Eling, 1983; Flowers, 1975; Peters, 1990) or the generation of force (e.g., grip strength; Borod et al., 1984; Eling, 1983; Peters, 1990; Provins and Magliaro, 1989; Steenhuis and Bryden, in preparation) and do not seem complex.

However, task complexity is rarely examined directly. Some investigators have unintentionally used tasks possibly differing in complexity (cf. Eling, 1983; Borod et al.,

1984). Manipulating task complexity has been the aim of other investigators. For instance, Provins and Magliaro (1989) compared the preferred and nonpreferred hands on a grip-strength task and a handwriting task because of their belief that these tasks differed in the level of skill required. As expected, there were larger intermanual differences [(P–NP/(P+NP)) × 100] for the handwriting task than for grip-strength. These investigators predicted that inducing fatigue would influence both hands equally during the unskilled task, (grip-strength) but with the skilled task (handwriting), the nonpreferred hand would be more affected than the preferred hand. The first prediction held. Both hands decreased equally in grip-strength during the fatigue condition. Contrary to their prediction, the preferred hand decreased about the same or more than the nonpreferred hand under the fatigue condition on the handwriting task. However, the achievement of the preferred hand under the fatigue condition remained well above that of the nonpreferred hand under the control condition. This finding caused the investigators to conclude that the skill requirement of the task was not the only variable in operation but that baseline ability level (or skill) of each hand might also be important.

Flowers (1975) examined a visually controlled aiming task and a rhythmical tapping task where the degree of control required to execute the movement was thought to differ. The preferred and nonpreferred hands had equivalent capacity on the tapping but not the aiming task, supporting Flowers' contention about the nature of the tasks. Watson and Kimura (1989) examined performance differences between the hands in right-handers for two tasks — throwing at a target and intercepting a projectile. Consistent with their prediction, the preferred hand was better at throwing but not intercepting. Overall, task complexity appears to have an influence in eliciting differences between the nonpreferred and preferred hands. Nevertheless, systematic evaluation of task complexity as a variable in hand preference has not occurred.

2.3.3.2 Learning in Handedness

The role that learning plays in handedness is not clear. Clues come from several sources. First, some report effects of age in children for some tasks but not others. Second, there are data about the effects of practice on hand preference in adults. Finally, the ability to adapt hand preferences to external factors has been evaluated.

Where age influences performance, a role for learning has been suggested. Krombholz (1989) looked at grip strength and dot-filling in children, measuring them at three intervals (beginning Year 1, end Year 1, and end Year 2; ages 81.5, 90.5, and 101.5 months, respectively). While facility at filling in dots and grip-strength both increased with age, the relative ability of the two hands was stable for grip strength but not for dot-filling. On dot-filling, a significant interaction between age and the performance of right and left hands stemmed from a substantial increase in the ability of the right hand between the beginning and the end of Year 1. This was interpreted as showing a role for learning in dot-filling but not grip strength. Similarly, Curt, Maccario, and Dellatolas (1992) have argued for an influence of learning on a dot-filling type of task (Graphic test), but not for peg-moving. The basis of this claim was their examination of over 700 preschool children. They found, in children less than 3.5 years of age, that a single distribution described the performance differences between the hands on the Graphic Test. For 3.5 to 4 year-olds, two distributions emerged — one distribution for left-handers and one for right-handers. Curt and colleagues speculated that this separation resulted from training of the preferred hand to use a pencil between ages 3 and 6.

Shimrat (1973) demonstrated an influence of experience with writing in a particular direction (right-left in Hebrew or left-right in English) in 8 to 9 year-olds. Children who experienced writing in both directions were faster and more accurate on a symbol transferring task. In adolescents (ages 10 to 17), Neiman (1989) notes with surprise some difficulties in motor performance in the nonpreferred hand of young musicians prior to receiving training for conducting skills. Systematic training took place to teach a variety of manual skills to both hands. Each hand plays an important role during conducting. The aim was to combine "the various continuous and punctuated, circular and linear movements using both hands simultaneously" (p. 848). Subjects drew figures simultaneously with both hands and practiced components and sequences of circular, vertical, and horizontal movements found in conducting with each hand. They were also asked to practice using their nonpreferred hand as much as possible for day-to-day activities. The goal was to achieve equal conducting skill in both hands. Three music teachers not involved in training the subjects rated their performance as "unsatisfactory," "satisfactory," or "good" on a monthly basis. At the end of the 9-month intensive training period, a majority of the students exhibited "satisfactory" performance of conducting skills in both hands. There was no information on the effect of this training on hand preferences.

In adults with well-established preferences, the opportunity to practice a particular task can lead to changes in ability in both hands. For example, Perelle, Ehrman, and Manowitz (1981) gave practice at a complex task involving sequencing to right- and left-handed subjects. Prior to practice, the preferred hand was better. Practice improved the proficiency of both the preferred and nonpreferred hands of right- and left-handers. The greatest improvement, however, occurred in the nonpreferred hand. Nevertheless, while both hands became very proficient, small differences favoring the preferred hand remained. Reddon and colleagues (Reddon, Stefanyk, Gill, and Renney, 1985) reported small improvements in grip strength over sessions. These findings were significant for men's nonpreferred and women's preferred hands. Thus, experience influences the proficiency of hands. However, how much increases in ability influence preference is not known.

Other factors had been examined in relation to altering hand preference. Porac, Rees, and Buller (1990) reviewed data showing that across a large number of studies: 8.9% of persons experienced pressure to alter their hand preference. Shifts occurred in both directions. However, they were qualitatively different. Persons who switched toward left hand preference did so at a later age because of self-interest in developing ambidexterity. These attempts rarely had an impact on handedness classification — most remained right-handed. In constrast, pressure toward right hand use was exerted by persons in authority at an early age and was successful much more often. As measured by current handedness, some 40.6% of switches to the right compared to 7.1% of switches to the left succeeded. The majority of switching attempts focused on writing. While writing hand is reliably reported, loads highly onto factor analyses (see Table 6.1), and probably underlies the performance measures showing the largest and most reliable differences between the hands, there is support from other sources for it being influenced by societal pressure (cf. Beukelaar and Kroonenberg, 1986). Because of this susceptibility to modification, the use of writing hand as a single or the best indicator of hand preference has long been controversial.

In sum, there is a lack of data on the influence of learning on the development of hand preferences. Learning in the form of environmental pressure to change hand preference is a more important factor in changing left-handers into right-handers than the converse. The limited success of later attempts to increase the usefulness of the nonpreferred hand to the extent of altering hand preference permanently suggests that learning does not play much of a role once hand preference has been established.

2.3.3.3 Summary

There are hints from different sources that skill is important with respect to handedness. As reviewed above, those hints come from primate research as well as from early and more recent human data. Consideration of how definitions of skill from the motor learning literature might relate to performance and preference data supports a role for skill in handedness. Skill is important both with regard to handedness tasks and to the relative ability of the preferred and nonpreferred hands.

The following data consider two hand preference factors representing skilled and less skilled activities in relation to observed hand use and to manual proficiency on various hand preference tasks. It was expected that skilled activities would be associated with stronger preferences reported on questionnaires and observed during hand use — basically, that observing hand use should give the same results as the questionnaire data, showing less preferred hand use for picking up an implement than for using it. Skilled activities (e.g., dot-filling and peg-moving) should be associated with larger differences between the hands and a more consistent relationship to preference than grip strength. These trends should be present in both right- and left-handers. However, right-handers and left-handers may differ in terms of specific relations between preference and performance.

3. CURRENT INVESTIGATION

The present experiment (see Steenhuis and Bryden, in preparation for more details) examined the relation between multidimensional hand preference, observed hand use, and hand proficiency on a range of manual tasks. The participants were 52 right-handed and 48 left-handed (50 males and 50 females) University of Waterloo students. Subjects had been prescreened for their handedness (both self-professed and questionnaire preference) and history of previous injury. Those who reported hand or arm injuries were not selected for further study. The mean age was 20.3 years.

3.1 METHOD

The performance tasks included pegboard (Annett, 1985) and dot-filling (Tapley and Bryden, 1985). Grip strength was measured using a dynamometer. Observations of hand use occurred for a large number of tasks (e.g., writing, cutting, throwing, batting, sewing, and opening a jar). Observations were made of both picking up and using the implements involved in doing a task. For example, hand use was recorded for picking up scissors and a piece of paper as well as cutting during the cutting out of a star. At an earlier time, a 60-item WHQ was administered (Steenhuis and Bryden, 1989). For the present analyses (converted from the five point (1 to 5) scale), a score of –1 indicated that the subject always used the right hand; a –.5 that they usually used the right hand; 0 that they used either hand equally; a .5 that they usually used the left hand; and a 1 that they always used the left hand. WHQ hand preference and factor scores were calculated in the same way as Bryden and Steenhuis (in preparation). Scores for all tasks were converted to a laterality ratio [(L – R)/(L + R)]. For most tasks, a negative ratio score reflected right handedness while a positive score reflected left-handedness. For the pegboard where the more proficient hand had a lower score (a faster time to move the pegs in seconds), a positive score reflected right-handedness. Thus, for the sake of consistency, the sign was reversed for the pegboard data so that again, a positive score demonstrated left-handedness. Scores of ±1.00 reflected complete use of or skill with the preferred hand.

3.2 RESULTS

There was an overall effect of handedness (F (1,90) = 333.12, $p < .0001$) and a task by hand interaction (F (6,85) = 156.42, $p < .0001$). As Figure 6.3 shows, the laterality quotients differed between right- and left-handers on all tasks, but the magnitude depended on the task (effect of task — F (6,85) = 7.31, $p < .0001$). The preferred hand of both self-professed left-handers (reflected by a positive laterality quotient) and right-handers (reflected by a negative laterality quotient) was more proficient (dot-filling, peg-moving). It was also reported to be used more often, and received more use than the nonpreferred hand but was stronger only in right-handers. For right-handers, all laterality quotients differed from zero (*ps* $< .05$). For left-handers, all but the laterality quotient for grip strength ($p > .05$) differed from zero.

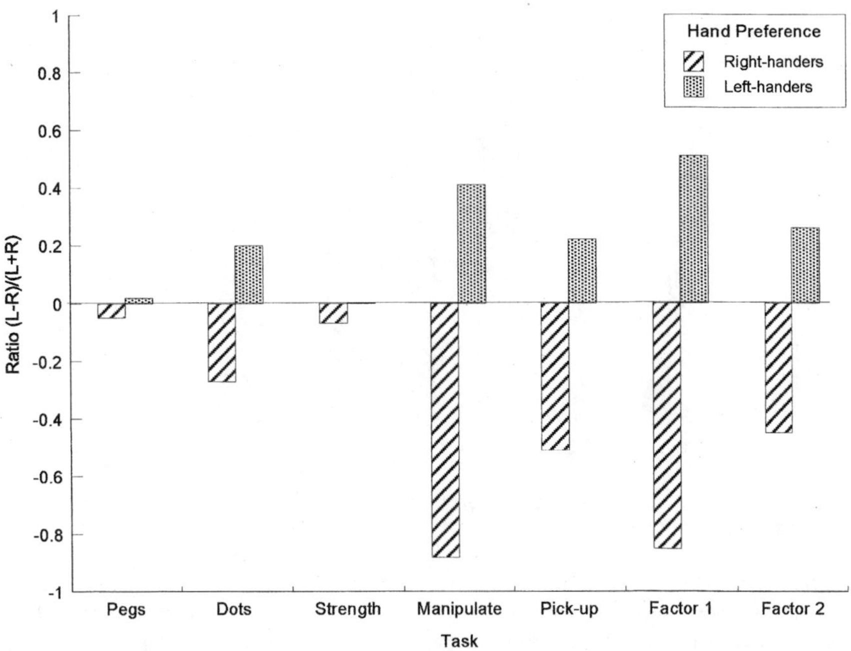

Figure 6.3 Mean laterality quotients on the skill, strength, and hand use tasks for left- and right-handers. Negative ratios indicate more right hand use or skill while positive ratios indicate more left hand use or skill.

Considering the degree of handedness (the absolute value of laterality quotients, Figure 6.4), right-handers were more strongly lateralized than left-handers (handedness effect; F (1,90) = 22.83, $p < .0001$), though there was a handedness by task interaction (F (6,85) = 6.86, $p < .0001$). Left-handers were less strongly lateralized on all measures (*ps* $< .05$), except grip strength and Factor 2 scores (*ps* $> .05$). For both left- and right-handers, the degree of handedness differed from zero (*ps* $< .05$) on all tasks. Some tasks were more strongly lateralized than others (effect of task — F (6,85) = 947.19, $p <$ .0001). There were clear differences in the degree of laterality between picking up and using implements. This was true for observed hand use and for the factor scores.

Table 6.2 shows the concordance between handedness determined by self-report and by the questionnaire data and handedness determined by the behavioral tasks (observed hand use, proficiency at filling dots and moving pegs, and grip-strength). The highest concordances are underlined for each preference measure for the whole sample, left-handers, and right-handers. For all groups, self-professed hand preferences (SRhand) were the same as handedness determined by dot-filling performance. That is, on dot-filling, all persons (100%) who said they were left-handed had better left hand proficiency while all persons who said they were right-handed had better right hand proficiency. For

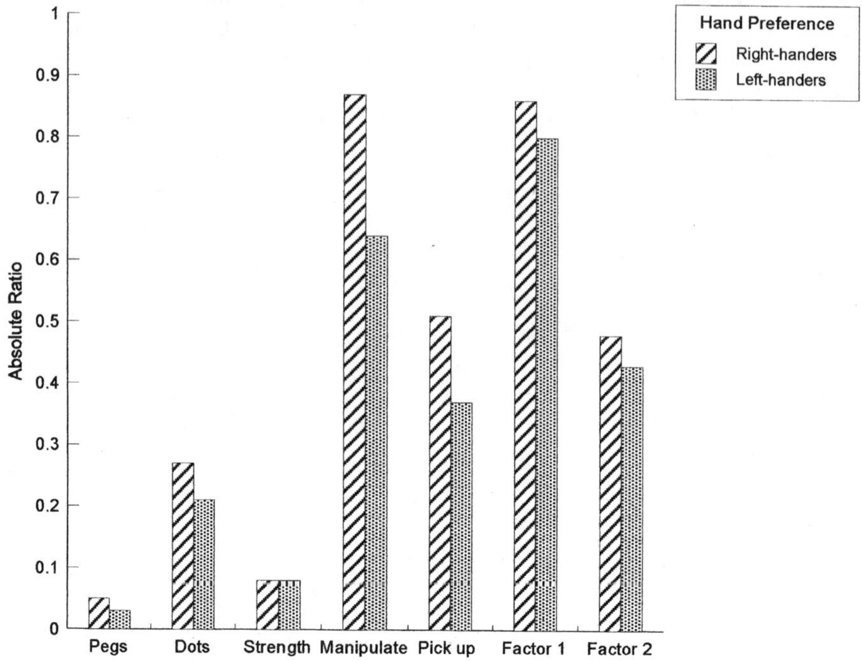

Figure 6.4 Mean absolute value of laterality quotients on the skill, strength, and hand use tasks for left- and right-handers.

the other methods of determining hand preference, left- and right-handers varied on which tasks showed optimal agreement. Determination of hand preference by total questionnaire responses (WHQ) related best to observed hand use for manipulating implements in the entire sample and in right-handers. For left-handers, manipulation gave a perfect outcome as did dot-filling. Factor 1 scores gave a similar pattern to the total questionnaire score, except now, picking up also classified the right-handers with equally high accuracy. Overall and for right-handers, picking up objects gave the best classification for Factor 2, but again dot-filling resulted in the best classification of left-handers.

For the dot-filling task, correct classification fell from 100% of self-professed right-handers to 79% with hand preference determined by the total questionnaire score and 84% by Factor 1 scores. This occurred because some subjects who called themselves left-handed and who had a superior left hand for dot-filling were right-handed according to their questionnaire score. Including these subjects with the right-handers lessened the agreement. Similarly, with the pegboard, classification agreement decreased slightly in right-handers for the questionnaire data over that obtained with self-professed hand preference (falling from 94 to 89%). It improved for left-handers from 71% with self-report to 88% with questionnaire classification. Grip strength gave adequate classification of right-handers but poor classification of left-handers. Across performance tasks, observed hand use for manipulation of objects related best to questionnaire preferences in right-handers. In left-handers, dot-filling related best. However, there were some persons who were left-handed for some activities and right-handed for others.

The direction of handedness correlated between measures. With the whole sample, correlations between the laterality quotients for all measures, except grip-strength, were

Table 6.2 Concordance Between Methods of Determining Handedness: Proportion of Subjects Classified as Left- or Right-Handed According to Self-Report and Questionnaire Preferences and Task Scores

		Hand use		Proficiency		
		Manip	**Pick-up**	**Dots**	**Pegs**	**Strength**
Srhand	Total	90%	86%	100%	83%	63%
	Left	78%	72%	100%	71%	47%
	Right	100%	98%	100%	94%	82%
WHQ	Total	97%	89%	86%	88%	72%
	Left	100%	84%	100%	88%	63%
	Right	95%	92%	79%	89%	77%
Factor 1	Total	99%	91%	90%	87%	71%
	Left	100%	83%	100%	83%	61%
	Right	97%	97%	84%	90%	77%
Factor 2	Total	91%	92%	88%	83%	69%
	Left	91%	88%	100%	79%	56%
	Right	92%	95%	81%	88%	75%

highly significant ($ps < .0001$). They ranged from .65 (peg-moving and dot-filling) to .97 (manipulate and factor 1). They were still significant ($ps < .01$) for grip-strength, but lower (ranging from .29 to .44). Table 6.3 shows the correlations between measures for the absolute value of the laterality quotients and indicates relations for the strength or degree of handedness, independent of the direction of handedness. The questionnaire preference for Factors 1 and 2 and hand use for picking up and manipulating objects were significantly correlated in both right and left-handers. Otherwise, there were few correlations between preference and performance, and the patterns differed in the two groups. Of interest is that overall, dot-filling correlated with manipulation while peg-moving correlated with picking up objects.

3.3 DISCUSSION

Overall, persons professing left-handedness were more proficient with, and more frequently used, their left hand while the converse was true for right-handers. Nevertheless, the relationships between preference, use, and proficiency differed in the two groups.

Questionnaire preference and observed use show large intermanual differences whereas differences between the hands-on proficiency tasks are not of the same magnitude. Even so, some proficiency tasks produce larger differences between the hands than others, with grip strength being weakly lateralized. This is a common finding (see Borod et al., 1984; Provins et al., 1982). Sometimes, the ability of the nonpreferred hand equals that of the preferred hand. In right-handers, Watson and Kimura (1989) demonstrated that the hands had equal ability for blocking (not catching) a projectile. In the same sample, they showed right hand superiority for throwing at a target. Similarly, Fischman and Sanders (1991) reported a high level of ability in both hands to catch a ball but not throw it.

People (even right-handers) use their nonpreferred hand (Bryden et al., 1994; Harris and Carlson, 1993; Verfaellie and Heilman, 1990). The present data shows that left-handers

Table 6.3 Correlation Between the Absolute Value of the Laterality Quotients for the Skill, Hand Use, Strength, and Questionnaire Preference Measures

	Dots	Pegs	Strength	Man	Pick up	Factor 1	Factor 2
				All subjects			
Dots	1.00	.14	.02	.23*	.14	–.11	.06
Pegs		1.00	–.04	.19	.29**	.22*	.18
Strength			1.00	–.01	–.02	.12	.16
Man				1.00	.45**	.25*	.25*
Pick up					1.00	.39**	.32**
Factor 1						1.00	.48**
Factor 2							1.00
				Right-handers			
Dots	1.00	–.03	.11	–.18	.08	–.34*	.01
Pegs		1.00	.08	.02	.20	.14	.13
Strength			1.00	.27	.08	.06	.17
Man				1.00	.29*	.34*	.29*
Pick up					1.00	.20	.28*
Factor 1						1.00	.43**
Factor 2							1.00
				Left-handers			
Dots	1.00	.22	–.08	.28	.00	–.09	.07
Pegs		1.00	–.16	.08	.25	.22	.20
Strength			1.00	–.14	–.10	.16	.15
Man				1.00	.37**	.09	.22
Pick up					1.00	.45**	.33*
Factor 1						1.00	.49**
Factor 2							1.00

* $p < .05$; ** $p < .01$.

generally do more with their nonpreferred hand than right-handers. The frequency of hand use depended on the task involved. Nonpreferred hand use increased for picking up implements compared to using those implements. This was apparent for both questionnaire data and observations of hand use. It was true of both right- and left-handers, providing strong support for the nature of Steenhuis and Bryden's two hand preference factors. One factor strongly lateralized, relating to the skilled action of manipulating an implement and one factor weakly lateralized, relating to less skilled actions like picking up objects.

Harris and Carlson (1993) measured the hand used to pick up objects in infants and adults. The adult subjects were 40 right- and left-handed college students selected on the basis of self-described handedness and confirmed by questionnaire responses (6 items). Subjects picked up a pellet, cube, or ball from one of three positions — at the midline or 12 inches to the right or left. The task was fast-paced and the position of the object could not be predicted. The results showed that 68 to 85% of midline reaches were with the preferred hand. About 90% of reaches to the dominant side involved the dominant hand and 60 to 75% of nondominant side reaches involved the nondominant hand. Their data resembled that presented here in that most of the time the preferred hand picked up objects but the nonpreferred hand was also used. Harris and Carlson's data suggested that to a great extent use of the nonpreferred hand depended on placing the object on that side of space, though this needs more systematic investigation.

In the present study, no single proficiency measure related perfectly to all aspects of hand preference. How well preference and performance related depended on both the proficiency and preference measures. It also depended on whether one considered the direction or the degree of handedness and whether the person was left- or right-handed. As has been reported by others, correlations between measures that included the direction of handedness were large but those looking at the degree or strength of handedness were not. Further, as predicted different patterns of correlations emerged for the two handedness groups.

A high correspondence between dot-filling and self-professed hand preference was also reported by Tapley and Bryden (1985). Steenhuis and Bryden (in preparation) note that for some left-handers asking for self-reported hand preference or using a dot-filling task to determine handedness will be misleading. These persons show mixed LH/RH handedness, with their preferences and proficiency split between tasks. They are equivalent to other left-handers in terms of describing themselves as left-handed and in the magnitude of left hand proficiency on dot-filling. Nevertheless, in the main, their right hand is stronger and they would be considered right-handed according to their questionnaire preference data. These persons represent a subset of the persons Peters and his colleagues (Peters, 1990a, 1990b; Peters and Servos, 1989) have described as "inconsistent left-handers."

4. SUMMARY AND CONCLUSIONS

Data from a variety of sources supports the presence of manual preferences that are weakly lateralized for picking up objects and preferences that are more strongly lateralized for manipulating those objects. Examples are found in early artwork (Spennemann, 1984), questionnaire preferences (Steenhuis and Bryden, 1989) and observed hand use (Steenhuis and Bryden, in preparation). Steenhuis and Bryden (1989) have postulated that it is the skill required to execute the task which produces this difference in strength of preference. While performance measures also vary in their ability to produce differences between the hands and it is often implied that the level of skill required might be an important moderating variable, this hypothesis is rarely examined. It seems reasonable to describe grip strength, which has weak lateralization and poor predictive power of handedness, as an unskilled task.

Describing tasks like peg-moving and dot-filling in terms of skill level is more problematic. Nevertheless, if one considers a definition of manual skill like the one put forward by Adams (1987), then dot-filling fulfills more of the criteria than peg-moving. Both tasks might be thought of as complex motor activities. Though it is difficult to determine how they equate in terms of the amount of skill required, dot-filling has larger laterality ratios and seems, at face value, to require greater dexterity. Evidence exists for an influence of learning in the preferred hand on dot-filling, but not on peg-moving (Curt et al., 1992). It is not clear whether a failure to demonstrate learning in peg-moving is because the "skill" was mastered at an earlier age (less than 3 years old). However, as noted above, self-reported hand preference and dot-filling performance in some left-handers provides misleading information about overall handedness. Finally, consideration also needs to be given to the possibility of an innate predisposition for lateralization as the substrate upon which learning might act. In order to access that predisposition, some would argue it is better to select tasks that are less skilled and therefore, less susceptible to societal pressure and overlearning.

Most handedness investigators seek to measure the unique qualities that can be ascribed to the preferred hand. However, we cannot understand what is unique about the preferred hand without understanding what the hands share in common, both in terms of their use and proficiency (see Chapter 9). Further work will be necessary to unravel the complex interactions between hand preference and the skills required to perform the tasks (both simple and complex) upon which those preferences act.

ACKNOWLEDGMENTS

The data presented here were collected at the University of Waterloo. This research was supported by a grant from the Natural Science and Engineering Research Council of Canada to Dr. M.P. Bryden. Thanks to Leslie MacRae and Kerri Bock for assistance with the data collection and to Cathy Gouchie, M.A., for reading the manuscript.

REFERENCES

Adams, J. A. (1987). Historical review and appraisal of research on the learning, retention, and transfer of human motor skills. *Psychol. Bull.*, 101, 41.

Annett, M. (1976). A coordination of hand preference and skill replicated. *Br. J. Psychol.*, 67, 587.

Annett, M. (1985). *Left, Right, Hand and Brain: The Right Shift Theory.* Hillsdale, NJ, Lawrence Erlbaum.

Annett, M. (1992). Five tests of hand skill. *Cortex*, 28, 583.

Annett, M. and Kilshaw, D. (1983). Right- and left-hand skill II: Estimating the parameters of the distribution of R-L differences in males and females. *Br. J. Psychol.*, 74, 269.

Beukelaar, L. J. and Kroonenberg, P. M. (1983). Towards a conceptualization of hand preference. *Br. J. Psychol.*, 74, 33.

Beukelaar, L. J. and Kroonenberg, P. M. (1986). Changes over time in the relationship between hand preference and writing hand among left-handers. *Neuropsychologia*, 24, 301.

Bishop, D. V. M. (1989). Does hand proficiency determine hand preference? *Br. J. Psychol.*, 80, 191.

Blau, A. (1946). *The Master Hand: A Study of the Origin and Meaning of Right and Left Sidedness and Its Relation to Personality and Language*. New York, The American Orthopsychiatric Association.

Borod, J. C., Caron, H. S., and Koff, E. (1984). Left-handers and right-handers compared on performance and preference measures of lateral dominance. *Br. J. Psychol.*, 75, 177.

Bradshaw, J. and Rogers, L. (1993). *The Evolution of Lateral Asymmetries, Language, Tool Use, and Intellect.* San Diego, Academic Press.

Bryden, M. P. (1977). Measuring handedness with questionnaires. *Neuropsychologia*, 15, 617.

Bryden, M. P., MacRae, L., and Steenhuis, R. E. (1991). Hand preference in school children. *Dev. Neuropsychol.*, 7, 477.

Bryden, M. P., Singh, M., Steenhuis, R. E., and Clarkson, K. L. (1994). A behavioral measure of hand preference as opposed to hand skill. *Neuropsychologia*, 32, 991.

Byrne, R. W. and Byrne, J. M. (1991). Hand preferences in the skilled gathering tasks of mountain gorillas (*Gorilla g. berengei*). *Cortex*, 27, 521.

Coren, S. and Porac, C. (1977). Fifty centuries of right-handedness: The historical record. *Science*. 198: 631.

Curt, F., Maccario, J., and Dellatolas, G. (1992). Distributions of hand preference and hand skill asymmetry in preschool children: Theoretical implications. *Neuropsychologia*, 30, 27.

Dean, R. S. (1978). Reliability and predictive validity of the Dean Laterality Preference Schedule with preadolescents. *Percept. Motor Skills*, 47, 1345.

Durost, W. N. (1934). The development of a battery of objective group tests of manual laterality, with the results of their application to 1300 children. *Gen. Psychol. Monogr.*, 16, 229.

Fabbro, F. (1994). Left and right in the bible from a neuropsychological perspective. *Brain Cognit.*, 24, 161.

Fischman, M. G. and Sanders, R. (1991). An empirical note on the bilateral use of a baseball glove by skilled catchers. *Percept. Motor Skills*, 72, 219.

Eling, P. (1983). Comparing different measures of laterality: Do they relate to a single mechanism. *J. Clin. Neuropsychol.*, 5, 135.

Flowers, K. (1975). Handedness and controlled movement. *Br. J. Psychol.*. 66, 39.

Harris, L. J. (1993). Handedness in apes and monkeys: Some views from the past. In J. P. Ward and W. D. Hopkins (Eds.), *Primate Laterality: Current Behavioral Evidence of Primate Asymmetries*, New York, Springer-Verlag, 1.

Harris, L. J. and Carlson, D. F. (1993). Hand preference for visually-guided reaching in human infants and adults. In J. P. Ward and W. D. Hopkins (Eds.), *Primate Laterality: Current Behavioral Evidence of Primate Asymmetries*, New York, Springer-Verlag, 285.

Healey, J. M., Liederman, J., and Geschwind, N. (1986). Handedness is not a unidimensional trait. *Cortex*, 22, 33.

Hopkins, W. D., Washburn, D. A., Berke, L., and Williams, M. (1992). Behavioral asymmetries of psychomotor performance in Rhesus monkeys (*Macaca mulatta)*: A dissociation between hand preference and skill. *J. Comp. Psychol.*, 106, 392.

Kilshaw, D. and Annett, M. (1983). Right- and left-hand skill I: Effects of age, sex and hand preference showing superior skill in left-handers. *Br. J. Psychol.*, 74, 253.

Koch, H. L. (1933). A study of the nature, measurement and determination of hand preference. *Gen. Psychol. Monogr.,* 13, 117.

Lawrence, D. G. and Kuypers, H. G. J. M. (1968a). The functional organization of the motor system in the monkey: I. The effects of bilateral pyramidal lesions. *Brain*, 91, 1.

Lawrence, D. G. and Kuypers, H. G. J. M. (1968b). The functional organization of the motor system in the monkey: II. The effect of lesions of the descending brain-stem pathways. *Brain*, 91, 15.

Lehman, R. A. W. (1993) Manual preferences in prosimians, monkeys and apes. In J. P. Ward and W. D. Hopkins (Eds.), *Primate Laterality: Current Behavioral Evidence of Primate Asymmetries*, New York, Springer-Verlag, 149.

Liederman, J. and Healey, J. M. (1986). Independent dimensions of hand preference: Reliability of the factor structure and the handedness inventory. *Arch. Clin. Neuropsychol.*, 1, 371.

Krombholz, H. (1989). Laterality and force of handgrip during the first two years at school. *Percept. Motor Skills*, 68, 955.

Magill, R. A. (1993). *Motor Learning: Concepts and Applications* (4th ed.). Madison, WI, Brown and Benchmark.

Marchant, L. F. and McGrew, W. C. (1994). Do chimpanzees show handedness or not? *Am. J. Phys. Anthropol.*, 94, 136.

McFarland, K. and Anderson, J. (1980). Factor stability of the Edinburgh Handedness Inventory as a function of test-retest performance, age and sex. *Br. J. Psychol.*, 71, 135.

McManus, I. C., Murray, B., Doyle, K., and Baron-Cohen, S. (1992). Handedness in childhood autism shows a dissociation of skill and preference. *Cortex*, 28, 373.

Neiman, Z. (1989). Teaching specific motor skills for conducting to young music students. *Percept. Motor Skills*, 68, 847.

Perelle, I. B., Ehrman, L., and Manowitz, J. W. (1981). Human handedness: The influence of learning. *Percept. Motor Skills*, 53, 967.

Peters, M. (1988). Footedness: Asymmetries in foot preference and skill and neuropsychological assessment of foot movement. *Psychol. Bull.*, 103, 179.

Peters, M. (1990a). Subclassification of non-pathological left-handers poses problems for theories of handedness. *Neuropsychologia*, 28, 279.

Peters, M. (1990b). Phenotype in normal left-handers: An understanding of phenotype is the basis for understanding mechanism and inheritance of handedness. In S. Coren (Ed.), *Left-Handedness: Behavioral Implications and Anomalies*, Amsterdam, Elsevier, 167.

Peters, M. and Servos, P. (1989). Performance of subgroups of left-handers and right-handers. *Can. J. Psychol.*, 43, 341.

Porac, C., Coren, S., Steiger, J. H., and Duncan, P. (1980). Human laterality: A multidimensional approach. *Can. J. Psychol.*, 34, 91.

Porac, C., Rees, L., and Buller, T. (1990). Switching hands: A place for left hand use in a right hand world. In S. Coren (Ed.), *Left-Handedness: Behavioral Implications and Anomalies*, Amsterdam, Elsevier, 259.

Provins, K. A., and Cunliffe, P. (1972). The reliability of some motor performance tests of handedness. *Neuropsychologia*, 10, 199.

Provins, K. A., Milner, A. D., and Kerr, P. (1982). Asymmetry of manual preference and performance. *Percept. Motor Skills*, 54, 179.

Provins, K. A. and Magliaro, J. (1989). Skill, strength, handedness, and fatigue. *J. Motor Behav.*, 21, 113.

Obrzut, J. E., Dalby, P. R., Boliek, C. A., and Cannon, G. E. (1992). Factorial Structure of the Waterloo Handedness Questionnaire for control and learning-disabled adults. *J. Clin. Exp. Neuropsychol.*, 14, 935.

Raczkowski. D., Kalat, J. W., and Nebes, R. (1974). Reliability and validity of some handedness questionnaire items. *Neuropsychologia*, 12, 43.

Reddon, J. R., Stefanyk, W. O., Gill, D. M., and Renney, C. (1985). Hand dynamometer: Effects of trials and sessions. *Percept. Motor Skills*, 61, 1195.

Roszkowski, M. J., Snelbecker, G. E., and Sacks, R. (1981). Children's, adolescents', and adults' reports of hand preference: Homogeneity and discriminating power of selected tasks. *J. Clin. Neuropsychol.*, 3, 199.

Shafer, D. D. (1993). Patterns of handedness: Comparative study of nursery school children and captive gorillas. In J. P. Ward and W. D. Hopkins (Eds.), *Primate Laterality: Current Behavioral Evidence of Primate Asymmetries*, New York, Springer-Verlag, 267.

Sherman, J. L., Kulhavy, R. W., and Bretzing, B. H. (1976). The Sherman-Kulhavy Laterality Assessment Inventory: Some validation data. *Percept. Motor Skills*, 42, 1314.

Shimrat, N. (1973). The impact of laterality and cultural background on the development of writing skill. *Neuropsychologia*, 11, 239.

Singh, M. and Bryden, M. P. (1994). The factor structure of handedness in India. *Int. J. Neurosci.*, 74, 33.

Spennemann, D. R. (1984). Right- and left-handedness in early South-East Asia: The graphic evidence of the Borobudar. *Bijdragen: Tot De Taal, Land -en Volkenkunde*, 140, 163.

Steenhuis, R. E. and Bryden, M. P. (1987). Handedness: A matter of direction and degree. *Can. Psychol.*, 28, N 586.

Steenhuis, R. E. and Bryden, M. P. (1988). Different dimensions of hand preference that relate to skilled and unskilled activities. *J. Clin. Exp. Neuropsychol.*, 10, 40.

Steenhuis, R. E. and Bryden, M. P. (1989). Different dimensions of hand preference that relate to skilled and unskilled activities. *Cortex*, 25, 289.

Steenhuis, R. E., Bryden, M. P., Schwartz, M., and Lawson, S. (1990). Reliability of hand preference items and factors. *J. Clin. Exp. Neuropsychol.*, 12, 921.

Steenhuis, R. E. and Bryden, M. P. (in preparation). The relation between hand preference and hand performance: What you get depends on what you measure.

Tan, U. (1992). The relation of hand preference to hand performance in left-handers: Importance of the left brain. *Int. J. Neurosci.*, 65, 1.

Tan, U. (1993). Normal distribution of hand preference and its bimodality. *Int. J. Neurosci.*, 68, 61.

Tapley, S. M. and Bryden, M. P. (1985). A group test for the assessment of performance between the hands. *Neuropsychologia*, 23, 215.

Todor, J. I. and Cisneros, J. (1985). Accommodation to increased accuracy demands by the right and left hands. *J. Motor Behav.*, 17, 355.

Vasconcelos, O. (1993). Asymmetries of manual motor response in relation to age, sex, handedness, and occupational activities. *Percept. Motor Skills*, 77, 691.

Verfaellie, M. and Heilman, K. M. (1990). Hemispheric asymmetries in attentional control: Implications for hand preference in sensorimotor tasks. *Brain Cognit.*, 14, 70.

Ward, J. P., Milliken, G. W., and Stafford, D. K. (1993). Patterns of lateralized behavior in Prosimians. In J. P. Ward and W. D. Hopkins (Eds.), *Primate Laterality: Current Behavioral Evidence of Primate Asymmetries*, New York, Springer-Verlag, 43.

Watson, N. V. and Kimura, D. (1989). Right-hand superiority for throwing but not for intercepting. *Neuropsychologia*, 27, 1399.

Woodworth, R. S. (1899). The accuracy of voluntary movement. *Psychol. Rev. Monogr. Suppl.*, 3, (2), 1.

Chapter 7

Manual Asymmetries in Goal-Directed Movement

Digby Elliott and Romeo Chua

CONTENTS

1. INTRODUCTION

Manual asymmetries in the performance of various motor tasks are typically attributed to the relative proficiency of the two cerebral hemispheres at particular types of perceptual-motor processing (Todor and Smiley, 1985). For right-handed individuals, the right hand exhibits superiority for tasks such as rapid finger-tapping (Todor, Kyprie, and Price, 1987), finger sequencing (Edwards and Elliott, 1987), and the execution of goal-directed aiming movements (Woodworth, 1899). This advantage is thought to reflect the special role the left cerebral hemisphere plays in the organization and execution of voluntary movement. By contrast, right-handed people often exhibit left hand superiority for tasks that have a large spatial component. Thus, left side advantages for tasks such as tactile matching (Benton, Varney, and deHamsher, 1978; Witelson, 1974) and the blind reproduction of a spatial position (Carnahan and Elliott, 1987; Roy and MacKenzie, 1978) are often attributed to a right hemisphere propensity for spatial processing. By default then, it has been argued that the absence of a hand difference reflects the failure of either cerebral hemisphere to play a more dominant role in task performance (Carson, Elliott, Goodman, and Dickinson, 1990).

0-8493-8999-2/96/$0.00+$.50

While globally useful, and to some degree consistent with the clinical neuropsychological literature on apraxia and agnosia (Roy, 1985), these *post hoc* characterizations of manual asymmetries usually obscure the overall complexity of the motor tasks being studied as well as the fact that even the simplest tasks require the cooperative interaction of different perceptual-motor systems (Luria, 1966). One approach to the study of manual asymmetries has been to examine not only the movement outcome but also the *process* by which a movement goal is achieved. By examining *how* the two hands accomplish a particular task under a variety of task conditions, movement scientists not only achieve a better understanding of manual asymmetries per se, but also how perceptual-motor systems subserved by the right and left cerebral hemispheres interact in the control of complex goal-directed movement.

In a review of the literature on performance asymmetries for tasks such as aiming, reaching, and finger-sequencing, we will attempt to identify the processing characteristics of the two cerebral hemispheres thought to underlie lateral performance advantages for simple motor tasks. As Hellige (1993, p. 29) points out, "even simple tasks consist of a number of components or subprocesses, and there is no guarantee that hemispheric asymmetry for one component is the same as that for another component." In studies of manual asymmetries, the involvement of different perceptual-motor systems in the performance of a task has been studied by manipulating the specific conditions under which the task is performed and/or the specific task requirements. By also examining a number of outcome and kinematic measures of task performance, recent work from our laboratory and elsewhere has focused on the specialized, but cooperative, contribution of the two cerebral hemispheres to overall task performance.

2. HISTORICAL OVERVIEW

2.1 WOODWORTH (1899)

One of the first investigators to examine the basis for lateral asymmetry in manual aiming was R.S. Woodworth (1899), who published his results in a classic monograph entitled "The accuracy of voluntary movement." In a seminal study, Woodworth had subjects perform a series of horizontal sliding movements with a pencil on paper. The paper was secured to a large drum which rotated at a constant speed. The subject's task on each attempt was to produce a movement with the same spatial endpoint as the previous movement. Thus, error was determined by measuring the difference between the lengths of consecutive lines on the paper. Woodworth manipulated the speed of the movements by having subjects perform to the beat of a metronome. On some trials, subjects were required to close their eyes while performing the aiming movements, while on other trials they were allowed full vision of the apparatus and the moving limb. Woodworth's results for the right and left hand performing this task are reproduced in Figure 7.1. While these same data have been used to estimate the time required to process visual feedback from an ongoing movement (see Carlton, 1992 for a review), probably the most striking characteristic of Figure 7.1 is the distinct superiority of the right hand in both visual conditions. Specifically, the left hand achieves comparable accuracy to the right hand only in the eyes open condition when subjects are moving extremely slowly (i.e., 20 beats/min or 3 s for each movement).

Woodworth (1899) suggested two possible reasons for the right hand advantage at manual aiming. Based on the fact that hand differences in accuracy increased in magnitude as the time for feedback utilization decreased (i.e., speed increased), he proposed that the "seat of superiority of the right hand is probably in the motor centers" (Woodworth, 1899, p. 34). Today this explanation of manual asymmetry may be linked to a left hemisphere propensity for movement organization or motor programming. Alternatively,

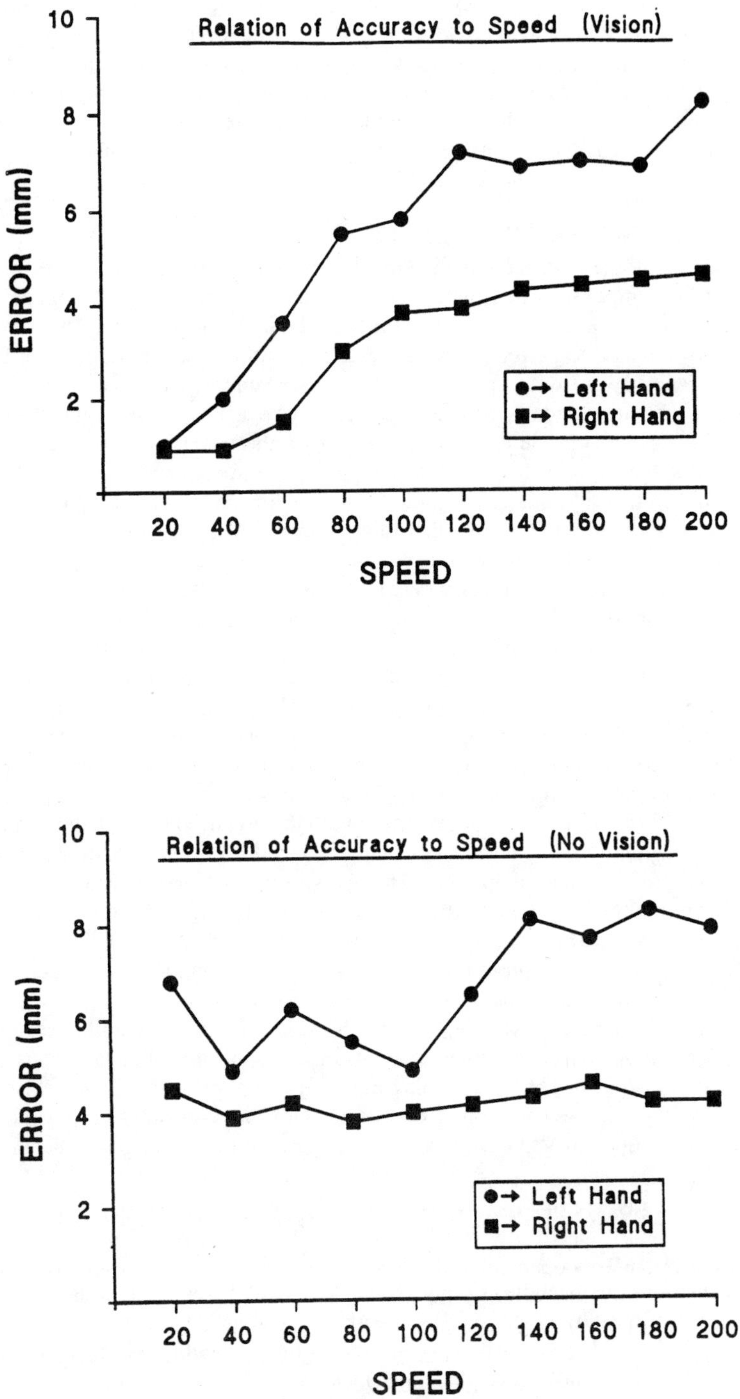

Figure 7.1 Movement error as a function of vision condition, hand, and speed. (From R.S. Woodworth, *Psychol. Rev.*, 3, (Monograph Supplement), 32, 1899. ©1899 by the American Psychological Association. Reprinted with permission.)

since hand differences in accuracy were still apparent even for very slow movements when the eyes were closed, Woodworth (1899, p. 34) conceded that "the muscle, joint and skin sensations from the right arm are probably more delicate than those from the left." That is, hand differences may be due to a right side superiority at kinesthetic feedback utilization. As will become evident in this review, these two positions, if somewhat expanded, have resurfaced repeatedly as possible explanations of manual asymmetries in motor control.

2.2 BETWEEN-TASK DIFFERENCES

A number of studies concerned with manual performance and skill have relied on between-task comparisons to isolate the processing determinants of asymmetries. For example, Provins (1956) compared the ability of the index finger on the "preferred" and "nonpreferred" hand to perform simple isometric contractions and rapid taps. Because hand differences were only apparent in the finger-tapping task (both for speed and consistency), he suggested that hand differences may be due to a preferred hand advantage in timing a series of muscle contractions. This hypothesis was also consistent with the finding that subjects were able to throw darts at a target more accurately with their right hand. Provins suggested that right hand advantages for the "timing" of muscle contractions may be more due to training than to any innate predisposition since asymmetries in timing were not evident in foot movements.

A number of years later, Flowers (1975) came to a very different conclusion regarding the basis for manual performance asymmetries based on another between-task comparison. Flowers examined the performance of strongly lateralized right-handers and left-handers on a rapid finger-tapping task and a visually monitored manual aiming task (Fitts, 1954). He characterized the tapping task as ballistic in nature, presumably because individual movements were completed too rapidly for kinesthetic or visual feedback utilization. In contrast, performance on the aiming task was deemed to be dependent on a corrective mode of control which involved continuous feedback monitoring. Since these strongly lateralized subjects performed better with the preferred hand on the aiming task, but not the tapping task, Flowers concluded that "the essential dexterity difference between the preferred and nonpreferred hands is in the sensory or feedback control of movement rather than in the motor function per se" (Flowers, 1975, p. 39). The fact that the preferred hand advantage increased as the accuracy demands of the aiming task increased suggests that the preferred hand advantage at aiming may be related to visual feedback utilization (Todor and Smiley, 1985; cf. Woodworth, 1899).

Flowers' (1975) failure to find a preferred hand advantage for rapid finger-tapping is somewhat of an anomaly (cf. Provins, 1956). In less controlled clinical testing (Reitan and Davison, 1974), a right hand tapping advantage of approximately 10% is expected in right-handers. This expectation is consistent with many of the more recent studies designed to examine manual asymmetries in finger-tapping and finger-sequencing.

3. ASYMMETRIES IN FINGER-TAPPING/SEQUENCING

3.1 PERFORMANCE RATE AND VARIABILITY

While many of the early studies simply examined overall finger-tapping rate, more recent work has partitioned each tap into its components, allowing the study of both mean performance for each component and finger-tapping variability. Using this approach, Todor and Kyprie (1980) found that right-handers not only exhibited an overall right hand advantage, but they also produced more consistent intertap intervals with the right hand (see also Peters and Durding, 1978, 1979). As well, the performance difference between the hands was more a function of the dwell or down time than the time at which the tapping key was released. This indicates that the right hand may be superior at modulating the muscular forces required to make the transition from flexion to extension. This suggestion is consistent with work by Peters (1980) who found preferred hand advantages for both the down-up and up-down finger-tapping transitions, but not the single-direction "up" and "down" components. As well, the advantage for the right hand was magnified when the precision of force modulation was increased by requiring the subjects to perform smaller, more subtle finger-tapping movements.

In addition to examining temporal variability in finger-tapping transitions, Todor and Smiley-Oyen (1987) measured the force levels directly and found that both mean force level and force-variability were greater for the nonpreferred hand. Because forces occur as a result of muscular contractions, it is difficult to know whether temporal differences between the two hands are the result of variability in the intensity or timing of neural bursts (i.e., optimal summation).

Although lateral asymmetries in finger-tapping appear to be a reasonably robust phenomenon, there has been some speculation that right hand superiority may reflect differential hand use or learning rather than any intrinsic property of the right hand/left hemisphere system. In order to examine this hypothesis, Peters (1976) conducted a single subject experiment involving 1300 10 s finger-tapping trials with each hand over the course of a number of weeks. While by the end of training and again after a 4-week retention period, the left hand was performing at the same overall rate as the right hand, it still exhibited greater variability in the intertap interval (see also Elliott, Weeks, and Jones, 1986). This asymmetry in tapping consistency was interpreted to reflect hand/hemisphere differences in the ability to precisely time the onset and offset of muscular contractions that are resistant to practice. The proposal that there are intrinsic differences in perceptual-motor processing between the hand systems is also consistent with the finding that right side advantages are exhibited for rapid foot tapping (Peters and Durding, 1979; Ruisel, 1970) where there is less possibility of different practice histories (cf. Provins, 1956).

Another approach that has been taken to examine the generalizability of lateral tapping advantages has been to compare the performance of various muscle groups to determine whether asymmetries are restricted to distal musculature for which only contralateral neural pathways are involved. For example, Todor, Kyprie, and Price (1982) examined finger, wrist, and arm tapping and found that right-handed subjects exhibit right side performance and consistency advantages independent of the primary joint involved in the movement. Thus, it appears that in the case of proximal musculature, the crossed pathways also have the primary role in motor control.

The asymmetries found in right-handed people for single finger-tapping are also evident when subjects are required to rapidly produce a sequence of movements involving two or more fingers. Specifically, right-handed children and adults are able to produce a predetermined sequence of movements more quickly and with greater temporal consistency when performing with the right hand (Edwards and Elliott, 1987, 1989; Taylor and Heilman, 1980). As with single finger-tapping, this finding has been taken to reflect a left hemisphere specialization for the temporal specification of muscular contractions. This explanation of manual performance asymmetries has received further support from studies of cross-hand transfer-of-training and motor overflow.

3.2 TRANSFER OF TRAINING

In experiments examining transfer of training, right-handed participants are required to learn a complex finger-sequencing task with either the right hand or left hand (e.g., Elliott, 1985; Edwards and Elliott, 1987; Taylor and Heilman, 1980). Following a period of unimanual training, intermanual transfer of training is examined by evaluating finger-sequencing in the untrained hand. Typically, transfer of training is asymmetric. That is, left-hand training results in greater transfer of training (to the right hand) than right-hand training (to the left hand). Taylor and Heilman (1980) have suggested that this asymmetric pattern of transfer reflects the special role that the left cerebral hemisphere plays in the organization and control of sequential movement. Specifically, while the contralateral cerebral hemisphere is always involved in finger-sequencing, when subjects are practicing with their left hand both cerebral hemispheres are involved (i.e., the left hemisphere is also involved because of its executive function). According to Taylor and Heilman (1980, p. 588) this provides the right hand with "direct access to skills learned by the left hand (and stored in the left hemisphere)." Presumably, following right hand training, the left hand only has indirect access to the acquired skills, via interhemispheric communication.

3.3 MOTOR OVERFLOW

A similar pattern of asymmetry exists for the nonfunctional, involuntary movements in one hand that often accompany performance of the other hand (i.e., motor overflow or mirror movements). Specifically, there is greater motor overflow when the left hand is active (i.e., to the right hand) than the reverse (Todor and Lazarus, 1986). The explanation for this asymmetry is similar to that of transfer of training — "due to the left-hemisphere's propensity for motor control and the activation of both hemispheres for left-hand performance, a greater spread of neural activity is generated in the other (right) hand. Conversely, because only the left hemisphere is involved in right-hand control, overflow to the left hand is minimal" (Edwards and Elliott, 1987, p. 301).

3.4 SUMMARY

Contrary to the findings of Flowers (1975), it thus appears that at least in right-handers, the preferred hand is not only faster and more consistent at finger-tapping, but also at finger-sequencing. These performance advantages, as well as asymmetries in intermanual transfer of training and motor overflow, suggest that the left cerebral hemisphere plays a special role in the organization and control of sequential finger movements, particularly in the temporal specification of muscular contractions. In terms of the original proposal of Woodworth (1899), the research on sequential finger movements suggests that the "seat of superiority of the right hand is probably in the motor centers."

4. ASYMMETRIES IN MANUAL AIMING

4.1 FEEDBACK PROCESSING VS. OUTPUT SPECIFICATION?

Certainly the most researched activity in the manual asymmetry literature is goal-directed reaching or aiming. From the time of Woodworth (1899), studies of manual target aiming have found right hand advantages, at least when target-aiming error and movement time have been the primary indices of performance (Todor and Smiley, 1985; see Chapter 8 for a discussion of left hand advantages in movement initiation). Until recently, the most popular position has been that right hand superiority at aiming reflects a right hand/left hemisphere propensity for closed-loop control; that is, the preferred hand system is either faster or more efficient at processing and utilizing response-produced feedback. This notion has been based primarily on the finding that hand differences in aiming performance increase along with the accuracy demands of the target-aiming task (Flowers, 1975).

Flowers' (1975) closed-loop explanation of manual asymmetries in aiming has been extended by Todor and Doane (1978) who found that for a given index of difficulty (Fitts,

1954), right hand advantages for movement time are more dependent on the size of the target than the amplitude of the target aiming movement.* Presumably, acquiring a small target puts greater demands on visual feedback processing for which the right hand system has an advantage.

Support for the position that the right hand/left hemisphere system enjoys an advantage in processing visual feedback also comes from Roy (1983), who approached the problem by manipulating subjects' instructional set rather than the accuracy demands of the movement. When subjects were given instructions emphasizing accuracy, the right hand exhibited a small, but reliable advantage. However, this advantage increased markedly when participants were instructed to move as rapidly as possible. According to Roy (1983) the temporal constraints in the *speed* condition allowed the "system most proficient at processing feedback regarding the relative positions of the pencil and the target(s)" to "experience an increased advantage."

Annett, Annett, Hudson, and Turner (1979) examined the ability of the two hands to rapidly place small pegs into target holes with different tolerances. As in the aiming work, they found that preferred hand advantages for movement time were most pronounced when the movement amplitudes were large and the target tolerances small. Based on film of the peg placement movements, Annett et al. suggested that the nonpreferred hand exhibited greater programming noise and thus required a greater number of time-consuming movements corrections while approaching the target. This explanation of manual asymmetry is consistent with the finger-tapping and finger-sequencing findings discussed earlier in that it emphasizes the differential ability of the right hand and left hand systems to select, specify, and time the muscular forces required for movement.

Todor and Cisneros (1985) attempted a more detailed kinematic analysis of goal-directed aiming by mounting an accelerometer on a stylus which subjects used to perform a discrete Fitts' aiming task. Since the longer movement times found for the left hand were primarily a result of the time spent after peak velocity when visual feedback processing is thought to be most important (Carlton, 1981), Todor and Cisneros concluded that in right-handers the right hand system is more efficient at processing response-produced visual feedback. Although their explanation of hand differences is consistent with Flowers' (1975) feedback processing hypothesis, their data can be interpreted from a different perspective. Specifically, it could be that greater programming noise associated with left hand performance results in the need for time-consuming adjustments late in the aiming movement (e.g., Annett et al., 1979). Further, the left hand system may be less able to specify and time the precise muscular forces required for fine adjustments. Once again, these latter two suggestions are more consistent with accounts for the tapping and sequencing data.

4.2 VISUAL FEEDBACK PROCESSING VS. OUTPUT VARIABILITY?

Although there has been speculation about the role of feedback processing in the expression of manual asymmetries since the time of Woodworth (1899), Roy and Elliott (1986, 1989) were the first investigators to approach the problem directly by manipulating visual feedback. In two experiments, Roy and Elliott (1986) had subjects aim a stylus at a small illuminated target in two different visual conditions. In a full-vision condition, subjects were able to see their limb and the stylus over the course of the movement, while in a no-vision condition the room lights were extinguished upon movement initiation and were not restored until after the movement was completed. This situation prevented the

* Index of difficulty = Log_2 (2 × Amplitude/Target Width)

subjects from processing visual information about the relative positions of the stylus and target during the movement. Subjects performed aiming movements in these two visual conditions with both the right and the left hands over a range of movement times (100 to 400 ms). As in previous studies, hand differences in movement error increased as movement time decreased. Although visual condition had a profound effect on movement accuracy, particularly when the movement times were long, the right hand advantage for movement accuracy did not depend upon the availability of visual feedback.

Based on suggestions by Honda (1982, 1984) that right hand advantages for manual aiming may reflect an attentional strategy related to preferential visual monitoring of the right hand, Roy and Elliott (1989) conducted two follow-up studies to determine whether manual aiming asymmetries were related to the differential use of visual information before movement initiation (see Elliott and Madalena, 1987). In these experiments, a condition was included in which visual information about the position of the limb and the target was eliminated 10 seconds before movement initiation. This manipulation resulted in a large overall increase in target-aiming error. As well, the no-vision delay before movement initiation caused a greater deterioration in performance in the left hand than the right hand. These findings are not entirely compatible with the notion that right hand performance advantages are related to the use of visual feedback/information about the relative positions of the target and the hand during the movement. Further, Carnahan, Roy, and Elliott (1993) have shown that when pointing with the left hand the eyes move toward the target before the hand even when movement speed is emphasized. If anything, this suggests an attentional bias in favor of left hand and not right hand movements (cf. Honda, 1982, 1984).

Questioning the viability of visual feedback accounts of manual asymmetries, Roy and Elliott (1986, 1989) suggested an alternative. Since hand differences in aiming error generally increase as movement speed increases, the extent of manual aiming asymmetries may be related to the absolute force requirements of the movement. As Schmidt, Zelaznik, Hawkins, Frank, and Quinn (1979) have demonstrated, force variability and movement end-point variability (error) increase proportionally with the absolute force requirements of a movement. Thus, "the lesser effect of movement speed on accuracy for the right hand may indicate that the right-hand system is less variable in generating force for a particular movement" extent (Roy and Elliott, 1989). However, this explanation is at odds with the finding that movement extent, a variable which affects the absolute force required to complete a movement in a given time, did not differentially influence aiming performance of the two hands (Roy and Elliott, 1989).

Other investigators examining a visual feedback based account of manual asymmetries have come to similar conclusions as Roy and Elliott (1989). Carson, Chua, Elliott, and Goodman (1990) conducted a manual aiming study in which they manipulated visual information about target and limb position independently. Although visual condition had a modest effect on movement time and a profound effect on movement accuracy, the pattern of results was similar for the two hands. In this study, reaction time was also included as a dependent variable and surprisingly subjects were faster initiating responses to targets with their left hand, particularly when the targets were presented to the left of the subjects midline. This type of finding will be discussed in more detail later (see also Chapter 8).

In a subsequent study Carson, Goodman, Chua, and Elliott (1993) examined the kinematics of right and left hand aiming movements in the same four visual conditions (i.e., full-vision, vision of limb, vision of target, no-vision). Once again, the right hand exhibited clear movement time and accuracy advantages that were independent of visual condition. The left hand was slightly faster at initiating a response. Like the performance findings, kinematic asymmetries were not mediated by visual condition. Overall the right hand achieved higher peak velocities than the left hand, and subjects exhibited a greater number of changes in acceleration following peak velocity when aiming with the left hand. Since discontinuities in acceleration following peak velocity are thought to reflect modifications to the initial movement trajectory, it is conceivable that the left hand is more dependent on nonvisual closed-loop regulation than the right hand. As suggested earlier, this type of regulation late in the movement could reflect less precise force specification or production during earlier stages of the movement (e.g., Annett et al., 1979).

Given that a visual feedback interpretation of Flowers' (1975) closed-loop explanation of manual asymmetries is difficult to reconcile with the results of studies in which visual feedback was manipulated directly, Carson, Elliott, Goodman, Thyer, Chua, and Roy (1993) decided to pursue an output variability hypothesis directly by manipulating the force requirements of the aiming movements. Rather than varying movement time and movement amplitude (cf. Roy and Elliott, 1989), Carson et al. (1993a) manipulated the mass of the limb by securing weights to a subject's wrist. Because force variability and thus the spatial variability about the movement endpoint increases with the absolute amount of force that must be produced (Schmidt et al., 1979), variable error was expected to increase with the mass secured to the limb. In terms of manual asymmetries, if the left hand/arm system is less able to specify and produce the required force for a particular movement then the disadvantage of that system should become more pronounced with the addition of an equivalent mass, that is, more mass requires greater muscular forces that will result in greater force variability, and therefore endpoint variability.

As expected, the right hand outperformed the left hand. Whereas the addition of mass to the right and left limbs did result in increased movement error, the two hands were not differentially affected. Moreover, the analysis of kinematic variables presumed to be sensitive to variation in force production, such as peak velocity, time to peak velocity, and variability in these two measures, failed to reveal any hand differences. Thus, Carson et al. (1993a, p. 298) concluded that "changes in impulse variability accruing from alterations in task demands were apparently independent of the factors that give rise to differences in endpoint variability of the hands." Moreover, the asymmetry in target-aiming error could not be attributed to visual feedback utilization, since in both experiments of Carson et al. vision of the limb was eliminated upon movement initiation.

4.3 KINESTHETIC FEEDBACK PROCESSING?

The finding that hand differences in manual aiming cannot be attributed to either visual feedback utilization or variability in the specification of the initial movement impulse has led investigators to consider other alternatives. One possibility is that the right hand system may be more proficient at the utilization of kinesthetic feedback, as Woodworth (1899) had originally proposed. This suggestion is compatible with findings by Roy, Kalbfleisch, and Elliott (1994) who have reported that movement time differences between the hands are primarily due to the time spent after peak velocity. The temporal advantage for the right hand occurred regardless of whether or not vision of the hand was permitted, and suggests that the right hand system may be more adept at using nonvisual sources of feedback to guide the limb to the target. That is, "the right system may take less time to detect and/or correct errors" based on proprioceptive feedback (Roy et al., 1994, p. 294). However, an alternative explanation may be that while the right hand system is no better at detecting error, it may be superior at producing the precise muscular forces necessary to correct a movement error when the limb is in the vicinity of the target.

4.4 OUTPUT SPECIFICATION: MOVEMENT MODIFICATIONS

While the kinematic studies discussed up to this point have failed to detect hand differences in force production (Carson et al., 1993a, 1993b; Roy et al., 1994), these experiments have been concerned primarily with variability in the initial movement impulse. In our most recent work, we have attempted to study the differential ability of the hands to rapidly adjust the movement trajectory by perturbing the target position (Elliott, Lyons, Chua, Goodman, and Carson, in press). In this study, we had subjects moving a mouse on a graphics tablet (away from the body) in order to move a cursor on a computer monitor (from bottom to top). The movements were initiated at the midline with the right or left hand to a target that was also on the midline. On the majority (60%) of trials the target remained stationary, but on other randomly placed trials it shifted 3 cm to the right (20%) or left (20%) when the subject had moved half the distance to the initial target position (cf. Paulignan, MacKenzie, Marteniuk, and Jeannerod, 1991). Of interest was how quickly and/or precisely the right and left hands could make the adjustment to this target perturbation.

Interestingly, when the target remained stationary there were no reliable differences between the hands either for movement time or any of the kinematic variables examined. This is similar to other studies we have conducted employing a graphics tablet (e.g., Maraj, Roy, Elliott, and Lyons, 1994), and may reflect the spatial and perceptual-motor translation that is required with this type of task (i.e., greater right hemisphere involvement; see Chapter 8). However, when the target position was perturbed the right hand was faster and less variable at completing the movement regardless of the direction of the perturbation.

Our kinematic analyzes revealed that the right hand advantage in the perturbation conditions was *not* due to the speed with which an initial adjustment to the perturbation was made. Rather, it was the case that the right hand spent less time near the new target position after peak velocity in the new trajectory was achieved. Once again, it appears reasonable to suppose that the right hand advantage reflects superiority at producing the small corrective changes necessary to acquire the final target position.

If it is assumed that when performing the aiming task, subjects fixate the initial target position; an unexpected but interesting finding in this study was a main effect for visual field in the "time-to-adjust" to a perturbation. Specifically, subjects initiated a correction to a perturbation in left space more quickly than to perturbations in right space regardless of the performing hand. This left space/right hemisphere advantage may reflect a propensity for spatial decision-making (e.g., Kimura, 1969) or the allocation of attention (e.g., Heilman and Valenstein, 1979). Alternatively, it could reflect the early involvement of the right cerebral hemisphere in the organization of spatial aspects of the movement (Chua, Carson, Goodman, and Elliott, 1992; Elliott, Roy, Goodman, Carson, Chua, and Maraj, 1993; see also Chapter 8).

4.5 SPATIAL ASYMMETRIES

Performance asymmetries related to hemispace are not confined to situations involving a target perturbation. Although there are typically overall right hand advantages for movement time and movement error and sometimes left hand advantages for reaction time, the two hands generally perform best when moving in their own hemispace (e.g., Bradshaw, Bradshaw, and Nettleton, 1990; Elliott et al., 1993; Fisk and Goodale, 1985; Van Der Staak, 1975; cf. Guiard, Diaz, and Beaubaton, 1983).* These ipsilateral performance advantages for target-aiming are assumed to occur because at least some aspects

* Bradshaw et al. (1990) have demonstrated that overall right hand advantages for movement time and left hand advantages for reaction time increase with the complexity of the response.

of the movement are better organized within a cerebral hemisphere (see Figure 7.2). Presumably when a hand is working in contralateral space the greater need for inter-hemispheric communications results in the loss, or at least degradation, of task relevant information. This position is consistent with kinematic findings which indicate greater variability in the time to achieve peak velocity when either the right or left hand is operating in contralateral space (Carson, Goodman, and Elliott, 1992). Interestingly, this asymmetry exists concurrently with an overall right hand advantage in temporal consistency which has the right hand performing as well as the left hand in left space (Carson et al., 1992). This type of data is compatible with the idea that the left hemisphere plays a special role in specifying, timing, and modulating the muscular forces required to move the performing limb to the target.

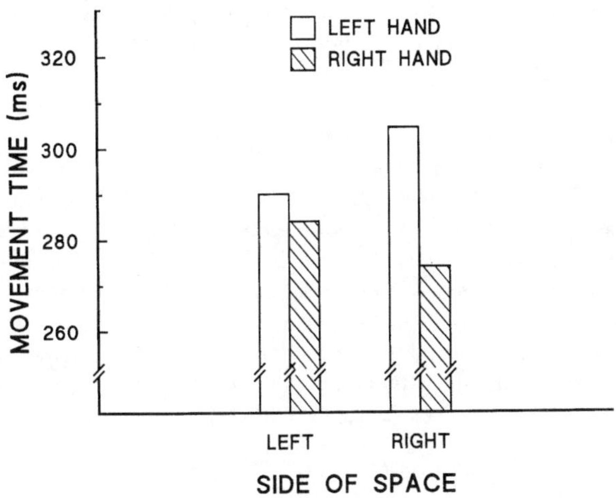

Figure 7.2 Movement time as a function of hand and side of space. (From D. Elliott, E.A. Roy, D. Goodman, R.G. Carson, R. Chua, and B.K.V. Maraj, *Can. J. Exp. Psychol.*, 47, 581, 1993. ©1993. Canadian Psychological Association. Reprinted with permission.)

In a very recent study, Morgan, Bradshaw, Phillips, Mattingley, Iansek, and Bradshaw (1994) also demonstrated that the right hand moves faster and more consistently than the left hand in right space. However, in line with the Elliott et al. (in press) perturbation study, both hands exhibited movement time advantages when moving leftward to targets in left hemispace. Morgan et al. (1994, p. 194) suggested that "a right-hemisphere mediation of visually directed movements into left hemispace, along with a left-hemisphere mediation of fast, precise, temporal sequencing may jointly determine" these more complex asymmetries. This proposal is certainly compatible with the position taken here that even relatively simple movement tasks require the cooperative interaction of different processing systems (see also Carson, 1989 and Hellige, 1993).

4.6 SUMMARY

Almost 100 years after Woodworth (1899), it is still difficult to decide whether manual performance asymmetries in target-aiming are the result of a right hand/left hemisphere propensity for organizing and implementing specific movement commands or in rapidly and efficiently evaluating response-produced feedback. This is in spite of the fact that current researchers have much more sophisticated ways of evaluating goal-directed movements than were available to Woodworth at the turn of the century.

4.6.1 Feedback Processing

The bulk of the evidence would seem to indicate that any feedback processing advantage enjoyed by the right hand system does not extend to the processing of visual feedback. A number of systematic studies in which visual response-produced feedback was manipulated directly have found that the right hand moves more rapidly, more accurately, and with less temporal and spatial variability regardless of the visual circumstance (e.g., Carson et al., 1990, 1993b; Roy and Elliott, 1986, 1989). However, a recent study by Elliott, Chua, and Pollock (1994) may provide a small footnote to this issue. In previous studies (e.g., Carson et al., 1990, 1993b), vision was always manipulated in essentially an all or none fashion. If one hand/hemisphere system is more proficient at processing and utilizing visual feedback, then visual mediation of manual asymmetries may emerge when visual feedback utilization is challenged under conditions of intermittent visual sampling. Indeed, Elliott et al. (1994) provided some data to suggest that right hand advantages may increase when the continuity of visual information during movement is perturbed and made intermittent.

The general failure to find evidence in favor of a visual feedback based account of the right hand advantage in manual aiming (cf. Elliott et al., 1994) leaves us with Woodworth's (1899, p. 34) proposal that "the muscle, joint and skin sensations from the right arm are probably more delicate than those from the left." That is to say that the right hand may be superior at processing kinesthetic feedback (e.g., Roy et al., 1994). However, a problem with this proposal emerges in the face of a number of other studies demonstrating left hand superiority of kinesthetic spatial judgments. For example, Benton et al. (1978) have shown that right-handers can judge the spatial orientation of small metal rods better with their left hand than their right hand. As well, Witelson (1974) has demonstrated that the left hand is better at matching nonsense shapes to a visual pattern. Even when the tactile task involves language such as reading braille the left hand in right-handers appears to enjoy an advantage (Smith, Chu, and Edmonston, 1977; see also Young and Ellis, 1979).

These left side advantages are not restricted to tasks involving finger manipulations. Roy and MacKenzie (1978) have demonstrated that when put in opposition, subjects are able to reproduce a kinesthetic spatial location better with their left thumb than their right thumb (see also Kimura and Vanderwolf, 1970). Similar asymmetries have been found for blind foot positioning (Carnahan and Elliott, 1987). If anything, then, the left hand/right hemisphere system appears to be superior at making kinesthetic spatial judgments.

Recent work alluded to earlier also indicates that the propensity of the right hemisphere at making spatial judgments is not restricted to the kinesthetic modality. Specifically, when an aiming task involves spatial uncertainty, there is often a left hand advantage, as well as a left field/hemispace advantage for movement initiation. That is, subjects are able to identify the spatial location of a target and initiate movement most quickly when the left hand is operating in left space. While this left hand advantage is discussed in detail in Chapter 8, it certainly appears that the right cerebral hemisphere may play a special role in allocating visual attention and/or organizing the spatial aspects of an upcoming movement.

4.6.2 Output Specification

The right hand advantage in movement execution appears to involve *production* rather than the *perception* of kinesthetic or visual-spatial relations. Examinations of impulse variability accounts of manual asymmetries have garnered little support for the hypothesis that performance asymmetries may be mediated by a differential ability of the hand/hemisphere systems to consistently specify the initial movement impulse (e.g., Carson et al., 1993a). However, hand differences seem to emerge during the latter portions of aiming movements, suggesting that the right hand may be more proficient at specifying and producing the precise muscular forces required to modify the terminal trajectory to achieve an exact movement endpoint.* Presumably, adjustments to the movement trajectory are made on the basis of whatever sensory (e.g., vision, kinesthesis) or motor (e.g., efference) information is available.

The notion that the right hand/left hemisphere system is better at precisely modulating muscular force is consistent with the finger-tapping and finger-sequencing data which indicate the most pronounced hand differences at the points of movement transitions, where timing the bursts of opposing muscles is crucial. Timing the interaction and relative contribution of various muscle groups is also important in tasks such as throwing for which the right hand in right-handers enjoys a distinct performance advantage (Calvin, 1983; Watson and Kimura, 1989). Moreover, the proposal that the left hemisphere has a particular propensity for coordinating the activity of various muscle groups is consistent with the idea that left hemisphere specialization for speech and language is at least partially due to preeminence in controlling the articulatory musculature (e.g., Goodale, 1988; Kimura, 1982; Wolf and Goodale, 1987). That is, the left hemisphere has an advantage at open-loop motor control (Haaland and Harrington, 1994; cf. Sussman and MacNeilage, 1975).

5. CONCLUSION

On the basis of some positive evidence, but partly by default, a century later it would appear that Woodworth (1899, p. 34) was correct in asserting that the "seat of superiority of the right hand is probably in the motor centers." Presumably manual performance asymmetries appear in tasks such as finger-sequencing, throwing, and manual aiming, because the ability of the hand/hemisphere system to precisely modulate muscular forces is the primary limiting factor. Overall performance differences between the hands, however, do not reflect the fact that one or the other cerebral hemisphere is responsible for that activity. Although the left hemisphere clearly plays a dominant role in tasks such as finger-sequencing, in tasks such as goal-directed aiming both cerebral hemispheres provide specialized contributions. By systematic manipulation of various aspects of a task, and examining the process by which a movement goal is achieved, experiments conducted in our laboratory and elsewhere suggest that the right cerebral hemisphere plays a role very early in the movement organization process (see Chapter 8). Specifically, it appears that the right cerebral hemisphere is involved "in either establishing the spatial location of the movement goal on the basis of environmentally derived information or in planning the goal directed spatial organization of the ensuing movement" (Elliott et al., 1993, p. 585). When the spatial coordinates of the movement goal must be translated into muscular forces operating at different joints at different times, the role of the left cerebral hemisphere emerges. Thus, a coordinated reaching or aiming movement typically involves the cooperative interaction of two specialized functional systems.

* This suggestion is consistent with work by Fisk and Goodale (1988) who demonstrated that patients with damage to the left cerebral hemisphere have problems in the final corrective phase of an aiming movement.

In summary, hand differences on specific aspects of manual performance, and in particular circumstances, provide us with a unique window into how cerebral systems interact in order to control complex goal-directed movements. Depending upon the nature of the activity, we might observe the predominant contribution of a single hemisphere or the complex interplay of both hemispheres.

ACKNOWLEDGMENTS

We would like to thank our friends and colleagues who collaborated with us on many of the studies reviewed in this chapter. These include Richard Carson, Eric Roy, David Goodman, Heather Carnahan, John Dickinson, Jim Lyons, Jackie Edwards, Brian Maraj, Winston Byblow, Dan Weeks, and Barb Pollock. We are indebted to Mary Cleland for her word processing skills which she used here, and in fact on the whole book.

The majority of the studies conducted in the McMaster, Simon Fraser and Waterloo laboratories were funded by the Natural Science and Engineering Research Council of Canada.

REFERENCES

Annett, J., Annett, M., Hudson, P.T.W., and Turner, A. (1979). The control of movement in the preferred and nonpreferred hands. *Q. J. Exp. Psychol.*, 31, 641.

Benton, A.L., Varney, N.R., and deHamsher, K.S. (1978). Lateral differences in tactile directional perception. *Neuropsychologia*, 16, 109.

Bradshaw, J.L., Bradshaw, J.A., and Nettleton, N.C. (1990). Abduction, adduction and hand differences in simple and serial movements. *Neuropsychologia*, 28, 917.

Calvin, W.H. (1983). A stone's throw and its launch window: timing precision and its implications for language and hominid brains. *J. Theor. Biol.*, 104, 121.

Carlton, L.G. (1981). Processing visual feedback information for movement control. *J. Exp. Psychol.: Hum. Percept. Perf.*, 7, 1019.

Carlton, L.G. (1992). Visual processing time and the control of movement. In L. Proteau and D. Elliott (Eds.), *Vision and Motor Control*, Amsterdam, North-Holland, 3.

Carnahan, H. and Elliott, D. (1987). Pedal asymmetry in the reproduction of spatial locations. *Cortex*, 23, 157.

Carnahan, H., Roy, E.A., and Elliott, D. (1993). Eye, head and hand coordination while pointing with the left and right hands. *J. Hum. Move. Stud.*, 25, 1.

Carson, R.G. (1989). Manual asymmetries: Feedback processing, output variability and spatial complexity. Resolving some inconsistencies. *J. Motor Behav.*, 21, 38.

Carson, R.G., Chua, R., Elliott, D., and Goodman, D. (1990a). The contribution of vision to asymmetries in manual aiming. *Neuropsychologia*, 28, 1215.

Carson, R.G., Elliott, D., Goodman, D., and Dickinson, J.D. (1990b). Manual asymmetries in the reproduction of a 3-dimensional spatial location. *Neuropsychologia*, 28, 99.

Carson, R.G., Elliott, D., Goodman, D., Thyer, L., Chua, R., and Roy, E.A. (1993a). The role of impulse variability in manual aiming asymmetries. *Psychol. Res.*, 55, 291.

Carson, R.G., Goodman, D., Chua, R., and Elliott, D. (1993b). Asymmetries in the regulation of visually guided aiming. *J. Motor Behav.*, 25, 21.

Carson, R.G., Goodman, D., and Elliott, D. (1992). Asymmetries in the discrete and pseudocontinuous regulation of visually guided reaching. *Brain Cognit.*, 18, 169.

Chua, R., Carson, R.G., Goodman, D., and Elliott, D. (1992). Asymmetries in the spatial localization of transformed targets. *Brain Cognit.*, 20, 227.

Edwards, J.M. and Elliott, D. (1987). The effect of unimanual training on contralateral motor overflow in children and adults. *Dev. Neuropsychol.*, 3, 299.

Edwards, J.M. and Elliott, D. (1989). Asymmetries in intermanual transfer of training and motor overflow in adults with Down's syndrome and nonhandicapped children. *J. Clin. Exp. Neuropsychol.*, 11, 959.

Elliott, D. (1985). Manual asymmetries in the performance of sequential movement by adolescents and adults with Down syndrome. *Am. J. Ment. Def.*, 90, 90.

Elliott, D. (1991). Human handedness reconsidered. *Behav. Brain Sci.*, 14, 341.

Elliott, D., Chua, R., and Pollock, B.J. (1994). The influence of intermittent vision on manual aiming. *Acta Psychol.*, 85, 1.

Elliott, D., Lyons, J., Chua, R., Goodman, D., and Carson, R.G. (in press). The influence of target perturbation on manual aiming asymmetries in right-handers. *Cortex*.

Elliott, D., and Madalena, J. (1987). The influence of premovement visual information on manual aiming. *Q. J. Exp. Psychol.*, 39A, 541.

Elliott, D. Roy, E.A., Goodman, D., Carson, R.G., Chua, R., and Maraj, B.K.V. (1993). Asymmetries in the preparation and control of manual aiming movements. *Can. J. Exp. Psychol.*, 47, 570.

Elliott, D., Weeks, D.J., and Jones, R. (1986). Lateral asymmetries in finger-tapping by adolescents and young adults with Down syndrome. *Am. J. Ment. Def.*, 90, 90.

Fisk, J.D. and Goodale, M.A. (1985). The organization of eye and limb movements during unrestricted reaching to targets in contralateral and ipsilateral visual space. *Exp. Brain Res.*, 60, 159.

Fisk, J.D. and Goodale, M.A. (1988). The effects of unilateral brain damage on visually guided reaching: Hemispheric differences in the nature of the deficit. *Exp. Brain Res.*, 72, 425.

Fitts, P.M. (1954). The information capacity of the human motor system in controlling the amplitude of movement. *J. Exp. Psychol.*, 47, 381.

Flowers, K. (1975). Handedness and controlled movement. *Br. J. Psychol.*, 66, 381.

Goodale, M.A. (1988). Hemispheric differences in motor control. *Behav. Brain Res.*, 30, 203.

Guiard, Y., Diaz, D., and Beaubaton, D. (1983). Left hand advantage for right handers for spatial constant error: Preliminary evidence in a unimanual ballistic aimed movement. *Neuropsychologia*, 21, 111.

Haaland, K.Y. and Harrington, D.L.(1994). Limb-sequencing deficits after left but not right hemisphere damage. *Brain Cognit.*, 24, 104.

Heilman, K.M. and Valenstein, E. (1979). Mechanisms underlying hemispatial neglect. *Ann. Neurol.*, 5, 166.

Hellige, J.B. (1993). *Hemispheric Asymmetry: What's Right and What's Left*. Cambridge, Harvard University Press.

Honda, H. (1982). Rightward superiority of eye movements in a bimanual aiming task. *Q. J. Exp. Psychol.*, 34A, 499.

Honda, H. (1984). Functional between-hand differences and outflow eye position information. *Q. J. Exp. Psychol.*, 36A, 75.

Kimura, D. (1969). Spatial localization in the left and right visual fields. *Can. J. Psychol.*, 23, 445.

Kimura, D. and Vanderwolf, C.H. (1970). The relation between hand preference and the performance of individual finger movements by left and right hands. *Brain*, 93, 769.

Kimura, D. (1982). Left-hemisphere control of oral and brachial movements and their relation to communication. *Phil. Trans. R. Soc.*, B298, 135.

Luria, A.R. (1966). *Higher Cortical Functions in Man*. New York, Basic Books.

Maraj, B.K.V., Roy, E.A., Elliott, D., and Lyons, J. (1994). The influence of spatial mapping on manual aiming asymmetries. Paper presented at the North American Society for the Psychology of Sport and Physical Activity Conference, Florida, June.

Morgan, M., Bradshaw, J.L., Phillips, J.G., Mattingley, J.B., Iansek, R., and Bradshaw, J.A. (1994). Effects of hand and age upon abductive and adductive movements: A kinematic analysis. *Brain Cognit.*, 25, 194.

Paulignan, Y., MacKenzie, C.L., Marteniuk, R.G., and Jeannerod, M. (1991). Selective perturbation of visual input during prehension movements. I. The effects of changing object position. *Exp. Brain Res.*, 83, 502.

Peters, M. (1976). Prolonged practice of a simple motor task by preferred and nonpreferred hands. *Percept. Motor Skills*, 43, 447.

Peters, M. (1980). Why the preferred hand taps more quickly than the nonpreferred hand: Three experiments on handedness. *Can. J. Psychol.*, 34, 62.

Peters, M. and Durding, B.M. (1978). Handedness measured by finger tapping: A continuous variable. *Can. J. Psychol.*, 32, 257.

Peters, M. and Durding, B.M. (1979). Left-handers and right-handers compared on a motor task. *J. Motor Behav.*, 11, 103.

Provins, K.A. (1956). Handedness and skill. *Q. J. Exp. Psychol.*, 8, 79.

Reitan, R. and Davison, L. (1974). *Clinical Neuropsychology: Current Status and Applications*. Washington, D.C., Winston and Sons.

Roy, E.A. (1983). Manual performance asymmetries and motor control processes: Subject-generated changes and response parameters. *Hum. Move. Sci.*, 2, 271.

Roy, E.A. (1985). (Ed.) *Neuropsychological Studies of Apraxia and Related Disorders*. Amsterdam, North-Holland.

Roy, E.A. and Elliott, D. (1986). Manual asymmetries in visually directed aiming. *Can. J. Psychol.*, 40, 109.

Roy, E.A. and Elliott, D. (1989). Manual asymmetries in aimed movements. *Q. J. Exp. Psychol.*, 41A, 501.

Roy, E.A., Kalbfleisch, L., and Elliott, D. (1994). Kinematic analysis of manual asymmetries in visual aiming movements. *Brain Cognit.*, 24, 289.

Roy, E.A. and MacKenzie, C.L. (1978). Handedness effects on kinesthetic spatial location judgments. *Cortex*, 14, 250.

Ruisel, I. (1970). Crossed laterality of the upper and lower extremities. *Studia Psychol.*, 17, 71.

Schmidt, R.A., Zelaznik, H.N., Hawkins, B., Frank, J.S., and Quinn, J.T. (1979). Motor output variability: A theory for the accuracy of rapid motor acts. *Psychol. Rev.*, 86, 415.

Smith, M.O., Chu, J., and Edmonston, W.E. (1977). Cerebral lateralization of haptic perception: Interaction of responses to Braille and music reveals a functional basis. *Science*, 197, 689.

Sussman, H.M. and MacNeilage, P.F. (1975). Studies of hemispheric specialization for speech production. *Brain Lang.*, 2, 131.

Taylor, H.G. and Heilman, K.M. (1980). Left-hemisphere motor dominance in right-handers. *Cortex*, 16, 587.

Todor, J.I. and Cisneros, J. (1985). Accommodation to increased accuracy demands by the right and left hands. *J. Motor Behav.*, 17, 355.

Todor, J.I. and Doane, T. (1978). Handedness and hemispheric asymmetry in the control of movements. *J. Motor Behav.*, 10, 295.

Todor, J.I., and Kyprie, P.M. (1980). Hand differences in the rate and variability of rapid tapping. *J. Motor Behav.*, 12, 57.

Todor, J.I. Kyprie, P.M., and Price, H.L. (1982). Lateral asymmetries in arm, wrist, and finger movements. *Cortex*, 18, 515.

Todor, J.I. and Lazarus, J.C. (1986). Exertion level and the intensity of associated movements. *Dev. Med. Child Neurol.*, 28, 205.

Todor, J.E. and Smiley, A. (1985). Manual asymmetries in motor control. In E.A. Roy (Ed.), *Neuropsychological Studies of Apraxia and Related Disorders*, Amsterdam, North-Holland, 309.

Todor, J.I. and Smiley-Oyen, A.L. (1987). Force modulation as a source of hand differences in rapid finger tapping. *Acta Psychol.*, 65, 65.

Van Der Staak, C. (1975). Intra- and interhemispheric visual-motor control of human arm movements. *Neuropsychologia*, 13, 439.

Watson, N.V. and Kimura, D. (1989). Right hand superiority for throwing but not for intercepting. *Neuropsychologia*, 27, 1399.

Witelson, S.F. (1974). Hemispheric specialization for linguistic and nonlinguistic tactual perception using a dichotomous stimulation technique. *Cortex*, 10, 3.

Wolf, M.E. and Goodale, M.A. (1987). Oral asymmetries during verbal and non-verbal movements of the mouth. *Neuropsychologia*, 25, 375.

Woodworth, R.S. (1899). The accuracy of voluntary movement. *Psychol. Rev.*, 3, (Monograph Supplement), 1.

Young, A.W. and Ellis, A.W. (1979). Perception of numerical stimuli felt by fingers of the left and right hands. *Q. J. Exp. Psychol.*, 31, 263.

Chapter 8

Putative Right Hemisphere Contributions to the Preparation of Reaching and Aiming Movements

Richard G. Carson

CONTENTS

1. PROLOGUE

Several cerebral cortical areas are now known to be involved in the control of reaching and aiming movements. Lesions in each area give rise to distinct motor dysfunctions. These deficits may range from spatiomotor coordination and misdirected reaching in the case of lesions to the parietal cortex, to disturbances in the learning and recall of motor patterns (prefrontal and premotor cortex), to varying degrees of paralysis (primary motor cortex) (Kalaska and Crammond, 1992).

While visual information mediates the appreciation of both an object's spatial location and its intrinsic properties, the neural bases of visual perception appear to be quite distinct from those which subserve the visual guidance of action (Ungerleider and Mishkin, 1982). Ventral pathways projecting from the striate cortex to the inferotemporal cortex are implicated in the perceptual designation of objects, whereas dorsal pathways projecting from the striate cortex to the posterior parietal cortex appear to subserve the "sensorimotor transformations" upon which visually guided reaching and aiming are based (Goodale and Milner, 1992). The behavioral deficiencies which result from damage to the posterior parietal region corroborate its importance in mediating spatial-motor transformations (e.g., Ghez, 1985).

The stereotypical behavioral outcomes which result from focal damage to the right hemisphere suggest that its visuospatial functions are also fractionated to an appreciable degree. It is now clear that vision and visual imagery do not share the same central (right hemisphere) mechanisms (Marshall and Halligan, 1993). Damage to the right fronto-temporal cortex generally has as its consequence disruption to visuospatial imagery. However, when the lesion is well circumscribed, the deficit does not usually extend to hemispatial neglect (Guariglla, Padovani, Pantano, and Pizzamiglio, 1993). In contrast, damage to the right parietal-lobe and right thalamus may result in left hemispatial neglect when drawing with vision, but not when guided by an internal image (Anderson, 1993). The visual agnosias are characterized by "seeing" without "recognizing" (e.g., Behrmann, Winocur, and Moscovitch, 1992; Jankowiak, Kinsbourne, Shalev, and Bachman, 1992),

0-8493-8999-2/96/$0.00+$.50

whereas their complement is a syndrome in which intact visual recognition is accompanied by a failure to generate images (Basso, Bisiach, and Luzzati, 1980; see also Gurd and Marshall, 1992).

Nonetheless, it is presently unclear how the fractionated visuospatial functions of the right hemisphere impinge upon the regulation of visually guided movements. The clinical data suggest that the variegated neural bases of visuospatial perception and visuospatial movement organization may find expression via clearly delineated behavioral outcomes. In this chapter it will be argued that given the appropriate stimulus and response contexts, the manifold contributions of right hemisphere to the regulation of goal directed movements in "normals" may also be revealed.

2. INTRODUCTION

As the chapters in the present volume attest, considerable attention has been devoted to the links between the functional attributes of the left cerebral hemisphere and the superiority of the preferred hand* for the *execution* of goal directed actions. As the generation of a spatial mapping between a target location and the position of an effector is thought to be a prerequisite for the initiation of these movements (e.g., Morasso and Tagliasco, 1986), it has been postulated that right hemisphere contributions will predominate during movement *preparation* (e.g., Carson, 1989a, 1989b; Guiard, Diaz, and Beaubaton, 1983).

Evidence derived from clinical populations comports with this proposal. Fisk and Goodale (1988) examined reaching movements to visual targets, executed by individuals with well circumscribed unilateral damage to either the left or right cerebral hemisphere. Patients with lesions to the right hemisphere generated reaches which preserved the kinematic characteristics of those made by normals. However, they required longer to prepare and initiate their movements. In contrast, movements made by the group with left hemisphere lesions were initiated with the same latency, yet executed more slowly than those made by their normal counterparts. Converging evidence has been provided by Haaland and Harrington (1989), who noted that only patients having suffered cardiovascular strokes to the right hemisphere exhibited slowed reaction times in a manual aiming task.

In neurologically intact individuals, when the rapid initiation of responses is emphasized, reaction times for aiming movements made by the left hand are generally shorter than those made by the right hand (e.g., Bradshaw, Bradshaw, and Nettleton, 1990; Brown et al., 1989; Carson, Chua, Elliott, and Goodman, 1990; Carson, Goodman, Chua, and Elliott, 1993; Goodman and Kelso, 1980; Haaland and Harrington, 1989). These differences are present in premotor reaction times and thus appear to be central rather than peripheral in origin (Elliott, Roy, Goodman, Carson, Chua, and Maraj, 1993). They are also not attributable to differences in speed-accuracy trade-off strategies (Carson, Chua, Goodman, Byblow, and Elliott, 1995; Chua, Carson, Goodman, and Elliott, 1992).

The presence of these asymmetries admits at least two possibilities. A right hemisphere advantage may exist for the localization of targets, prior to the organization of the movement, arising from greater degree of engagement in spatial coordinate processing (Kosslyn, 1987). An alternative explanation is that the left hand advantage reflects a greater degree of right hemisphere engagement in the "spatial parameterization" of the movement itself. This process is conceived of as the integration and feedforward of information about the position, orientation, and movement of the body as a whole, or part of the body, relative to the environment. It is presumed to occur prior to the initiation of movement (Carson et al., 1995).

* In this paper, any reference to hand advantage is with respect to right handers.

3. ASYMMETRIES IN SPATIAL COORDINATE PROCESSING?

If the left hand advantage for reaction time in manual aiming arises from right hemisphere involvement in spatial coordinate transformations, it would be anticipated that the extent of this asymmetry would covary with the complexity of the processing required to establish the position of a visual target in extrapersonal space (cf. Hellige, 1983). However, in order to assess this proposal, one must necessarily manipulate visuospatial complexity independently of the required response movement (Carson, 1989a; cf. Watson and Kimura, 1989).

Most of the experimental tasks which have been employed to document right hemisphere involvement in the appreciation of visuospatial configurations have employed tachistoscopic presentations, involved simple keypress responses, and have been static rather than dynamic.* In a spatial task of a dynamic nature, Eals (1987) required that subjects predict the final location of a dot array from a series of brief presentations simulating a pattern transition. Individuals were required to predict the spatial array which would occupy the next position in the sequence. Response accuracy was found to be superior for those sequences presented to the left hemi-field, and thus initially to the right hemisphere.

Carson, Goodman, and Elliott (1992) devised an extension of this task, in which the required endpoints of aiming movements were not explicitly defined but were obtained by extrapolating from briefly presented geometric patterns. Four patterns were used, consisting respectively of five point linear, quadratic, cubic, and quartic functions (Figure 8.1). It was assumed that the spatial complexity of each pattern was related to the number of reversals in the function. Having been given prior knowledge of the patterns, the subjects' task was to predict and to move to the position of the final "phantom" point, on the basis of a sequential presentation of the first four points. The display coordinates were chosen to ensure that the actual position of the target was equivalent across all patterns.

An assessment of the time taken to initiate reaches to the target location indicated that movements of the left hand were, on average, 11 ms faster than those of the right hand. The two hands were equally accurate in acquiring the target, although movements of the right hand were executed more rapidly. Contrary to expectations, the manipulation of pattern complexity was without influence upon terminal accuracy or upon the time taken to initiate the movements. Response accuracy and reaction times were also equivalent for sequences displayed in the left and the right visual fields.

As such, the data failed to support Kosslyn's (1987) prediction of a right hemisphere (left visual field or left hand) superiority in establishing the metric spatial coordinates of visual stimuli. However, the manipulation of spatial complexity used by Carson et al. (1992) included a number of possible confounds. The pattern presentation sequence had a strong temporal component. A large body of theoretical work has been based explicitly upon the assumption that the left hemisphere assumes some privileged role in the execution of timing functions (e.g., Bradshaw and Nettleton, 1981; Ojemann, 1984; Tzeng and Wang, 1984). Furthermore, subjects were required to distinguish between four possible spatial configurations. Therefore, the task involved a categorization component in addition to the extraction of metric spatial information. Kosslyn (1987) has proposed that the evaluation of categorical spatial relations is primarily the domain of the left hemisphere (cf., Sergent, 1991). Therefore, the task may have favored the processing propensities of both hemispheres.

* In this context, "dynamic" refers to a spatial configuration which evolves over time.

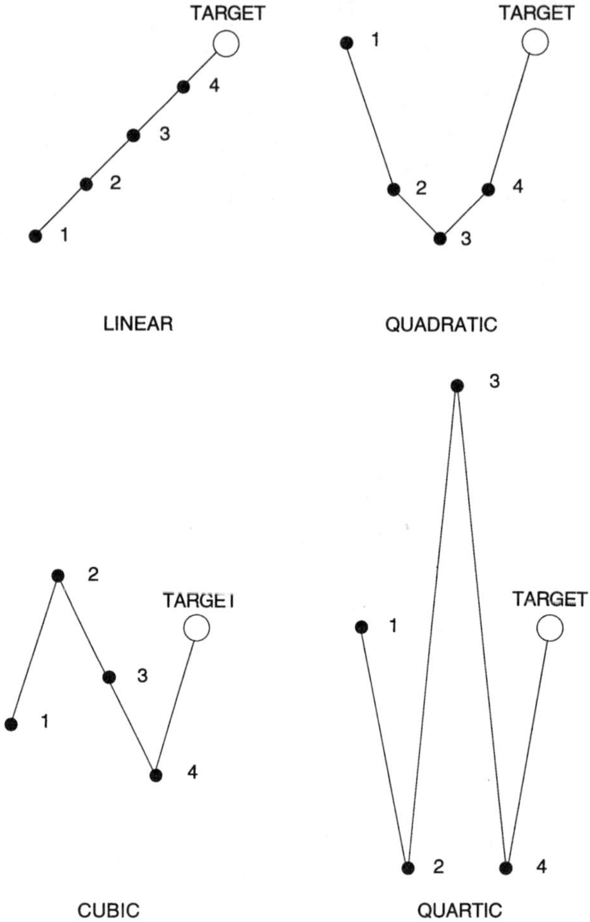

Figure 8.1 Schematic representing the pattern display sequences. (From R.G. Carson, D. Goodman, and D. Elliott, *Brain Cognit.*, 18, 174, 1992. ©1992 by Academic Press, Inc. Reprinted with permission.)

In an attempt to overcome these limitations Chua et al. (1992) utilized a target localization task which had neither strong temporal nor categorization components. Rather than reach directly to targets, subjects were required to make a response movement in a direction other than straight to a visual stimulus. It has been hypothesized that individuals solve tasks of this nature by performing a mental rotation of "an imagined movement vector" from the direction of the visual stimulus to the direction of the required response (Georgopoulous and Massey, 1987). The spatial components of such tasks appear to be lateralized to a greater degree to the right hemisphere (e.g., Corballis and McLaren, 1984; Ratcliffe, 1979). These conjectures have been supported by *direct* physiological measures (Deutsch, Bourbon, Papanicolau, and Eisenberg, 1988; Osaka, 1984; Papanicolau, Deutsch, Bourbon, Will, Loring, and Eisenberg, 1987). Chua et al. (1992) argued that if the left hand advantage for reaction time reflects the engagement of the right hemisphere in establishing the position of a target prior to the initiation of a movement, this advantage would be accentuated in conditions in which the *difficulty* of obtaining the target position was increased. Specifically, greater left hand advantages for reaction time would be anticipated when subjects are required to perform a mental rotation to establish the position of a target, relative to conditions in which the target is presented directly.

In an attempt to evaluate this hypothesis, Chua et al. (1992) required that their subjects make aiming movements in two experimental conditions. In the first (mirror) condition, a stimulus was presented in either the left or the right visual field. Subjects were required to conduct a transformation or mental rotation of the stimulus position about a virtual line dividing the left and right visual fields. The spatial position which resulted from this transformation constituted the target. The target was thus the mirror image of the stimulus position. Subjects were required to move to this target position. In a second (control) condition, subjects were required to move directly to the stimulus position.

As one might have anticipated, movements made directly to the visual stimulus were more accurate, were initiated more rapidly, and also tended to be of shorter duration than those executed in the mirror condition. Consistent with prior expectations, left hand movements were initiated 9 ms more rapidly than right hand movements. However, the extent of this left hand advantage was equivalent in both experimental conditions. Although the mirror transformation appeared to require the representation of spatial relations using a metric coordinate scheme, reaction times were equivalent for responses directed to the left and the right visual fields. The data thus failed to provide support for the hypothesis that there is right hemisphere mediation of these processes.

In a further effort to evaluate the proposition that the left hand advantage in initiating aiming movements arises from right hemisphere involvement in spatial coordinate transformations, Elliott et al. (1993) used an alternative means of manipulating the complexity of the task. They required that their subjects estimate the position of a movement goal by interpolating the center of a 6 cm diameter circle (e.g., Mace, 1931). In a control condition, a small dot served as a target to which subjects were to move directly. Elliott et al. proposed that in the interpolation condition, establishing the location of the target would necessarily require a spatial transformation of the available visual information. It was reasoned that if transformations of this nature are mediated more efficiently by the right hemisphere, the asymmetry will find expression in a left hand advantage for movement preparation.

The results obtained by Elliott et al. (1993) indicated that movements of the left hand were initiated more rapidly than those of the right hand. The left hand advantage for movement initiation was most pronounced when movements were directed into left space. However, the extent of the left hand superiority was equivalent in the interpolation and the control conditions. Movements made by the right hand were executed both more rapidly and more accurately than those made by the left hand, thereby confirming the superiority of the right hand for movement execution.

In each of the studies detailed above, the visuospatial complexity of the aiming task was manipulated independently of the nature of the required response movement. The outcomes of these experiments indicated that increasing the complexity of the transformations necessary to establish the position of targets had little influence upon the magnitude of the left hand advantage for reaction time. Clearly, if the left hand advantage indexes right hemisphere involvement during movement preparation, it does not arise from an engagement in spatial coordinate processing.

4. ASYMMETRIES IN SPATIAL PARAMETERIZATION?

While all movements have a spatial dimension, it is at present unclear how this is encapsulated within a regulatory scheme for movement (cf. Georgopoulous, Schwartz, and Kettner, 1986). It has largely been assumed that a cogent representation of task space is both the initial step for the motor control system and the final step for the vision system (Morasso and Tagliasco, 1986). This presumption has as its corollary the axiom that the influence of spatial localization is confined to neural systems prior to those concerned with motor output (e.g., Fisk and Goodale, 1985). However, evidence from both clinical (Joanette and Brouchon, 1984) and normal (Carson et al., 1992) populations indicates that these processes are not only intermingled but interdependent.

Carson et al. (1992) noted that the integration of information relating the spatial location of a target continues to define the organization of a movement in the period following its initiation. These observations corroborate the supposition that visuospatial localization also impinges upon neural systems which subserve motor output. On the basis of this premise, Carson et al. (1995) examined whether the left hand advantage for reaction time reflects a greater degree of right hemisphere engagement in the spatial parameterization of the movements themselves. In order to do this, they used a variation of the movement precue technique (Goodman and Kelso, 1980; Rosenbaum, 1980). Their rationale was as follows: when provided with advance information regarding the spatial position of a target, subjects may partially prepare their movement to the target in advance of the "go" signal. In circumstances in which no advance information is provided, subjects are unable to accrue the benefit of partial preparation. In these situations, preparation may only commence upon presentation of the imperative stimulus. It was reasoned that if the left hand advantage for reaction time reduces to an advantage in preparing the movement itself, this advantage would be eliminated if the provision of a precue permitted this preparatory activity to take place prior to the reaction time period.

In the first of a series of three experiments, Carson et al. (1995) required that their subjects make aiming movements to visual targets in one of three cue conditions. In the first (SRT8) condition, a simple reaction time paradigm was employed using eight targets. The second (CRT4) condition was a choice reaction time protocol utilizing two sets of four targets. The third (CRT8) condition was also a choice protocol, in this instance using eight targets. In the SRT8 condition, subjects were precued with complete information concerning the target position. In the CRT4 condition, subjects were precued with partial information indicating a subset of four possible target positions. In the CRT8 condition, advance information regarding the target position was entirely ambiguous (Figure 8.2).

Consistent with previous findings, movements made by the left hand were initiated more rapidly than those made by the right hand. More interesting was the observation that the magnitude of the left hand advantage decreased as a function of the amount of advance information which was provided. When the number of target position alternatives was sufficiently large as to prevent advance preparation (in the CRT8 condition), a reliable left hand advantage for reaction time was obtained. However, when subjects were precued as to the exact spatial position of the target in advance of stimulus presentation (in the SRT8 condition) and could therefore complete some portion of movement preparation in advance, the left hand advantage was effectively eliminated.

It was conceivable that the left hand advantage in the choice precue condition indexed a nonspecific difference in the speed with which cued parameters per se could be integrated during movement preparation. Therefore, a second experiment was conducted in which response hand rather than target location was cued (by an auditory signal) either prior to, or simultaneously with, the presentation of the imperative stimulus. The results of this experiment were unambiguous. When subjects were cued as to response hand in advance of target presentation, responses were initiated more rapidly than when hand was cued simultaneously. In the precue condition, left hand movements were initiated more rapidly than right hand movements. In contrast, in the simultaneous cue condition, movements made by the right hand were initiated more rapidly than those made by the left hand.

In the precue condition, the aiming task was analogous to that of the choice conditions of Experiment 1. Subjects were able to select the response hand in advance and thus were required to parameterize the movement primarily along spatial dimensions during the reaction time period. In these circumstances a left hand advantage for speed of preparation was obtained. However, when subjects were forced to parameterize the movement along an additional dimension during this period, in selecting the appropriate response hand, this advantage was reversed. These data suggest that the left hand advantage for reaction time does not reduce to a greater efficiency in integrating movement parameters per se, but rather may be specific to the organization of movement with respect to spatial parameters.

There exists a large body of evidence to support the assertion that reaction times increase with the involution of a response movement (Henry and Rogers, 1960). This outcome is manifested most clearly when subjects are required to both initiate and complete their movements as rapidly as possible. When maximal speeds of execution are not emphasized, reaction times do not necessarily increase across levels of movement complexity, but may remain invariant (e.g., Garcia-Colera and Semjen, 1988). Recently, van Donkelaar and Franks (1991) have argued that when response accuracy is stressed, an execution sequence may be prepared in part during the movement, rather than entirely in advance. This is referred to as "on-line" preparation (van Donkelaar and Franks, 1991).

Carson et al. (1995) argued that the left hand advantage for reaction time reflects a right hemisphere involvement in the *advance* preparation of movement, which is specific to the spatial parameters of the movement. It was thus predicted that the left hand advantage would be reduced or eliminated in circumstances in which on-line preparation was permitted to occur. In order to test this postulate, Carson et al. (1995) conducted a third experiment in which subjects made aiming movements in the three precue conditions employed in their Experiment 1. They also employed two instructional conditions which stressed, respectively, the speed and the accuracy with which the response movements were to be *executed*.

In the fast instructional condition in which on-line preparation was less opportune, a left hand advantage for reaction time was obtained. This asymmetry was substantially reduced in the simple reaction time condition in which subjects could complete some portion of their movement preparation in advance of the imperative stimulus. These outcomes thus replicated those obtained in their Experiment 1. In contrast, in the accurate instructional condition in which subjects were presumably able to engage in some degree of on-line preparation (van Donkelaar and Franks, 1991), reaction times for the left and right hand were equivalent.

The results obtained by Carson et al. (1995) are consistent with the proposal that the left hand advantage for reaction time reflects a greater degree of right hemisphere engagement in the spatial parameterization of aiming movements. However, their data also illustrate that the asymmetry is present only in response contexts in which the speeded initiation and execution of responses is emphasized. If subjects are afforded the opportunity to undertake movement preparation in advance of the reaction time period (as when precued), or if on-line preparation is promoted, the left hand advantage for movement initiation is extinguished.

5. RESPONSE CONTEXT

Asymmetries in reaction time favoring the left hand have been remarkably consistent, in terms of scale, across studies which have varied appreciably in their *stimulus* context

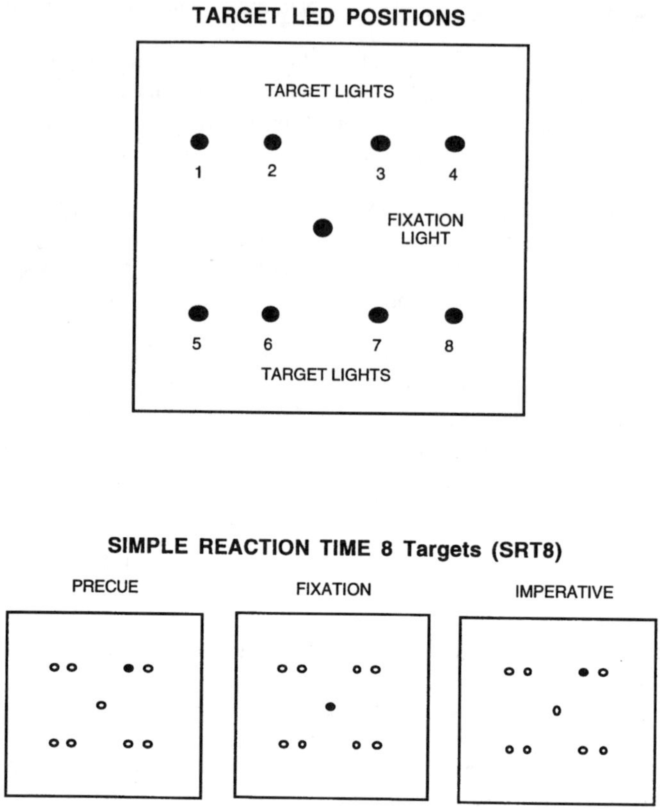

Figure 8.2 Schematic representing the precue-fixation-imperative sequence for the SRT8, CRT4, and CRT8 cue conditions. (From R.G. Carson, R. Chua, D. Goodman, W.D. Byblow, and D. Elliott, *Brain Cognit.*, 28, 136, 1995. ©1995 by Academic Press, Inc. Reprinted with permission.)

(Bradshaw et al., 1990 [12 ms]; Carson et al.,1990 [17 ms]; Carson et al., 1993 [10 ms]; Carson et al., 1995 [7.5 ms, 9 ms and 12.8 ms]; Chua et al., 1992 [9 ms]; Elliott et al., 1993 [12 ms]; Goodman and Kelso, 1980 [21 ms and 11 ms]). The magnitude of this difference also appears to increase with age (Haaland and Harrington, 1989 [155 ms for elderly]; Chua, Pollock, Elliott, Swanson, and Carnahan, 1995 [28 ms for elderly, 11 ms for young and middle aged]). In the majority of these studies, aiming movements requiring flexion of the shoulder joint and extension of the elbow joint (cf. Bradshaw et al., 1990), were directed to distant targets located either in the transverse plane or on a surface perpendicular to the mid-sagittal plane (cf. Haaland and Harrington, 1989). The similarity of the *response* contexts across tasks supports the view that the asymmetries in reaction time are intimately associated with preparation of the aiming response, rather than the perceptual localization of movement targets. The observation that the left hand advantage for reaction time can be eliminated or reversed (Carson et al., 1995) emphasizes that this effect is not simply of structural origin.

However, left hand advantages of another kind can be elicited in quite different response contexts. In slow positioning studies in which spatial accuracy is the sole

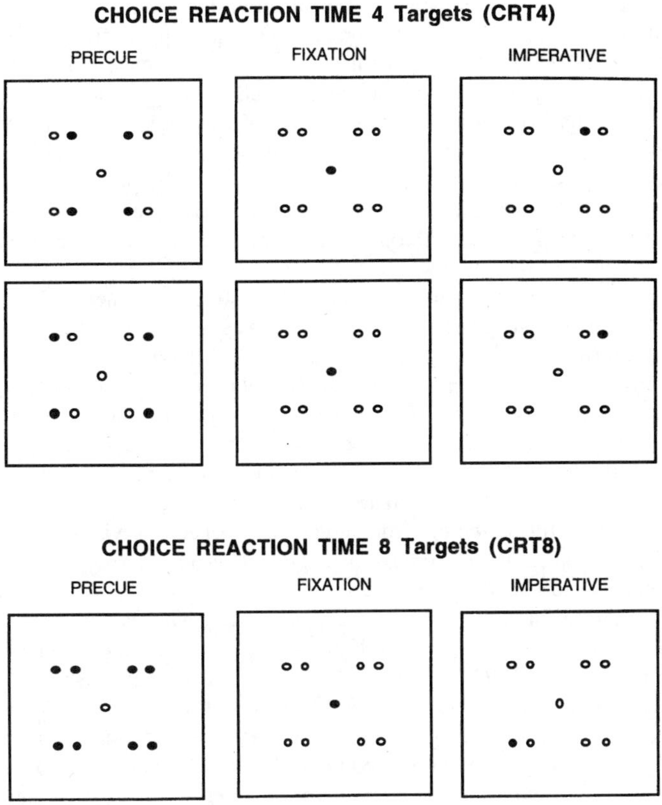

Figure 8.2 (continued)

response criterion, left hand or left side superiority is often observed (e.g., Carnahan and Elliott, 1987; Roy and MacKenzie, 1978). Moreover, Carson, Elliott, Goodman, and Dickinson (1990) found no hand differences in two studies in which subjects were required to reproduce a preselected arm position in 3-dimensional space (see also Watson and Kimura, 1989). In addition, Guiard et al. (1983) obtained a left hand and left field advantage for spatial accuracy in a task requiring rapid positioning. The Guiard et al. data are, however, somewhat anomalous, and conflict with a large body of research suggesting right hand advantages for the execution of *rapid* aiming tasks (Elliott, 1991; Chapter 7).

6. A DESCRIPTIVE FRAMEWORK

Dissociations in the expression of manual asymmetries favoring the nondominant hand support the assertion that the diverse manifestations of right hemisphere involvement in visuomotor processing do not draw upon identical neural substrates. The fractionation of visuospatial functions within the parietal lobe proposed by Goodale and Milner (1992), between the "what" and the "how" of reaching, suggests a descriptive framework within which consideration may also be given to the disparate contributions of the right cerebral hemisphere to visuomotor function. In particular, a distinction between the "where" and the "where to" of visually guided reaching and aiming is promoted.

There are indications of hemispheric specialization for a number of basic perceptual functions. It has been proposed that the processing of low spatial frequencies is accomplished more effectively in the right hemisphere, whereas the processing of high spatial frequencies is more rapid and more accurately discharged by the left hemisphere (e.g., Sergent, 1983). This hypothesis has been supported by studies which have selectively reduced the availability of higher rather than lower spatial frequencies, by increasing in retinal eccentricity, stimulus size, or blur/degradation, and by decreasing luminance or exposure duration (Christman, 1989, 1993; but see also Peterzell, 1991). Additional corroboration has been provided through related research examining evoked potentials (EP) and brain-injured patients (Mecacci, 1993).

In addition, there is a large body of evidence suggesting a right hemisphere advantage, expressed as a left visual field superiority for the establishment of the spatial position of visual stimuli (e.g., Hellige et al., 1994; Hellige and Michimata, 1989; Kosslyn et al., 1989). Recent studies also suggest a left visual field advantage for the acquisition of visual targets, expressed in terms of the spatial accuracy of eye movements (Bracewell, Husain, and Stein, 1990), and for the localization of visual targets in grasping space (MacKenzie, Sivak, and Elliott, 1988). The conclusion may be drawn that right hemisphere advantages for spatial coordinate processing (Kosslyn, 1987) and thus for the localization and transformation of visual targets (the "where" of visually guided action) will, in the appropriate *stimulus* context, be expressed as a *left visual field* advantage for speed or accuracy measures (Sergent, 1991).

Yet visual field asymmetries for the localization of visual targets are not typically exhibited in studies of reaching and aiming movements (e.g., Carson et al., 1992; Chua et al., 1992; Elliott et al., 1993). It is likely that the exemplar aiming task does not provide a stimulus context commensurate with the elicitation of visual field asymmetries. The retinal eccentricities and durations of visual input employed in studies of manual aiming are often beyond those required in divided visual half-field experimentation. In addition, asymmetries in spatial coordinate processing are likely to be most prominent when the task requirements emphasize the determination of perceptual features rather than either the operation of simple sensory processes or the execution of complex cognitive or motor functions. The motor demands of a reaching or aiming task may simply overwhelm and obscure any behavioral asymmetries attributable to perceptual factors (cf. Christman, 1989).

However, robust manual asymmetries exist that favor the left hand which, in protocols requiring speeded initiation of responses are manifested as shorter reaction times, and in protocols requiring the slow positioning of limb segments are evident as enhanced spatial accuracy. It is therefore proposed that there exists a qualitatively distinct right hemisphere advantage for the translation of limb segments through extrapersonal space (the "where to" of visually guided action) which is, in the appropriate *response* context, expressed as a *left hand* advantage for speed or accuracy measures.

While these asymmetries appear to be intimately linked to the spatial parameterization of the response movement, there is no *a priori* metric which permits quantitative specification of a movement's spatial complexity. The relative spatial locations of limb segments and movements goals are succinctly described using a Cartesian coordinate system and may be conceived of in terms of "joint angle coordinates" and "muscle coordinates" (e.g., Hollerbach, 1990). Yet, the extent to which these systems form the organizational bases for the neuromuscular system is not apparent (cf. Turvey and Carello, 1986).

There is presently a limited body of clinical data which speaks to the possible loci of these fractionated functions of the right hemisphere. Harvey, Milner, and Roberts

(1995) have proposed that it is possible to tease apart those aspects of spatial neglect which are of perceptual origin from those which are action-related. Furthermore, it has been demonstrated that the relative contribution of these perceptual and motor factors is directly related to lesion location (Bisiach, Geminiani, Berti, and Rusconi, 1990; Tegnér and Levander, 1991). The etiology of directional hypokinesia (spatially misdirected actions) is generally damage to anterior regions of the right cerebral hemisphere, whereas perceptually based neglect seems to be associated with more posterior, including parietal, lesions (Harvey et al., 1995; Ladavas, Umilta, Ziani, Brogi, and Minarini, 1993; Tegnér and Levander, 1991).

On the basis of these domain specific forms of neglect, it has been argued that the functional architecture of goal directed action is necessarily modular in nature (Umiltà, 1995). The observation that the directional motor form of neglect typically follows disruption of the right frontal lobe, while the perceptual form results from more posterior damage, suggests closely related anatomical dissociations.

Domain specific asymmetries in the organization of manual aiming are also emblematic of modularity of function. Yet, in the absence of clinical correlates, the neuroanatomical bases of these dissociations remain abstruse. Furthermore, domain specific processing modules are also necessarily constituted by networks of neurons which are capable of long range interactions with other areas of the brain (e.g., Bressler, 1995). Studies of oscillatory responses in the visual cortex have demonstrated phase- and frequency-locking in spatially separate neurons within (Gray, König, Engel, and Singer, 1989) and between hemispheres (Engel, König, Kreiter, and Singer, 1991). If the anatomical concomitants of right hemisphere contributions to goal directed movement are to be established, it may be necessary to employ techniques, such as electroencephalography and magnetoencephalography, which are sensitive to temporal and spatial coherence across large areas of cortex.

REFERENCES

Anderson, B. (1993). Spared awareness for the left side of internal visual images in patients with left-sided extrapersonal neglect. *Neurology*, 43, 213.

Basso, A., Bisiach, E., and Luzzati, C. (1980). Loss of mental imagery: A case study. *Neuropsychologia*, 18, 435.

Behrmann, M., Winocur, G., and Moscovitch, M. (1992). *Nature*, 359, 636.

Bisiach, E., Geminiani, G., Berti, A., and Rusconi, M.L. (1990). Perceptual and premotor factors of unilateral neglect. *Neurology*, 40, 1278.

Bracewell, R.M. Husain, M. and Stein, J.F. (1990). Specialization of the right hemisphere for visuomotor control. *Neuropsychologia*, 28, 763.

Bradshaw, J.L., Bradshaw, J.A., and Nettleton, N.C. (1990). Abduction, adduction and hand differences in simple and serial movements. *Neuropsychologia*, 28, 917.

Bradshaw, J.L. and Nettleton, N.C. (1981). The nature of hemispheric specialization in man. *Behav. Brain Sci.*, 4, 51.

Bressler, S.L. (1995). Large-scale cortical networks and cognition. *Brain Res. Reviews*, 20, 288.

Brown, J.V., Schumacker, V., Rohlmann, A., Ettlinger, G., Schmidt, R.C., and Skreczek, W. (1989). Aimed movements to visual targets in hemiplegic and normal children: Is the "good" hand of children with infantile hemiplegia also normal?. *Neuropsychologia*, 27, 283.

Carnahan, H. and Elliott, D. (1987). Pedal asymmetry in the reproduction of spatial locations, *Cortex*, 23, 157.

Carson, R.G. (1989a). Manual asymmetries: feedback processing, output variability and spatial complexity. Resolving some inconsistencies. *J. Motor Behav.*, 21, 38.

Carson, R.G. (1989b). Manual asymmetries: in defense of a multifactorial account. *J. Motor Behav.*, 21, 157.

Carson, R.G., Chua, R., Goodman, D., Byblow, W.D., and Elliott, D. (1995). The preparation of aiming movements. *Brain Cognit.*, 28, 133.

Carson, R.G., Chua, R., Elliott, D., and Goodman, D. (1990). The contribution of vision to asymmetries in manual aiming. *Neuropsychologia*, 28, 1215.

Carson, R.G., Elliott, D., Goodman, D., and Dickinson, J. (1990). Manual asymmetries in the reproduction of a 3-dimensional spatial location. *Neuropsychologia*, 28, 99.

Carson, R.G., Goodman, D., Elliott, D., and Chua, R. (1993). Asymmetries in the regulation of visually guided aiming. *J. Motor Behav.*, 25, 21.

Carson, R.G., Goodman, D., and Elliott, D. (1992) Asymmetries in the discrete and pseudocontinuous regulation of visually guided reaching. *Brain Cognit.*, 18, 169.

Christman, S.D. (1989). Perceptual characteristics and visual laterality research. *Brain Cognit.*, 11, 238.

Christman, S.D. (1993). On the complex relation between perceptual characteristics and hemispheric asymmetry. *Brain Cognit.*, 21, 123.

Chua, R., Carson, R.G., Goodman, D., and Elliott, D. (1992). Asymmetries in the spatial localization of transformed targets. *Brain Cognit.*, 20, 227.

Chua, R., Pollock, B.J., Elliott, D., Swanson, L.R., and Carnahan, H. (1995). The influence of age on manual asymmetries in movement preparation and execution. *Dev. Neuropsychol.*, 11, 129.

Corballis, M.C. and McLaren, R. (1984). Minding one's Ps and Qs: Mental rotation and mirror image discrimination. *J. Exp. Psychol.: Hum. Percept. Perf.*, 10, 318.

Deutsch, G., Bourbon, W.T., Papanicolaou, A.C., and Eisenberg, H.M. (1988). Visuospatial tasks compared via activation of regional cerebral blood flow. *Neuropsychologia*, 26, 445.

Eals, M. (1987). Asymmetric processing in perception of apparent movement. *Neuropsychologia*, 25, 429.

Elliott, D. (1991). Human handedness reconsidered. *Behav. Brain Sci.*, 14, 341.

Elliott, D., Roy, E.A., Goodman, D., Carson, R.G., Chua, R., and Maraj, B.K.V. (1993). Asymmetries in the preparation and control of manual aiming movements. *Can. J. Exp. Psychol.*, 47, 570.

Engel, A.K., König, P., Kreiter, A.K., and Singer, W. (1991). Interhemispheric synchronization of oscillatory neuronal responses in cat visual cortex. *Science*, 252, 1177.

Fisk, J.D. and Goodale, M.A. (1985). The organization of eye and limb movements during unrestricted reaching to targets in contralateral and ipsilateral visual space. *Exp. Brain Res.*, 60, 159.

Fisk, J.D. and Goodale, M.A. (1988). The effects of unilateral brain damage on visually guided reaching:hemispheric differences in the nature of the deficit. *Exp. Brain Res.*, 72, 425.

Garcia-Colera, A. and Semjen, A. (1988). Distributed planning of movement sequences. *J. Motor Behav.*, 20, 341.

Georgopoulous, A.P. and Massey, J.T. (1987). Cognitive spatial-motor processes. 1. The making of movements at various angles from a stimulus direction. *Exp. Brain Res.*, 65, 361.

Georgopoulous, A.P., Schwartz, A.B., and Kettner, R.E. (1986). Neuronal population coding of movement direction. *Science*, 233, 1416.

Ghez, C. (1985). Voluntary movement. In E.R. Kandel and J.H. Schwartz (Eds.), *Principles of Neural Science*, New York, Elsevier, 487.

Goodale, M.A. and Milner, D.A. (1992). Separate visual pathways for perception and action. *Trends Neurosci.*, 15, 20.

Goodman, D. and Kelso, J.A.S. (1980). Are movements prepared in parts? Not under compatible (naturalized) conditions. *J. Exp. Psychol.: Gen.*, 109, 475.

Gray, C.M., König, P., Engel, A.K., and Singer, W. (1989). Oscillatory responses in cat visual cortex exhibit inter-columnar synchronization which reflects global stimulus properties. *Nature*, 338, 334.

Guariglla, C., Padovani, A., Pantano, P., and Pizzamiglio, L. (1993). Unilateral neglect restricted to visual imagery. *Nature*, 364, 235.

Guiard, Y., Diaz, D., and Beaubaton, D. (1983). Left hand advantage for right handers for spatial constant error: Preliminary evidence in a unimanual ballistic aimed movement. *Neuropsychologia*, 21, 111.

Gurd, J.M. and Marshall, J.C. (1992). Drawing upon the mind's eye. *Nature*, 359, 590.

Haaland, K.Y. and Harrington, D. (1989). The role of the hemispheres in closed loop movements. *Brain Cognit.*, 9, 158.

Harvey, M., Milner, A.D., and Roberts, R.C. (1995). An investigation of hemispatial neglect using the landmark task. *Brain Cognit.*, 27, 59.

Hellige, J.B. (1983). Hemisphere × task interaction and the study of laterality. In J.B. Hellige (Ed.), *Cerebral Hemisphere Asymmetry*, New York, Praeger, 411.

Hellige, J.B., Bloch, M.I., Cowin, E.L., Lee Eng, T., Eviatar, Z., and Sergent, V. (1994). Individual variation in hemispheric asymmetry: Multitask study of effects related to handedness and sex. *J. Exp. Psychol.: Gen.*, 123, 235.

Hellige, J.B. and Michimata, C. (1989). Categorization vs. distance: Hemispheric differences for processing spatial information. *Mem. Cognit.*, 17, 770.

Henry, F.M. and Rogers, D.E. (1960). Increased response latency for complicated movements and a "memory drum" theory of neuromotor reaction. *Res. Q.*, 31, 621.

Hollerbach, J.M. (1990). Planning of arm movements. In D.N. Osherson, S.M. Kosslyn, and J.M. Hollerbach, (Eds.), *Visual Cognition and Action: An Invitation to Cognitive Science: Vol. 2*, Cambridge, MA, MIT Press, 183.

Jankowiak, J., Kinsbourne, M., Shalev, R.S., and Bachman, D.L. (1992). *J. Cognit. Neurosci.*, 4, 119.

Joanette, Y., and Brouchon, M. (1984). Visual allesthesia in manual pointing: Some evidence for sensorimotor cerebral organization. *Brain Cognit.*, 3, 152.

Kalaska, J.F. and Crammond, D.J. (1992). Cerebral cortical mechanisms of reaching movements. *Science*, 255, 1517.

Kosslyn, S.M. (1987). Seeing and imagining in the cerebral hemispheres: a computational approach. *Psychol. Rev.*, 94, 148.

Kosslyn, S.M., Koenig, O., Barrett, A., Cave, C.B., Tang, J., and Gabrieli, J.D.E. (1989). Evidence for two types of spatial representations: Hemispheric specialization for categorical and coordinate relations. *J. Exp. Psychol.: Hum. Percept. Perf.*, 15, 723.

Ladavas, E., Umilta, C., Ziani, P., Brogi, A., and Minarini, M. (1993). The role of right side objects in left side neglect: A dissociation between perceptual and directional motor neglect. *Neuropsychologia*, 31, 761.

MacKenzie, C.L., Sivak, B., and Elliott, D. (1988). Manual localization of lateralized visual targets. *J. Motor Behav.*, 20, 443.

Mace, C.A. (1931). The influence of indirect incentives upon the accuracy of skilled movements. *J. Psychol.*, 22, 101.

Marshall J.C. and Halligan, P.W. (1993). Imagine only the half of it. *Nature*, 364, 193.

Mecacci, L. (1993). On spatial frequencies and cerebral hemispheres: Some remarks from the electrophysiological and neuropsychological points of view. *Brain Cognit.*, 22, 199.

Morasso, P. and Tagliasco, V. (1986). *Human Movement Understanding: From Computational Geometry to Artificial Intelligence*. Amsterdam, North Holland.

Ojemann, G.A. (1984). Common cortical and thalamic mechanisms for language and motor functions. *Am. J. Physiol.*, 246, R901.

Osaka, M. (1984). Peak alpha frequency of EEG during a mental task: task difficulty and hemispheric differences. *Psychophysiology*, 21, 101.

Papanicolau, A.C., Deutsch, G., Bourbon, W.T., Will, K.W., Loring, D.W., and Eisenberg, H.M. (1987). Convergent evoked potential and cerebral blood flow evidence of task-specific hemispheric differences. *Electroenceph. Clin. Neuropsychol.*, 66, 515.

Peterzell, D.H. (1991). On the nonrelation between spatial frequency and cerebral competence. *Brain Cognit.*, 15, 62.

Ratcliffe, G. (1979). Spatial thought, mental rotation and the right cerebral hemisphere. *Neuropsychologia*, 17, 49.

Rosenbaum, D.A. (1980). Human movement initiation: Specification of arm, direction, and extent. *J. Exp. Psychol.: Gen.*, 109, 444.

Roy, E.A. and MacKenzie, C.L. (1978). Handedness effects in kinesthetic spatial location judgments. *Cortex*, 14, 250.

Sergent, J. (1983). Role of the input in visual hemispheric asymmetries. *Psychol. Bull.*, 93, 481.

Sergent, J. (1991). Judgments of relative position and distance on representations of spatial relations. *J. Exp. Psychol.: Hum. Percept. Perf.*, 91, 762.

Tegnér, R. and Levander, M. (1991). Through the looking glass: A new technique to demonstrate directional hypokinesia in unilateral neglect. *Brain*, 114, 1943.

Turvey, M.T. and Carello, C. (1986). The ecological approach to perceiving-acting: A pictorial essay. *Acta Psychol.*, 63, 133.

Tzeng, O.J.L. and Wang, W.S.-Y. (1984). Search for a common neurocognitive mechanism for language and movements. *Am. J. Physiol.*, 246, R904.

Umiltà, C. (1995). Domain-specific forms of neglect. *J. Clin. Exp. Neuropsychol.*, 17, 209.

Ungerleider, L.G. and Mishkin, M. (1982). In In D. Ingle, M.A. Goodale, and R.J.W. Mansfield (Eds.) *Analysis of Visual Behavior*, Cambridge, MA, M.I.T. Press, 549.

van Donkelaar, P. and Franks, I.M. (1991). The effects of changing movement velocity and complexity on response preparation: evidence from latency, kinematic, and EMG measures. *Exp. Brain Res.*, 83, 618.

Watson, N.V. and Kimura, D. (1989). Right-hand superiority for throwing but not for intercepting. *Neuropsychologia*, 27, 1399.

Section IV

The Implications *of* Asymmetric Motor Function

Chapter 9

Asymmetry in Bimanual Skills

Yves Guiard and Thierry Ferrand

CONTENTS

0-8493-8999-2/96/$0.00+$.50

1. INTRODUCTION

In their spontaneous motor behavior, humans exhibit innumerable instances of lateral asymmetry. The manual gestures of humans appear to violate repeatedly the symmetry principle which otherwise governs their muscular and skeletal anatomy, either because a single upper limb is recruited in action or because, both upper limbs being involved, their roles differ markedly.

1.1 HUMAN TWO-HANDEDNESS AND THE IDEA OF HAND DOMINANCE

It has been many decades since neuropsychologists realized that a theory assigning complementary cognitive functions to the two halves of the brain should have a better explanatory power than one assuming that the contribution of one hemisphere is more important or more sophisticated than that of the other. Indeed, the study of cerebral dominance, as initiated by Broca (1860), was gradually replaced during the second half of this century by the study of hemispheric specialization (e.g., Brain, 1941; Hécaen and Ajuriaguerra, 1964; see Hellige, 1993, for recent references).

To date, despite the strict formal analogy and the functional links that relate the bihemispheric and the bimanual systems, a conceptual transition from lateral dominance to lateral specialization has not really taken place in the field of manual skills. Even though the frequency of occurrence of the term "dominance" is more limited in the contemporary literature on human manual asymmetry than it used to be, research in the field remains heavily influenced by the postulate that one side dominates the other in the expression of motor behavior.

Most basic research on manual asymmetries thus far has revolved about two basic issues, hand preference and hand performance asymmetry, which correspond to the two major aspects of handedness. *Hand preference* refers to the fact that an individual usually chooses one hand with little hesitation to execute a unimanual task such as throwing a dart. By recording the proportion of right- and left-hand preferences in standardized questionnaires, one obtains a global estimate of the individuals' manual lateralization and it becomes possible to classify them as more or less right- or left-handed. Questionnaire studies have shown that human individuals tend to exhibit consistency of hand preference across the variety of unimanual acts of everyday life, even though a number of puzzles remain, particularly among left-handers — for example, almost 50% of left-handed writers prefer to use their right hand for throwing (Gilbert and Wisocki, 1992).

Hand superiority, the other classical approach to handedness, is assessed experimentally by submitting subjects to unimanual performance tests and comparing the scores obtained with the left and right hands. Much research has been aimed at understanding the relation between hand preference and hand superiority as an attempt to characterize handedness in general, an enterprise that turned out to be unexpectedly difficult (Peters, 1994).

Recourse to the traditional concept of handedness,* still so pervasive in the motor asymmetry literature, logically implies adherence to the assumption of hand dominance, regardless of whether one refers to hand preference (the subjective aspect of handedness), hand superiority (the objective aspect of handedness), or both. Importantly, the hand-

---

* Note incidentally that the word "handedness," by ordinary morphological rules, should normally designate the mere possession of hands — i.e., the fact, specific to the primate, of being handed. Quite interestingly, the word has come to stand for left- vs. right-handedness (a factor specific to the human) and to denote, more technically, a continuous between-individual variable with left- and right-handedness as its extrema. The fact that the laterality attribute proper (left vs. right) is implicit in this term is somewhat puzzling given that laterality is a concern central to those who have coined it.

dominance concept implies a *competitive* representation of the bimanual relationship, in the sense that the assessment of either hand preference or hand superiority requires a left-right confrontation. This will appear more and more clearly, by contrast, as the reader proceeds in this chapter aimed at outlining an alternative, *cooperative* approach to upper-limb motor asymmetry.

A fact of central importance in our view, but still reluctantly acknowledged in the handedness literature, is that the vast majority of human manual activities involve the two hands concurrently (for recent exceptions to this reluctance, see Baecker, Grudin, Buxton, and Greenberg, 1995; Kabbash, Buxton, and Sellen, 1994; Peters, 1994; Treffner and Turvey, 1995, in press). Perhaps the most straightforward argument for this statement is to be found in the composition of current hand-preference questionnaires (Guiard, 1987). By definition, the function of such questionnaires is to record answers to a set of left- or right-hand, *exclusive-or* questions. Because the issue of hand preference is a nonsense for truly bimanual activities like, say, swinging a golf club or playing the violin, logically bimanual activities should *not* be mentioned in the lists. Rather surprisingly, however, current hand-preference questionnaires have the majority of their items refer to undoubtedly bimanual acts, as can be readily illustrated with a few classical examples. In the eight-item questionnaire of Annett (1967), there are five references to bimanual activities (sweeping, shoveling, striking a match, using scissors, and threading a needle) and only three to (conceivably) unimanual activities (writing, drawing, throwing). Likewise, 11 of the 20 items of Oldfield's (1971) once famous questionnaire refer to bimanual activities. Finally, the more copious 75-item questionnaire of Provins, Milner, and Kerr (1982) has at least 45 bimanual items.

In a sense it is a trick that makes it possible to record exclusive-or responses with bimanual items. Respondents are requested to indicate, of course not the hand they prefer to use, but rather the hand they prefer to assign to one manual post specified within parentheses. Typical formulations will be of the form: "Dealing cards (dealing)," "sweeping the floor (indicate the hand placed at the end of the broom handle)," "opening a jar (lid)," and so forth.

Although this practice does introduce a left/right forced choice in the context of bimanual behavior, this forced choice is rather artificial. On theoretical grounds it has the fundamental weakness that there is no principled justification to the conversion into hand preferences of the responses recorded with reference to bimanual activities. In the case of the broom item, for example, to register the "right-hand" response (i.e., the preference for placing the right hand at the top of the handle) as an indication of right-*hand* preference is quite arbitrary for lack of an explicit theory of manual specialization for bimanual action in general, or at least of a hypothesis on manual roles in the particular instance considered. In fact, the only (implicit) justification for the conversion seems to be that right-handers are (informally) known to preferentially use that grip for that particular implement. Such a justification, however, must be rejected as circular: handedness is something that the hand-preference questionnaire must assess, not assume.

This common practice has the consequence of keeping alive the old belief that hand dominance features at the heart of human motor lateralization. Beneath the striking difficulty met by designers of handedness questionnaires in finding instances of truly unimanual activities, we believe it is the importance of *two-handedness* in the repertoire of human everyday manual gestures that conspicuously shows through.

1.2 THE LATERALITY PROBLEM IN THE CONTEXT OF BIMANUAL COOPERATION

From the moment it is recognized that in general human manual skills involve both hands and that intermanual competition should give way to bimanual cooperation in our theoretical representations, the relevance of the classical handedness concept becomes questionable. The cooperation viewpoint suggests that hand preference is an artifact of forced-choice procedures and hand superiority an artifact of performance confrontation. From this viewpoint, therefore, handedness is a nonissue.

There is a constructive side, however, as new avenues open up for research. The stimulating questions that arise pertain to the differentiated partition of labor between the two upper limbs in human bimanual activities. Accounting for the very existence of bilateral manual specialization and identifying the fundamental logic that underlies it — if there is one (Bertelson, 1981) — becomes our major concern. Why should the two hands contribute different parts to motor action in humans? Our assumption is that there must be similar reasons to the emergence of between-hand differentiation of function in the natural history of humans and, at a shorter time scale, to the emergence of division of labor in the history of the industrial world: differentiation increases the adaptive power of working structures.

Obviously, the issues of hand preference and hand superiority have to be reformulated. There remains one inevitable laterality-related forced choice in the face of real-life two-handed activities, namely, the choice between the two possible ways of assigning a pair of different roles to a pair of hands. For instance, one can either deal cards with the right hand while manipulating the pack with the left or proceed the other way round, but there is no room for a compromise. As will be illustrated below with some data, the preferences people exhibit for one of the two mirror-image approaches to two-handed action problems are apparently just as definite as the hand preferences they exhibit in the context of one-handed acts. To avoid any confusion with hand preference, we will designate these observables as *lateral preferences* (Guiard, 1987, 1988).

Just as lateral preference, as just defined, is the bimanual counterpart to hand preference, there is an obvious bimanual counterpart to hand superiority, which we will term *lateral superiority*. Below we report experiments that tested individuals at performing a bimanual task with the two alternative assignments of roles to hands — the preferred and the nonpreferred. In sum, whereas hand-preference and hand-superiority effects are the two major observables for one-handed tasks, lateral-preference and lateral-superiority effects constitute our two major observables now that we are considering bimanual motor behavior.

Below we progress in two steps. In Section 2, which represents an attempt to elaborate the matter theoretically, we start with a few principles of asymmetric bimanual cooperation in humans as suggested by observation and end with the exposition of the kinematic-chain model (Guiard, 1987, 1988), an analogical model aimed at accounting for the principles in question. In Section 3, we present a new experimental paradigm for the study of bimanual cooperation based on the two-handed manipulation of rods in the context of aiming tasks and report some fresh data.

2. TOWARD A MODEL OF ASYMMETRICAL BIMANUAL COOPERATION

2.1 PRINCIPLES OF BIMANUAL COOPERATION AS SUGGESTED BY OBSERVATION

2.1.1 Right-to-Left Reference

A general principle that appears to govern bimanual activities in humans is the *frame-content* relationship that links the left and the right manual roles (MacNeilage, Studdert-Kennedy, and Lindblom, 1987). That is, the contribution of the right, preferred hand typically inserts itself in the reference frame provided by the left, nonpreferred hand. In peeling an apple, for example, this principle may show through the simple fact that during the manipulation the mobility of the fruit is limited in comparison with that of the knife, which reveals that the person tends to move the latter *relative to* the former. Such a principle, which we call right-to-left reference, seems to be valid across an impressive diversity of two-handed tasks, including instances as different as graphic activities and the two-handed manipulation of long-handled tools (Guiard, 1987).

2.1.2 Left-Right Scale Differentiation

Perhaps the most striking fact that emerges from a survey of the vast catalogue of human bimanual activities is that the roles played by the two hands differ in terms of their spatiotemporal scale. It is quite a common observation that movements of the right, preferred hand are usually much finer than those of the left. Notice, however, that the familiar notion of "fineness" suffers from a contamination of the concept of *level of resolution* by a pernicious connotation of *level of skill*. Even though it is often the case that the coarser role attributed to the left hand is less difficult to learn (this is most notably the case in graphic tasks), there is no compelling reason to assume that this must necessarily be the case: the fact that hummingbirds control the oscillations of their wings with a finer grain of spatiotemporal resolution than albatrosses does not imply a higher level of skill in the former species.

2.1.3 Left-Hand Precedence

A third general principle of human bimanual cooperation is that the contribution of the left, nonpreferred hand tends to precede that of the right. For example, one first places the nail before hitting it with the hammer, one positions and orients the page before starting to write or draw, etc. This is not to say, however, that the left-hand precedence principle applies exclusively to the case of a static/dynamic or postural/manipulative partition of labor between the hands — the principle seems to enjoy a much broader domain of validity. Below we will report evidence that it also governs the two-handed manipulation of rods in tasks that demand truly dynamic contributions on the part of the two hands.

2.1.4 Right-Hand Dominance

Obviously, this list must not omit the fact that most human individuals express a marked subjective preference for one of their hands. The venerable, but we believe unreasonable, assumption that only one hand really counts — despite the overwhelming evidence that the two hands are normally needed in human action — has pervaded the scientific domain, with most of the research to date constituting a theory of hand dominance, as already noted in Section 1.

2.2 ACCOUNTS PROVIDED BY THE KINEMATIC CHAIN MODEL

To account synthetically for the above four principles, Guiard (1987) has proposed to use the *kinematic chain* (KC) as an analogical model. The term "kinematic chain," borrowed from an old subdomain of mechanics (Reuleaux, 1877), denotes generically any concrete structure formed by the serial assembly of a number of rigid links — we may take an *arm* as an exemplary case. We will include in the KC category larger-scale structures built according to a similar hierarchical organization (e.g., a mountaineering expedition).

We now present a summary of how the KC concept may serve to model bimanual cooperation and how it accounts for the basic facts, considering the four above-listed principles successively (see Guiard, 1986, 1987, 1988, 1990, 1991, for more detailed presentations of the model).

2.2.1 Modeling Right-to-Left Reference as Distal-to-Proximal Reference

A KC is a serially assembled structure with each of its components mounted on top of its proximal neighbor and moving relative to it thanks to a specialized device called a joint. In a primate arm, for example, fingers rotate about their first knuckle relative to the hand palm, which in turn rotates about the wrist relative to the forearm, which in turn rotates about the elbow relative to the upper arm, which in turn rotates about the shoulder relative to the trunk.* A compelling reason in an arm for a principle of distal-to-proximal reference rather than the reverse is because an arm, like any KC, constitutes an *oriented* structure with a free (distal) extremity and a grounded (proximal) extremity, and with an increasing inertia in the proximal direction (Guiard, in press).

Thus, it is a criterial property of KCs that they obey a distal-to-proximal reference principle. The central proposal contained in the KC model is to liken the (nonpreferred) *left* and the (preferred) *right* of bimanual cooperation respectively to the *proximal* and the *distal* of the cooperation that takes place in a KC between two contiguous elements. As suggested in the beginning of Section 2, such an analogy seems quite viable in light of the evidence. Our next step will be to show that it helps to understand the other aspects of asymmetrical bimanual cooperation.

2.2.2 Accounting for Left-Right Scale Differentiation

To sketch an explanation of why the movements of the right, preferred hand generally have a finer grain of resolution than those of the left hand is an easy matter in the light of the KC model. An invariant law of this world is that the higher the inertia of a body, the longer its natural period — simultaneously in the temporal and spatial domain, owing to allometric constraints (Kugler and Turvey, 1987). This may be readily experienced by trying to establish a comfortable oscillatory tempo at the wrist, the elbow, and the shoulder. It will be immediately apparent that the more proximal the joint (i.e., the longer the KC segment mobilized), the slower the oscillation, reflecting both mass recruitment from joint to joint and the accelerated increase of rotation radius (Guiard, 1986, in press). The lesson is that a KC constitutes a *hierarchical* structure not only because of its serial organization (with links and joints that can be ranked), but also in the sense that its different components contribute to overall action at different levels of resolution.

Then, from the moment it is assumed that the left and right hands cooperate in humans like two contiguous elements of a KC, one must predict that the contribution of the hand corresponding to the more distal element (the right hand) will be characterized by a finer granularity.

2.2.3 Accounting for Left-Hand Precedence: Relative-Phase Effects

A functional property of KCs is that they exhibit a phase gradient: the more proximal a component in the structure, the earlier its contribution, a fact that derives from the scale gradient along the KC. Because the contribution of the proximal is macrometric in comparison with that of the distal, the former must operate first, in keeping with a ball-park or funnel principle. For example, kinematic analyses have shown that in reaching movements, the contribution of the shoulder and elbow takes place before that of the wrist and fingers (e.g., Jeannerod, 1981).

We have seen that the contribution of the left hand tends to precede that of the right. Indeed, such a temporal patterning appears to represent a fairly general invariant for

* Of course, at a local level, a 2- or 3-phalanx finger is itself a KC. Likewise, at a higher level, the whole skeletal system constitutes a KC whose distal component is the arm. That is, KCs can be and are often composed of serially assembled KCs.

tasks that involve qualitatively differentiated manual contributions. In the light of the KC analogy, this is what should be expected.

A stimulating challenge for the KC model has been the demonstration, by dynamically oriented students of bimanual coordination, of a slight phase lead of the right, preferred hand in a variety of frequency-locked bimanual oscillatory tasks (Carson, 1993; Collins, 1995; Kugler and Turvey, 1987). That is, the right hand precedes the left, apparently in contradiction with the just-mentioned prediction of the KC model. It must be noted, however, that symmetrical oscillatory tasks such as those most popular in the dynamic study of bimanual coordination (e.g., swinging a pair of pendulums at a common frequency) squarely ignore the differential specialization of the two hands. Because such tasks are invitations to use one's hands as two equivalent oscillators, rather than in accordance with their familiar differentiated logic, there is no reason to predict the left-hand precedence effect of common observation in asymmetrical tasks.

In the coupled-oscillators paradigm with 1:1 frequency locking, it has been established that relative phase is strongly linked to the difference in eigenfrequency between the two components. If one of the two oscillators is given a higher eigenfrequency than the other (e.g., by reducing pendulum length or mass in Kugler and Turvey's (1987) wrist-pendulum paradigm), this oscillator will systematically lead regardless of the prescribed relative phase (0° or 180°). It has been further demonstrated that the larger the eigenfrequency difference between the two component oscillators, the larger the spontaneous phase difference between them (Schmidt, Carello, and Turvey, 1990; Treffner and Turvey, 1995). Assuming, as the KC model does, that the right hand's specialized role is to contribute the higher frequency components to ongoing activity implies that the right upper limb should have a higher eigenfrequency than the left. The observed phase lead of the right hand in symmetrical bimanual oscillatory tasks is therefore consistent with the KC model's prediction.

2.2.4 Accounting for Right-Hand Dominance: The Metonymy Hypothesis*

In the introductory section, we critically discussed the general concept of hand dominance in terms of its implications for research on human motor lateralization. Beyond our theoretical position, it remains intriguing that the idea of hand-dominance is so ubiquitous across time and human cultures. If, as we postulate, humans have developed a truly bimanual specialization with neither of the two manual contributions being of negligible importance, how can it be that in their most current representations of manual roles humans persistently view one of their hands as dominant?

Although this question looks rather complex (see Hertz, 1960, for a classic anthropological text), the KC model does suggest something of potential relevance. It is often the case that the terminal element of a hierarchical structure — the element whose contribution to the structure's action has the highest level of resolution — constitutes the structure's privileged point of interaction with the external environment, as noted by Saltzman and Kelso (1987). This is the case of complex biological machines like articulated appendages: although a KC generally uses most of its components to execute an act, only the terminal organ (the foot or the hand in the case of the primate limb) will usually get in contact with the world. This may also be the case of quite different structures. Imagine a Himalayan mountaineering expedition: all teams are needed but

* A metonymy, broadly speaking, is a rather common rhetorical figure whereby a locutor designates x implicitly by saying y, with x and y bearing some obvious relationship such as part-whole or cause-effect. For example, by saying that there is no *sail* in view, one means that no *boat* is visible.

only one, the smallest, with the shortest distance to cover, will actually reach the summit in the final attack.

The noteworthy fact is that such hierarchical structures tend to be designated by their sole *terminal* element according to a *metonymy* process. Here are a few examples. A throwing gesture will be often classified, even possibly in scientific parlance, as a hand movement — ignoring the role of the other links of the limb.* Hitting a ball in soccer is currently considered to involve the foot (hence the term football), as though a foot alone made up an effector. Turning to artificial structures, the whole vehicle mounted on caterpillars and made up of an arm ended with a shovel is commonly called a (mechanical) shovel. Finally, the Everest is known to have been first conquered by just two men, a British mountaineer and a Sherpa. In all these cases, the terminal high-resolution component works, for both the observers of action and the actors themselves, as the representative of the whole structure.

If we make the KC analogy more specific and admit that in humans the left and right hands usually cooperate like the penultimate and the ultimate link of a KC, we will not be surprised that the right hand, which plays the role of the chain's terminal element, is considered with special care — at the cost of some unfairness with regard to the left upper limb and all other effectors inevitably involved in the simplest "manual" gesture. From the moment this favoring process is recognized as the law for KCs (whatever may be the reasons for this fact), the hand-dominance phenomenon, as well as perhaps the *attentional* bias that favors the right-hand side in the continuous stream of motor action (Peters, 1981), becomes a prediction of the KC model.

3. THE TWO-HANDED ROD PARADIGM

To study phenomena, scientists must elaborate simple observational or experimental protocols that make operational definitions possible while still capturing the features of reality they believe to be essential. One possible reason for the competitive tradition in the field of human motor lateralization has been that one-sidedness apparently offers a simpler framework for the study of asymmetry than two-sidedness. We contend, however, that asymmetry can be studied quite parsimoniously in the context of bimanual action. In this section we introduce a simple new paradigm designed for the study of asymmetrical bimanual cooperation, the two-handed rod paradigm, and we report some fresh data.

The reason for choosing the manipulation of long, bimanually held rods for the study of bimanual cooperation is basically twofold. First, we believe that rod manipulation constitutes a promising paradigm for research on asymmetry in bimanual skills. A rod is a simple machine (a long rigid object, i.e., a lever) which imposes tight geometrical constraints on its manipulation. As a consequence, the field of behavioral possibilities open to the researcher's exploration is limited. This field has structure, however: we will present below a simple two-class taxonomy of rod manipulations allowing, for either class, a tentative identification of the two complementary manual roles.

The second reason is that the rod undoubtedly represents the basic prototype of an impressive variety of human tools, with hosts of instances in virtually every domain of traditional human activity such as craft, housework, gardening, and sports. So we believe that an accurate characterization of differentiated bimanual cooperation within the simple framework of the rod paradigm should improve our understanding of human motor lateralization in general.

* A phrase like "manual asymmetries" (in the place of upper-limb asymmetries), which figures in the very title of this book, obviously involves a metonymical process of this sort.

3.1 EXPERIMENT 1: PATTERNS OF GRIP PREFERENCES IN THE TWO-HANDED MANIPULATION OF TOOLS

The aim of this experiment was to assess lateral preferences for the manipulation of a sample of current bimanual implements. Rather than resorting to the questionnaire method, we decided to have participants actually manipulate the tools. Therefore, the experiment was run outdoors, on a working site next to the Department of Experimental Psychology of the University of Oxford.

3.1.1 Method

The equipment consisted of the 13 implements listed in Table 9.1, most of which represented everyday-life tools hired for the experiment. Handles were marked with colored adhesive tape every 10 cm to facilitate the recording of spontaneous hand placement during manipulation.

Table 9.1 The Sample of Implements Used in Experiment 1

Implement	Total Length (cm)	Task Instructions
Pointer	150	Touch specified wall mark with the tip
Telescope	150	Aim at specified target through the tube
Blow Pipe	150	Aim at specified target with tube in mouth
Garden Fork	101	Drive in sand and move
Window Cleaner	152	Rub wall surface at 23 m height
Scrubbing Brush	131	Rub the floor
Broom	125	Sweep the floor
Rake	138	Gather imaginary dead leaves on the ground
Shovel	100	Drive in sand and carry
Hoe	78	Hit the ground to cut imaginary roots
Bludgeon	92	Hit imaginary target (hard, downward)
Sledge Hammer	76	Hit the ground (hard)
Pick Ax	92	Hit the ground (hard)

Note: The same object, a 150-cm tube with a diameter of 3 cm, served to represent the first three implements.

In this study, 30 male students with definite right-handedness participated and were paid for their service. Handedness was assessed with a specially designed hand-preference questionnaire derived from Oldfield's (1971) inventory.

Participants were provided with all 13 implements in a balanced order. For each implement, they were asked to perform the appropriate utilization gesture as many times as desired while alternating between the two possible bimanual grips (i.e., with the left hand placed at the extremity of the handle and the right in the forward position and vice versa) to evaluate their preference. Lateral preferences were scored in terms of their direction and strength: a negative (positive) score denoted preference for placing the right hand (the left hand) at the extremity of the handle, and preference strength was scored from 0 (no preference) to 3 (very strong preference).

The spontaneous positioning of the two hands, measured form handle extremity, was noted for each implement handled with the preferred grip. As it was found that the extremity of the handle was always occupied by one hand (be it the left or the right), a single measure indicating hand spacing turned out to be sufficient.

3.1.2 Results and Discussion

The distribution of preference scores obtained with the 30 participants for each of the 13 implements is illustrated in Figure 9.1.

First, note that all distributions display both kurtosis and skewness, in comparison with the shape of the normal distribution (no-preference hypothesis). Concerning kurtosis, several distributions are bimodal: on average, over all participants and implements, the no-preference score was the one with the far lowest probability ($p = .03$), while ±1 and ±2 scores ($p = .32$ and .31, respectively) were less probable than a ±3 score ($p = .35$). As for skewness, chi square tests on the frequency of positive vs. negative scores revealed a statistically significant deviation from symmetry in all 13 distributions. To our knowledge, these results constitute one of the few empirical demonstrations of lateral preferences, as distinct from hand preferences, in (right-handed) humans (see Ibbotson and Morton, 1981, and Peters, 1985, 1994).

Fortunately, given the arbitrary nature of our sample of implements, the two possible lateral preferences were represented in the experiment. This offered some information for a preliminary taxonomy of the human manipulation of rod-like tools. Note that all three instances with a predominance of positive scores (nonpreferred left hand at the end of the handle, black-bars in Figure 9.1) correspond to the case of hitting — more specifically, to *hitting in rotation*. Clearly, this observation is consistent with known prescriptions and practice in the various sports that use bimanual hitting implements (e.g., golf, cricket, baseball, and field hockey).

A characteristic common to the remaining ten implements, for which the preference was opposite (preferred right hand at handle end, gray-bars in Figure 9.1) is that their utilization gesture culminates in an *axial translation*, rather than in a rotation. Although these implements obviously need to be oriented in the initial phase of the movement, the terminal phase consists of either an axial push (e.g., scrubbing brush) or an axial pull (e.g., broom, hoe) at various force levels ranging from a gentle contact (e.g., pointer) to a hard thrust (e.g., shovel). Note incidentally that the hoe, which at first glance might be classified in the first category, but which was in fact preferentially grasped like the rake, actually constitutes an ambiguous tool with regard to the above criterion. Hitting the ground with a hoe, whose blade is tilted at about 45°, implies a combination of a hard rotation and a hard pull. The distribution of preferences we obtained suggests that the pull component predominated for this tool in most of our participants.

For convenience, we will designate the two emerging categories of gestures as the *cut* and the *thrust*, using the old martial terminology suggested by Guiard (1987).

The data on hand spacing, illustrated in Figure 9.2, nicely complete the picture. They show a clearly bimodal distribution with a much smaller between-hand distance in the case of a cut than thrust implement.*

In sum, the results of Experiment 1 suggest that cut implements, whose utilization culminates in a fast rotational movement, are preferentially held and manipulated with the two hands placed close to each other and with the *left*, nonpreferred hand occupying the extremity of the handle. In contrast, thrust implements, whose axial translation typically represents the terminal phase of the movement, are preferentially grasped with a large between-hand gap and with the *right*, preferred hand occupying the handle extremity.

* It must be mentioned that with tools such as the sledgehammer and the pickax, which have rather high moments of inertia, the preparatory backswing cannot be initiated without the two hands placed at a large distance (40 to 50 cm) from each other. At the end of this phase, however, the right hand slides downward and forward with a drastic reduction of between-hand distance. In this experiment, hand spacing was estimated during the second, downward phase of the swing.

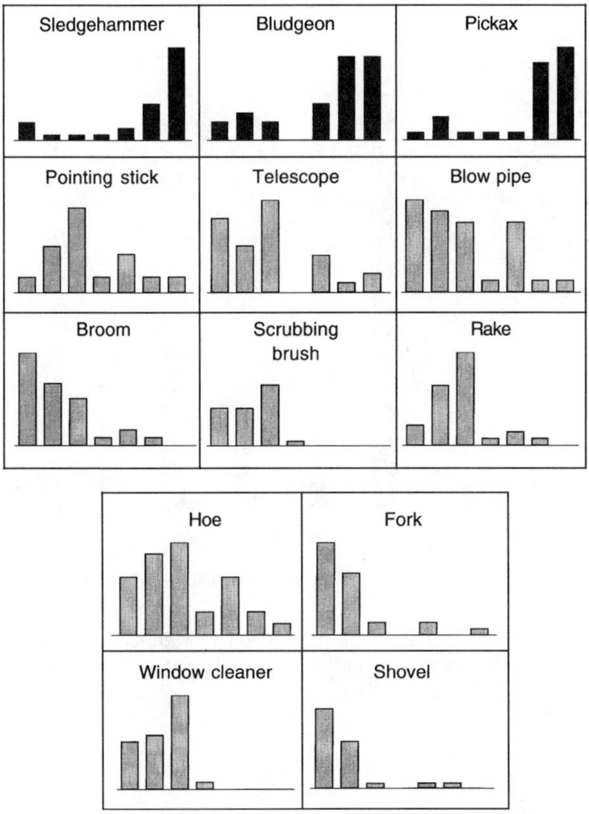

Figure 9.1 Distributions of preference scores obtained for each of the 13 implements with the 30 right-handers of Experiment 1. Scores range from –3 (very strong preference for placing the right hand at the handle extremity) to +3 (very strong preference for the inverse grip), with scores of ±2, ±1, and 0 corresponding to decreasing levels of preference strength (definite, weak, and no preference).

3.2 EXPERIMENT 2: THE EFFECT OF GRIP ON AIMING PERFORMANCE WITH A POINTER

Moving from preference to performance without leaving the realm of two-handedness, we now consider the actual dexterity of right-handers at manipulating rods. In Experiments 2, 3, and 4 we had recourse to several variants of a pointing task derived from Fitts' (1954) reciprocal tapping task, with the participants having to tap with the tip of a long, bimanually held stick alternatively on two targets of width W separated by a distance D. Fitts' tapping paradigm was chosen because it allows performance assessment at well controlled levels of difficulty.

The main goal of Experiment 2 was to evaluate the effect on level of performance of holding the pointer with the preferred vs. nonpreferred bimanual grip at several levels of difficulty.

3.2.1 Method

The pointing implement was a 130-cm long wooden rod with a pointed tip. The two targets consisted of metal strips 4 cm wide × 40 cm high fixed to the left and to the right of a wooden panel attached to a wall.

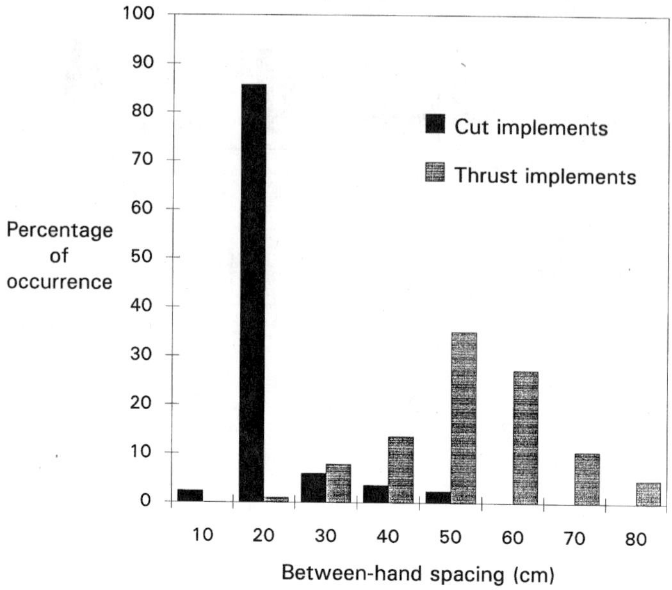

Figure 9.2 Distribution of between-hand spacing on tool handle, averaged over the 3 cut implements and over the 10 thrust implements of Experiment 1.

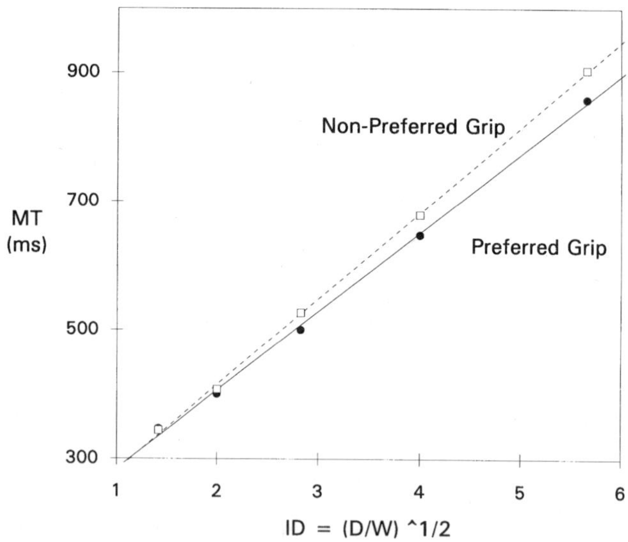

Figure 9.3 Mean *MT* as a function of task difficulty, using Meyer et al.'s (1988) power index of difficulty, for the preferred and the nonpreferred grip (Experiment 2).

Participants were ten male students of the University of Oxford, selected on the basis of their having both a strong right-hand preference and a strong preference for placing their right hand at the proximal end of the experimental pointer. They were asked to keep standing in front of the target setup and to tap alternatively on the left and right targets with the tip of the implement as quickly as possible, while keeping error rate to a minimum. The main independent variables were between-target distance ($D = 8, 16, 32, 64$, and 128 cm), the factor responsible for task difficulty, and grip (preferred vs. nonpreferred). There were two subsidiary factors, target-panel elevation (90 vs. 166 cm from the floor, imposing in the pitch plane a horizontal vs. oblique orientation of the pointer, respectively) and between-hand spacing on the pointer (one half vs. one third of pointer length).

3.2.2 Results and Discussion

A 5 × 2 × 2 × 2 ANOVA with repeated measures on the factors of distance, grip, hand spacing, and target elevation was carried out on movement time (*MT*). The main effect of distance was highly significant ($F(4, 36) = 258.27, p < .001$), as predicted by Fitts' Law. So was the effect of hand spacing ($F(1, 9) = 33.23, p < .001$), with a shorter *MT* for the larger between-hand distance. Elevation also influenced performance significantly ($F(1, 9) = 11.08, p < .01$), with a shorter *MT* for the target panel fixed at 166 rather than 90 cm. Finally, *MT* was shorter on average with the preferred than nonpreferred grip (551 vs. 573 ms, respectively), but this effect was not significant statistically ($F(1, 9) = 3.18, p > .10$).

The latter null result must be qualified in the light of two considerations. First, there was a consistent preferred-grip advantage for aiming *accuracy*: mean error rate was 2.0% for the preferred grip and 2.8% for the nonpreferred grip, a significant difference by the sign test ($p < .05$) as nine of the ten participants exhibited an advantage of the same sign. Thus, the laterality variable influenced performance accuracy rather than performance speed.

Second, the ANOVA* revealed a highly significant grip × distance interaction on *MT* ($F(4, 36) = 10.18, p < .001$), reflecting the fact that the preferred-grip advantage increased linearly with between-target distance, with an advantage of –3, 7, 27, 35, and 45 ms for $D = 8$, 16, 32, 64, and 128 cm, respectively ($r^2 = .920$ for the linear regression). An illustration of this finding is given in Figure 9.3, with *MT* plotted, separately for the preferred and the nonpreferred grip, as a function of $(D/W)^{1/2}$, the index of difficulty proposed by Meyer, Abrams, Kornblum, Wright, and Smith (1988), which provides excellent fits ($r^2 = .999$ in either case). Indeed, the preferred-grip advantage on *MT* became significant at $D = 128$ cm ($F(1, 9) = 14.25, p < .01$). So the greater the difficulty of the aiming, the larger the lateral superiority effect.

3.3 EXPERIMENT 3: THE GEOMETRY OF LEFT-RIGHT PARTITION OF LABOR IN POINTER MANIPULATION

A rod, the prototype of many everyday-life implements, can be characterized as a (more or less elastic) rigid object of oblong shape, generally with a simple morphology (e.g., a constant cross section from end to end). A rod, by definition, has considerable relative extension in a single dimension (its length). Hence the rotations of a rod-like tool — especially in the yaw and pitch planes — always have critical consequences for the person that manipulates it.

Perhaps the simplest and most basic distinction here is whether the tool must be brought to some *angular position* or to some *angular velocity*: a thrust implement such as a lecturer's pointing stick or a picador's pike must be *oriented,* but a cut implement like a golf club or a kendo saber must be *swung*. These two rather different types of rotation appear to have the same axis, roughly speaking the wrist of the hand positioned at the end of the handle. How then can we explain that in most right-handers this axis is offered by the left hand for hitting with the implement, but by the right for orienting it?

* The only other interaction that reached significance in this ANOVA was that between distance and target elevation ($F(4,36) = 7.17, p<.001$), reflecting a steeper slope of *MT* as a function of *D* in the 90 cm than 166 cm condition.

It must be noticed that angular motion contributes quite differently to the manipulation in the cut and in the thrust. Whereas to swing a cut implement is to *execute* the required gesture, to orient a thrust implement amounts to *initiating* an act whose execution proper is to follow: as already noted, the terminal, truly executory phase of a thrust consists of an axial translation, either a pull (e.g., the broom or the rake) or a push (e.g., the pointer, the garden fork, or the shovel).

Experiment 3 involved right-handers tapping at targets with the tip of a long pointer (a thrust act), using their preferred bimanual grip, to test a third-class lever hypothesis suggested by our observations.* To orient the pointer during the target-approach phase, people seem to use predominantly their nonpreferred hand, the one they have spontaneously placed at the greatest distance from the body when grasping the implement. It is the nonpreferred limb apparently that provides the effort, with the right hand, placed at the proximal end of the implement, providing a relatively stationary axis of rotation. To test this, we used a specially designed device, fixed to the ground, which imposed a fixed rotation axis to the implement. In different conditions, the pointer was forced to rotate either about a point close to the left hand, or about a point close to the right hand — without affecting the push-pull control (see Figure 9.4). When the forced rotation axis took place close to the position of one hand on the handle, this hand could no longer participate in the orientation of the implement. So, relative to a free-orientation condition, we predicted a larger performance impairment with exclusion from rotational control of the left-distal hand than with exclusion of the right-proximal hand.

Our second hypothesis was that the right, preferred hand predominates in the control of the pointer's axial translations, and in particular in the production of the quick push leading to target percussion in our tapping task. We had participants hold in one hand a light, 20 cm long plastic tube whose internal diameter fit the external diameter of the pointer while allowing the latter to slide through with little friction. When held in one hand, this simple device selectively prevented this hand from participating in the control of the implement's axial translation, for lack of the necessary friction, and hence forced the other hand to assume this control all on its own. Relative to a control condition with no slider, a larger performance impairment was expected with the slider held in the right-proximal than left-distal hand. Importantly, the equipment made it possible to manipulate this second factor independently of the first.

Finally, hypothesizing that the rotational and the translational controls of implement motion are relatively independent, we predicted an additive relation between the effects of these experimental manipulations.

3.3.1 Method

The target setup in Experiment 3 was invariant. The two targets, electrically connected to a microcomputer and placed one above the other at a constant D of 16 cm, were 30 cm wide × 4 cm high metal strips fixed to a wooden panel attached to a wall. Target panel elevation was such that the participant could easily reach the two targets while seated (with the lower target located about 60 cm from the floor). Error areas were covered with metal plates also connected to the computer, so that hits and misses could be recorded, along with *MT*s. The pointer, an aluminum rod with a rubber tip flush-mounted with copper threads, had its own connection wire.

It was soon realized that the task was almost impracticable with a fixed axis of rotation imposed about the forward, left-hand position (a constraint shown in Figure 9.4B).

* Recall that levers are conventionally classified according to the spatial-order relation born by the fulcrum, the resistance, and the effort. The lever is said to belong to the first, the second, or the third class if the intermediate position is occupied by the fulcrum, the resistance, or the effort, respectively.

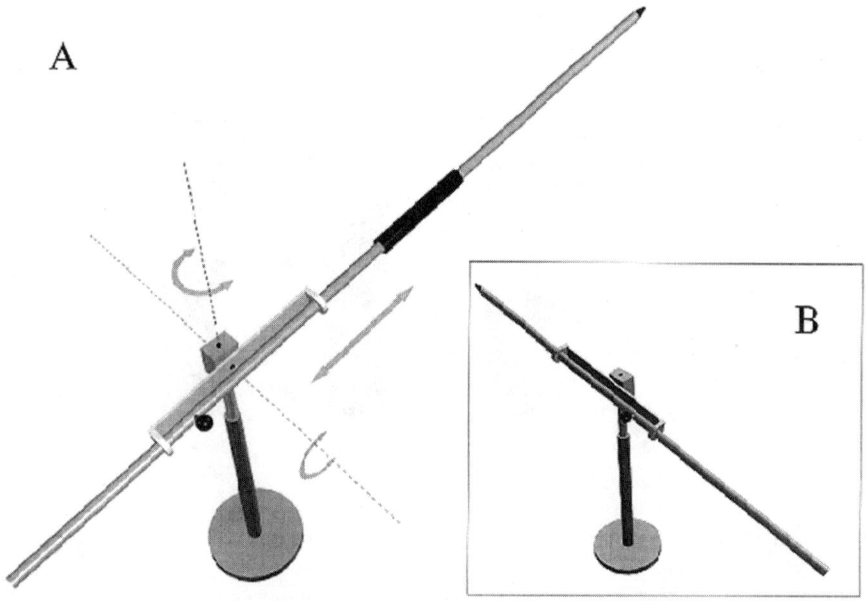

Figure 9.4 A representation of the mechanical apparatus that served to selectively constrain the translational and rotational components of pointer motion (Experiment 3). Panel A shows the combination of constraints that turned out to minimize performance impairment. The slider (in black) is shown at the position where it was grasped by the left hand; the rotation axis was fixed close to the right hand, with which the small spherical handle (in black) had to be grasped. In this condition, the control of axial push-pull motion relied entirely on the right hand, while the left hand had exclusive control over pointer rotations in the pitch and yaw plane, as illustrated with circular arrows. Panel B shows the rotational constraint that was so detrimental to performance that it had to be abandoned in the experiment.

Aiming performance was so poor with this constraint that this modality of the rotation factor had to be abandoned. Thus, only six of the nine initially planned conditions were run (two rotation conditions × three translation conditions). Six paid right-handed students participated in three 1-hour sessions, with condition order balanced within session.

3.3.2 Results and Discussion

The first and perhaps the most striking finding of Experiment 3 was that participants were extremely poor at coordinating rotations and axial translations of the pointer when constrained to orient the implement about a rotation axis passing through their left, distal hand — that is, when they were forced to manipulate the implement as a first-class lever. In contrast, they all performed smoothly with their right hand totally deprived of rotational control. This is clear-cut evidence for our third-class lever hypothesis: apparently, the natural way of controlling the orientation of a pointing stick is to produce the effort with one's nonpreferred limb while using the wrist of one's preferred limb as the rotation axis.

An ANOVA was carried out on *MT* with repeated measures on both experimental factors, translational constraint (no slider, slider in the left hand, slider in the right hand) and rotational constraint (free axis vs. forced axis in the right hand). Not surprisingly, given the familiarity reduction and the introduction of some friction, *MT* was lengthened

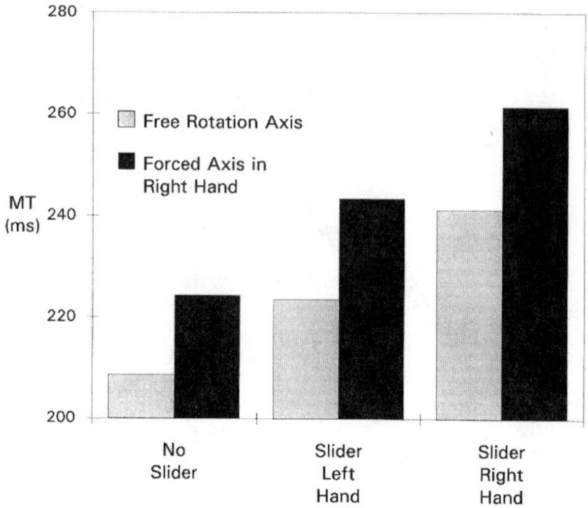

Figure 9.5 Mean *MT* as functions of the translational and rotational factors of Experiment 3.

both by the slider ($F(2, 10) = 18.77, p < .001$) and by the device used to fix the rotation axis ($F(1, 5) = 21.71, p < .01$). The pattern, however, was as predicted (see Figure 9.5). First, performance impairment was larger with the slider placed in the right hand than in the left (35 and 17 ms, respectively, $F(1, 5) = 6.97, p < .05$), and second, there was no sign of an interaction between the rotational and the translational factors ($F(2, 10) < 1$), with quite similar mean slider effects with and without the fixed axis (37 ms and 33 ms, respectively).

In sum, performance impairment was found to be minimal when the left hand alone was forced to take charge of the rotations of the pointer about the right hand used as a fulcrum and when the right hand had to assume all on its own the responsibility for the pointer's axial translations, an outcome consistent with our hypothesis on between-hand specialization for the manipulation of this sort of implement. Importantly, the apparent additivity between the two experimental factors suggests that the orientation and the translation of the implement are controlled by the two hands quite independently, with a neat between-hand partition of labor.

3.4 EXPERIMENT 4: THE PREPARATORY VS. EXECUTORY ROLE OF ROTATION AND TRANSLATION IN AIMING WITH A POINTER

The above experimental results lend support to the view that when they use a bimanual stick for pointing, right-handers control implement rotations predominantly with their distal-left hand and axial translations predominantly with their proximal-right hand. However, because in the task of Experiment 3 the rotation always preceded the translation in the tapping movement, it cannot be decided which dimension of between-hand partition of labor, rotation/translation, or preparation/execution, was critical to performance. Experiment 4 was aimed at disentangling these two factors thanks to a new variant of the tapping task in which the translation played a preparatory role and the rotation an executory role.

3.4.1 Method

Two pointing conditions were explored using the target panel and the computerized equipment of Experiment 3. In the *control* condition, the target panel was fixed vertically to the wall with the two targets now presented on the left- and right-hand sides, as shown

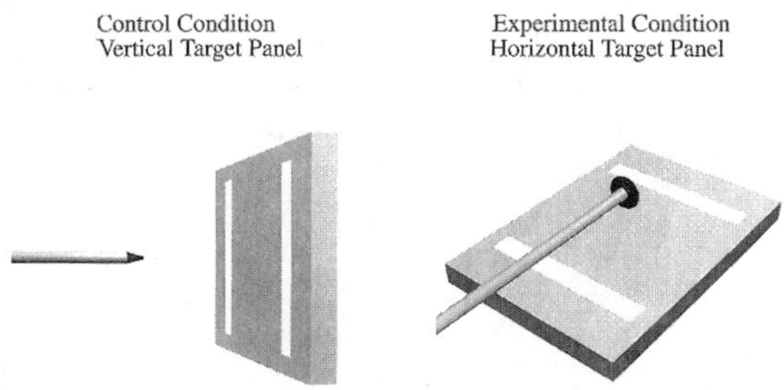

Figure 9.6 A representation of the two tapping conditions of Experiment 4.

in Figure 9.6 (left), at about 1.1 m above the floor. To hit the targets with the pointer tip while standing, participants had to keep the implement roughly horizontal, perpendicular to the target panel. Note that target approach in this condition required a rotation of the pointer about its proximal end, alternately in the clockwise and counterclockwise direction, while the final percussion required an axial push.

In the *experimental* condition, the target panel was fixed horizontally to the surface of a table and oriented with its two targets located near and far relative to the standing participant, as shown in Figure 9.6 (right). The implement was still oriented horizontally — but now parallel to the target panel. To make the tapping possible, the pointer was fitted at its distal end with a rubber disk, similar to the head of a reflex hammer, flush-mounted with copper threads to insure electrical conductance. Target approach took the form of an axial translation (alternately an axial push to bring the implement's head above the far target and an axial pull to bring it back over the near target) while the final percussion required a rotation (about the proximal end of the implement, in the pitch plane). Thus, the crucial characteristic of this condition was to permute the preparatory and executory roles played by rotation and translation in aiming.

There were two additional independent variables, the bimanual grip (preferred vs. nonpreferred) and between-target distance (D = 8, 16, and 32 cm).

The experiment involved 12 paid right-handers, the 6 well-practiced students of Experiment 3 plus 6 fresh unpracticed students. Each participated in two 1-hour sessions successively dedicated to the control and to the experimental condition, with the 6 combinations of grip and D presented in a balanced order within each session.

3.4.2 Results and Discussion

An ANOVA was performed on *MT* with group (practiced vs. nonpracticed) as a between-participant factor and distance (8, 16, 32 cm), grip (preferred vs. nonpreferred), and condition (control vs. experimental) as within-participant factors. Not surprisingly, the main effects of group (practice effect) and D (Fitts' law) were quite pronounced and highly significant. *MT* also turned out to be significantly faster overall with the horizontal target panel of the experimental condition (274 ms) than with the vertical target panel of the control condition (315 ms) ($F(1, 10) = 16.12, p < .002$).

There were only two significant interactions, both quite eloquent. The first was a grip × condition interaction ($F(1, 10) = 7.72, p < .025$) reflecting that whereas in the control condition performance was faster with the preferred grip (307 vs. 322 ms) — a replication of the result of Experiment 2 — in the experimental condition the *non*preferred grip was the most efficient (270 vs. 278 ms). However, the other significant interaction, a 3-term group × grip × condition interaction ($F(1, 10) = 8.24, p < .02$), indicated that the above interaction was specific to the practiced group, as clearly shown in Table 9.2. In fact, no grip effect was apparent in the unpracticed group.

Table 9.2 Main Results of Experiment 4

	Mean *MT* (ms)		Mean Error Rate (%)	
	Preferred Grip	Nonpreferred Grip	Preferred Grip	Nonpreferred Grip
Unpracticed Participants				
Control Task	341.4	341.6	8.7	7.8
Experimental Task	295.7	296.7	8.3	7.4
Practiced Participants				
Control Task	272.7	302.7	8.1	8.8
Experimental Task	261.3	243.8	9.7	8.4

In the analysis of error rates (see Table 9.2), no effect was found to run counter to any of the above *MT* effects. The main patterns for performance accuracy mimicked those for performance speed, adding reliability to the findings.

It seems worth mentioning that when asked for their impression on performing the (rather unusual) experimental task with one and the other grip, all 12 participants anticipated they would perform better with the grip they preferred for thrust actions (right hand proximal). So the superior performance that 5 of the 6 practiced participants actually displayed with the left hand placed at the proximal end of the pointer occurred despite their firm belief that they were less skilled with this grip.

In sum, Experiment 4 yielded clear-cut evidence in favor of the KC model. Right-handers manipulate tapping rods more efficiently, in terms of both speed and accuracy of aiming, with the grip that allows them to *initiate* the tapping movement with the left hand and to *terminate* it with the right, irrespective of the manual distribution of the rotational and translational roles that have to be played. So a single criterion, the one dictated by the principle of left-hand precedence, apparently accounts for the observed lateral superiority effect, in keeping with the KC model.

The experiment also revealed that in the context of a two-handed activity a lateral superiority effect need not necessarily match a lateral preference. This somewhat puzzling outcome is reminiscent of a common finding in the handedness domain (e.g., Annett, 1985).

4. OVERVIEW AND PERSPECTIVES

The foregoing was an attempt to outline a new perspective for the study of manual lateralization with the main concern of doing justice to the fundamental two-handedness of humans. We criticized the classical concept of (right- vs. left-) handedness, which we argued implies a competitive approach to human laterality, on the grounds that in real-life activities the two hands of human beings *cooperate*, rather than compete, with each other in the service of motor action.

Contrary to the often expressed view that emergence of a dominant hand for motor action has represented a most decisive step in the evolution of the human kind (see Calvin, 1982, for an extreme position), our data on lateral preference and superiority effects in tool manipulation would rather suggest that the characteristic that has come to genuinely distinguish humans from other primates is bimanual specialization. Although many primate species have been reported to use rods as tools (see MacNeilage et al., 1987), it is quite unlikely that bilateral patterns as consistent as those we observed in human right-handers will ever be observed in monkeys or apes.

The above reported preliminary results look reassuring. They show that the study of human motor asymmetry is not necessarily more complex in the context of normal two-handed action than it is in the context of single-handed action — on which much research has been focused somewhat artificially. Not only is it the case that right-handers, in the face of long tools that must be grasped bimanually in one of two ways, exhibit clear-cut lateral preference and superiority effects, but also the data show that these effects depend on tool type in an intelligible manner. Overall, our data on rod manipulation in simple aiming tasks support the KC hypothesis of a hierarchical partition of labor in humans, showing that the left, nonpreferred hand is in charge of the initial, relatively low-resolution component of the act and the right in charge of the terminal, relatively high-resolution component.

Why should a hierarchical specialization of this sort be adaptive? The KC analogy, we believe, suggests an answer. Partitioning a manipulation task into two (or more) hierarchical levels makes it possible for action to overcome, so to speak, the limitations imposed by Weber's law. That is, thanks to the contrasted contributions of its proximal and distal element(s), the KC can produce movements that have a remarkably high level of spatiotemporal resolution given their magnitude (Guiard, 1988). The level of skill exhibited by our participants at the various tapping tasks they had to carry out was impressive. An interesting questions that arises is to what extent, within the rod tapping paradigm, bimanual aiming performance surpasses unimanual performance.

This research on rod manipulation leads to numerous possible developments. We have started to explore the relation between lateral preference and performance in the sports domain. In a statistical investigation on baseball, we have shown that while almost 60% of players who bat left (clockwise) are right-handed, these right-handed players are less likely to hit with power and to strike out than left-handed players batting left, in keeping with the prediction of the KC model (Grondin, Koren, Ivry, and Guiard, submitted).

To broaden our methodology, we have developed an alternative aiming paradigm for the study of bimanual cooperation in which individuals have their two hands cooperate in moving a pointer with one hand and a pair of targets with the other hand, relative to one another. This paradigm designed to study the kinematics of within-person bimanual cooperation also makes it possible to have two different individuals perform one and the same aiming task cooperatively, as is the case in a handshake. We have recently shown that Fitts' Law remains perfectly valid in the between-person version of the task (Ferrand and Guiard, 1995).

When it is fully realized that the manual effector system of humans is basically a compound effector with a specialized role for each hand, we believe substantial changes will occur in the design of human-machine interfaces in general, and notably in the field of computer design. So far designers of input to computer systems have implicitly assumed that users do best with just one hand, and hence *either* a trackball *or* a mouse has been made available to them, an assumption and a practice well in line with traditional thinking in the handedness domain. Recently, however, convincing demonstrations have been offered by the Input Research Group of Toronto that when operators are provided with a pair of input devices such as a trackball and a mouse their performance at familiar computer tasks greatly improves (Kabbash et al., 1994; Baecker et al., 1995). Importantly, Kabbash et al. (1994) showed that the benefit of a two-handed input was maximal when the software allowed the right hand to act relative to the left, in keeping with expectations from the KC model.

Sooner or later, we believe that the functional relation between a two-sided brain system and a two-sided hand system should become one of the most important basic-research questions in the field of human functional lateralization. Our guess is that some of the enduring puzzles that have been met since Broca (1860) in attempts to account jointly for hemispheric specialization and hand dominance will vanish as soon as it is recognized that the two hands of humans, and not only their cerebral hemispheres, behave cooperatively with each other.

ACKNOWLEDGMENTS

Experiments 1 and 2 were run in 1985, during a 1-year visit of the first author in the Department of Experimental Psychology of the University of Oxford, jointly supported by the Royal Society and the French *Centre National de la Recherche Scientifique*. He is indebted to late Donald Broadbent, as well as to Alan Allport, Peter McLeod, and Michel Treisman for helpful discussions. Experiments 3 and 4, performed later in Marseilles, would not have been possible without the technical assistance of Monique Chiambretto (computer programming), Raymond Fayolle (electronics), and Bernard Arnaud (mechanical design and construction), whom the authors wish to warmly thank. Finally, thanks are due to Richard Ivry for carefully reading a preliminary version of this chapter and offering insightful suggestions.

REFERENCES

Annett, M. (1967). The binomial distribution of right, mixed, and left handedness. *Q. J. Exp. Psychol.*, 29, 327.

Annett, M. (1985). *Left, Right, Hand and Brain: The Right Shift Theory.* Hillsdale, NJ, Erlbaum.

Baecker, R., Grudin, J., Buxton, W., and Greenberg, S. (Eds.) (1995). *Readings in Human-Computer Interactions: towards the Year 2000.* San Francisco, CA, Morgan Kaufmann Inc.

Bertelson, P. (1981). The nature of hemispheric specialization: why should there be a single principle? *Behav. Brain Sci.*, 4, 63.

Brain, R. (1941). Visual disorientation with special reference to the lesions of the right cerebral hemisphere. *Brain*, 64, 244.

Broca, P. (1860). Sur le siège de la faculté de la parole articulée. *Bull. Soc. Anthropol. Paris*, 6, 377.

Calvin, W. H. (1982). Did throwing stones shape hominid brain evolution? *Ethol. Sociobiol.*, 3, 115.

Carson, R. G. (1993). Manual asymmetries: old problems and new directions. *Hum. Move. Sci.*, 12, 479.

Collins, D. R. (1995). The detuning factor in elementary coordination dynamics. In B. G. Bardy, R. J. Bootsma, and Y. Guiard (Eds.), *Studies in Perception and Action III*, Hillsdale, NJ, Lawrence Erlbaum, 45.

Ferrand, T. and Guiard, Y. (1995). Fitts' law in cooperative two-person aiming. In B. G. Bardy, R. J. Bootsma, and Y. Guiard (Eds.), *Studies in Perception and Action III*, Hillsdale, NJ, Lawrence Erlbaum, 65.

Fitts, P. M. (1954). The information capacity of the human motor system in controlling the amplitude of movement. *J. Exp. Psychol.*, 47, 381.

Gilbert, A. N. and Wisocki, C. J. (1992). Hand preference and age in the United States. *Neuropsychologia*, 30, 601.

Grondin, S., Koren, S., Ivry, R. D., and Guiard, Y. (1995). *Hand and Lateral Preferences in Relation to Hitting Performance in the History of Major League Baseball.* Manuscript submitted for publication.

Guiard, Y. (1986). *Latéralisation Manuelle et Spécialisation Hémisphérique chez l'Homme: Réflexions Théoriques et Contributions Expérimentales.* Unpublished doctoral thesis, University of Aix-Marseille.

Guiard, Y. (1987). Asymmetric division of labor in human skilled bimanual action: The kinematic chain as a model. *J. Motor Behav.*, 19, 486.

Guiard, Y. (1988). The kinematic chain as a model for human asymmetrical bimanual cooperation. In A. Colley and J. Beech (Eds.), *Cognition and Action in Skilled Behavior*, Amsterdam, North-Holland, 205.

Guiard, Y. (1990). Bimanual cooperation in human motor action: A reformulation of the laterality problem. In H. Bloch and B. Berthental (Eds.), *Sensory-Motor Organization and Development in Infancy and Early Childhood*, Berlin, Kluwer Academic Publishers, 345.

Guiard, Y. (1991). Several effectors for a single act: coordination in the context of cooperation. In J. Requin and G. Stelmach (Eds.), *Tutorials in motor neuroscience*, Dordrecht, Kluwer Academic Publishers, 297.

Guiard, Y. (in press). The distal-to-proximal increase of link length along the human kinematic chain: An exponential progression of workspace extension. *Ann. Sci. Nat. (Zool.).*

Hécaen, H. and Ajuriaguerra, J. (1964). *Left Handedness: Manual Superiority and Cerebral Dominance.* New York, Grune and Stratton.

Hellige, J. B. (1993). *Hemispheric Asymmetry: What's Right and What's Left.* Cambridge, MA, Harvard University Press.

Hertz, R. (1960). The pre-eminence of the right hand: A study in religious polarity (translated from the French). In R. Hertz, *Death and the Right Hand.* Aberdeen: The University Press.

Ibbotson, N. R. and Morton, J. (1981). Rhythm and dominance. *Cognition*, 9, 125.

Jeannerod, M. (1981). Intersegmental coordination during reaching at natural visual objects. In J. Long and A. Baddeley (Eds.), *Attention and Performance IX*, Hillsdale, NJ, Erlbaum, 153.

Kabbash, P., Buxton, W., and Sellen, A. (1994). Two-handed input in a compound task. *Proceedings of the CHI '94*, 417.

Kugler, P. N. and Turvey, M. T. (1987). *Information, Natural Law, and the Self-Assembly of Rhythmic Movement.* Hillsdale. Lawrence Erlbaum.

MacNeilage, P. F., Studdert-Kennedy, M. G., and Lindblom, B. (1987). Primate handedness reconsidered. *Behav. Brain Sci.*, 10, 1.

Meyer, D. E., Abrams, R. A., Kornblum, S., Wright, C. E., and Smith, K. J. E. (1988). Optimality in human motor performance: ideal control of rapid aimed movements. *Psychol. Rev.*, 95, 340.

Oldfield, R. C. (1971). The assessment and analysis of handedness. *Neuropsychologia*, 9, 97.

Peters, M. (1981). Attentional asymmetries during concurrent bimanual performance. *Q. J. Exp. Psychol.*, 33, 95.

Peters, M. (1985). Constraints in the performance of bimanual tasks and their expression in unskilled and skilled subjects. *Q. J. Exp. Psychol.*, 37A, 171.

Peters, M. (1994). Does handedness play a role in the coordination of bimanual movement? In S. Swinnen, H. Heuer, J. Massion, and P. Casaer (Eds.), *Interlimb Coordination*, New York, Academic Press, 595.

Provins, K. A., Milner, A. D., and Kerr, P. (1982). Asymmetry of manual preference and performance. *Percep. Motor Skills*, 54, 179.

Reuleaux, F. (1877). *Cinématique: Principes fondamentaux d'une théorie générale des machines* (translated from the German). Paris: Librairie F. Savy.

Saltzman, E. and Kelso, J. A. S. (1987). Skilled actions: A task-dynamic approach. *Psychol. Rev.*, 94, 84.

Schmidt, R. C., Carello, C., and Turvey, M. T. (1990). Phase transitions and critical fluctuations in the visual coordination of rhythmic movement between people. *J. Exp. Psychol.: Hum. Percep. Perform.*, 16, 227.

Treffner, P. J. and Turvey, M. T. (1995). Handedness and the asymmetric dynamics of bimanual rhythmic coordination. *J. Exp. Psychol.: Hum. Percept. Perform.*, 21, 318.

Chapter 10

Manual Asymmetries in Children with Developmental Disabilities

Deborah Dewey

CONTENTS

1. INTRODUCTION

In recent years there has been increased interest in asymmetries of human behavior and cerebral lateralization of function. One area of particular interest has been that of manual asymmetries. However, what are manual asymmetries and how can they be examined? Manual asymmetries in their most general form can be defined as the differences between the two hands and they can be examined in a number of different ways. At the most basic level, manual asymmetries can involve the investigation of actual structural differences between hands. For example, is one hand bigger than the other?

Measurements of hand preference have also been used to assess manual asymmetries. Preference inventories typically ask the person which hand they prefer to use for specific unimanual actions listed on a questionnaire. This self-report method is normally used with adults. For children and special populations (i.e., autistic, mentally retarded), materials are presented and the individuals are asked to demonstrate hand use. However, a recent study by Bryden, MacRae, and Steenhuis (1991) indicated that preference inventories can be reliably used with primary school children. Many different hand preference inventories have been developed (e.g., Crovitz and Zener, 1962; Oldfield, 1971; Provins, Milner, and Kerr, 1982; Steenhuis and Bryden, 1989). These inventories differ in terms of their length, the type of actions that are examined (common acts vs. less common acts), and their focus (predominantly unimanual acts vs. unimanual and bimanual acts). However, all of the inventories emphasize actions that require a moderate to high level of skill (e.g., writing, drawing, using a scissors, batting) over unskilled acts (reaching and picking up an object). Hand performance has also been used as a means of assessing manual asymmetries. The tests that have been used to measure hand performance are tests of actual skill. However, the skills that are assessed are not those listed in preference

0-8493-8999-2/96/$0.00+$.50

inventories. Rather, they are usually nonpracticed or less practiced acts such as peg moving (Annett, 1970), square drawing (Bishop, 1990a), dot-marking (Tapley and Bryden, 1985) and finger tapping (Peters and During, 1978, 1979).

Research investigating motor asymmetries in infants and children has been spurred on by a number of factors. First, with infants there is need for physicians to distinguish as early as possible those that show asymmetrical behaviors that are of pathological significance and those that display asymmetries that are expected as part of normal infant development (Cohen and Duffner, 1981; Prechl, 1977). Second is the view that the motor asymmetries demonstrated by infants and children may be the earliest signs of the functional specialization of the cerebral hemispheres (Kinsbourne and Hiscock, 1983; Witelson, 1985). Handedness is often used as an indirect index of cerebral lateralization of function. Further, research indicates strong and significant associations between handedness and other measures of cerebral specialization in group data. However, in individuals, hand preference remains an unreliable indicator of lateralization (Satz, 1977).

In this chapter, manual asymmetries in children are examined from various perspectives. The first section discusses structural asymmetries in the size of the hands. Structural asymmetries of the hands in terms of directional asymmetries (i.e., where one hand is larger than the other hand) and fluctuating asymmetries (i.e., the degree of difference between bone pairs without one hand being consistently larger than the other) are examined. In addition, research that has measured structural asymmetries in left- and right-handers and in different populations of children (e.g., cerebral palsy, developmental dyspraxia, low birth weight) is presented. The next section of this chapter discusses functional asymmetries from a developmental perspective. Literature pertaining to the development of hand preference and hand skill in infants, preschool children, and school-age children is reviewed. Finally, research that has investigated manual asymmetries in children with developmental disabilities, particularly children with developmental coordination disorder is presented.

2. STRUCTURAL ASYMMETRIES

Although the human body is bilaterally symmetrical, there are distinct structural asymmetries found in children and adults (Van Dusen, 1939; Wolanski, 1972). For example, the internal organs of the human are asymmetrically organized. Also, asymmetries in fingerprints, hair whorls, and other ectodermal structures have been found (Coren, 1994; Livshits and Kobyliansky, 1987; and Ortiz De Zarate and Ortiz De Zarate, 1991). Research that has specifically examined structural asymmetries in children and adults has found that the bodies of right-handers and left-handers display subtle asymmetries.

The hands are developmentally complex structures that are each composed of 19 metacarpals and phalanges. Research has shown that the metacarpophalangeal profile across the two hands does not change appreciably with age (McLeod and Dewey, in preparation; Poznanski, 1984; Walker and Ashcroft, 1978). Thus, hand asymmetry seems to be established *in utero*. Ingelmark (1947 cited in Peters 1988), in a comprehensive study that examined both arm and leg length in relation to handedness, reported that for all right-handed subjects between the ages of 6 and 20 years, the right arm was longer, and for all left-handed subjects the left arm was longer. Studies that have specifically investigated lateral asymmetries in hand size have also reported that the right hand of right-handers is significantly larger than the left (Purves, White, and Andrews cited in White, Lucas, Richards, and Purves, 1994). For left-handers, however, studies of arm and hand asymmetries have not reported consistent results. Kimura and Konishi (1981), reported only minor left-right differences in radiogrammetric dimensions of the hands of left-handers, while Garn, Mayor, and Shaw (1976) found larger radiogrammetric dimensions of the second metacarpal in the right hands of left-handed individuals. Colburne, Kaplan, Crawford and Mcleod (1993), using the Computer Automated Metacarpophalangeal Profile System (CAMPS; Coupland, McLeod, Wesenberg, and Lowry, 1985) which measures the length of each metacarpal and phalangeal bone in the hands from radiographs, found that extreme left-handers had significantly larger left than right hands, while extreme right-handers had significantly larger right than left hands. In a follow-up study, Hoffer and Kaplan (1993) divided their left-handed subjects into two groups: one with a family history of left-handedness and a second without a family history of left-handedness. Examination of the hand asymmetries of these two groups indicated that the left-handers with a family history of left-handedness had significantly larger left than right hands, while the hands of left-handers without a family history of left-handedness were symmetrical. In other words, in the nonfamilial left-handers the right and the left hands did not differ in terms of hand size. Thus, in left-handed individuals there appears to be a more variable pattern of lateralized structural asymmetries of the hands than in right-handed individuals.

It has long been recognized that children with early unilateral brain lesions may develop trophic limb changes resulting in limb asymmetries (Aram, Elkelman, and Satz, 1986; Hiscock, Hiscock, Benjamins, and Hillman, 1989; Satz, Yanowitz, and Willmore, 1984). Although there has been much research to suggest that children with certain developmental disabilities (e.g., dyslexia, autism) may also have subtle cerebral abnormalities that may be the result of perinatal stress, little research on structural limb asymmetries has been reported. However, Iloeje (1988) found a higher incidence of pathological limb asymmetry (i.e., one limb being significantly larger than the other limb) among children with developmental dyspraxia compared to normal control children. Also, Dewey, McLeod, and Kaplan (1993) reported that children with developmental motor deficits demonstrate a trend towards significant left-right differences in hand asymmetries compared to normal controls.

As indicated by the above discussion, most of the research that has investigated structural hand asymmetries in children has looked at directional asymmetries, that is, whether one hand is larger than the other (e.g., Aram et al., 1986; Hiscock et al., 1989; White et al., 1994). However, a second type of hand asymmetry that can been investigated is fluctuating asymmetry which reflects the inability of organisms to develop perfect symmetry. It can be defined as the measure of random differences in bone pairs (McLeod and Coupland, 1992). Thus, in the case of the hands, a high degree of fluctuating asymmetry would reflect a large size difference between bone pairs but without one side (i.e., right or left) being consistently larger than the other.

In the genetics literature, the magnitude of fluctuating asymmetry in a population is felt to be an indicator of genetic, developmental, or environmental stress (Clarke, Brand, and Whitten, 1986; Livshits, David, Kobyliansky, Ben-Amital, Levi, and Merlob, 1988; Livshits and Kobyliansky, 1987; Malina and Buschang, 1984). Research with humans has found that premature infants (Livshits et al., 1988), individuals with cleft lip and/or palate (Woolf and Gianas, 1976), Down's syndrome (Barden, 1980), and Fragile X syndrome (Peretz, Ever-Hadani, Casamassimo, Eidelman, Shellhart, and Hagerman, 1988) show increased fluctuating asymmetry. Dewey et al. (1993) also reported that children with developmental motor deficits displayed a trend towards increased fluctuating asymmetry of the hands compared to normal controls. This finding was accompanied by a reported trend towards greater perinatal complications among the motor deficit group.

Some investigators have suggested that left-handedness is the consequence of stressful prenatal and/or birth conditions (Bakan, Dibb, and Reed, 1973; Beaton, 1985; Harris and Carlson, 1988). As fluctuating asymmetry is thought to be the result of increased developmental stress, left-handers should demonstrate higher levels of fluctuating asymmetry than right-handers if they have experienced prenatal and/or birth stress. However, two studies that have investigated fluctuating asymmetry in the hands of right- and left-handers found no significant differences (Colburne et al., 1993; Hoffer and Kaplan, 1993).

In conclusion, the above studies indicate that among right-handers the right hand is larger than the left hand. With left-handers, however, there appears to be a more variable pattern of directional asymmetry. Research findings have indicated that left-handers with a family history of left-handedness have a larger left than right hand, while left-handers without a family history of left-handedness do not demonstrate any directional asymmetries in terms of hand size. Studies with children and adults with developmental disabilities suggest that these different populations may demonstrate different types of hand asymmetries (i.e., directional, fluctuating). Therefore, studies of structural hand asymmetries should look not only at directional asymmetry as many previous investigators have done (i.e., Aram et al., 1986; Iloeje, 1988) but also at fluctuating asymmetry.

3. DEVELOPMENT OF MANUAL ASYMMETRIES

Infants are not capable of the motor activities that have been used to investigate manual performance and to determine manual preference in more mature individuals. However, studies have attempted to investigate manual asymmetries in infants by looking at spontaneous limb movements (e.g., Valentine and Wagner, 1934), infant grasp (e.g., Caplan and Kinsbourne, 1976) and object-oriented movements (e.g., Difranco, Muir, and Dodwell, 1978). Valentine and Wagner (1934) recorded the spontaneous movements of 100 newborn infants for 5 to 20 minutes each day over a 10-day period following birth. They reported significantly more movements with the right arm than the left arm. Specifically, they found that 12 of the infants showed a predominance of right arm activity for the 10-day period, while 2 showed a predominance of left arm activity. The majority of infants, however, displayed a fluctuating predominance of activity from one side to the other from day to day. Giesecke (1936) in a study that investigated differences in the spontaneous activity of the right and left hands in seven infants during the first 6 months of life found greater overall activity in the right hand for four subjects and a similar predominance of left hand activity in the other three. Consistent with Valentine and Wagner (1934), Giesecke also reported that there was considerable variation in the dominance of the right and left hand from one time to another for all of the subjects involved in the study. A more recent study that examined newborns' spontaneous movements that bring the hand to the mouth (Hopkins, Lems, Janssen, and Butterworth, 1987) found that hand-mouth contacts were much more common with the right hand. In this study, 10 of the 12 infants showed a right hand preference, while 2 displayed a definite left hand preference. Of note was the finding that in these infants no predominance for the right or left hand was noted for hand-face contacts. Butterworth and Hopkins (1988) suggested that these differences in lateral hand preference for hand-mouth vs. hand-face movements may be due to the intention of the movement. They stated that hand-mouth movements appear to be intentional, rather than random, as the mouth opened before the hand reached it.

Although the above studies reported lateral differences in spontaneous hand movement in early infancy, other studies have not found such differences. Korczyn, Sage, and Karplus (1978) investigated differences between the right and left sides in the initiation of movements of the arms and legs in 150 infants aged 24 hours to 3 days. Results indicated no difference in the number of babies initiating a movement with the right arm or the right leg. Korczyn et al. also tested another group of 15 infants five times at 12-hour intervals. Results of this serially tested sample were similar to the previous finding.

Further, none of the these infants showed a consistent preference for either the right or the left side. Eaton, McKeen, and Lam (1988) also reported finding no differences between sides in the total number of spontaneous movements for upper and lower limbs in infants with a mean age of 6.7 weeks. However, no data were published for the upper and lower limbs separately.

A number of studies have investigated lateral asymmetries in how long infants grasp a rattle. Caplan and Kinsbourne (1976) studied 21 infants aged 1 to 4 months and reported that grasp was maintained for longer with the right hand than with the left. Similar results were recorded by Petrie and Peters (1980) and Hawn and Harris (1983) for 2-month-old infants. However, other investigations that have attempted to replicate these experiments have failed to find any manual asymmetries in the performance of this task (Strauss, 1982; Yu-Yan, Cun-Ren, and Over, 1983).

Investigations of manual asymmetries in the object-oriented movements of infants have also reported inconsistent results. For example, von Hofsten (1982, 1984) and Ottaviano, Guidette, Allemand, Spinetoli, and Seri (1989) reported right hand biases for object-oriented movements, while Difranco et al. (1978) and McDonnell, Anderson, and Abraham (1983) reported left hand biases.

The results of the above studies indicate that lateral inconsistencies are characteristic of the limb movements of infants. Further, analyses confined to group trends conceal the considerable variability in the manual preference that infants demonstrate within groups and over time (Carlson and Harris, 1985). Finally, it should be noted that the manual behaviors (i.e., grip strength endurance, spontaneous movements that involve simple extension and flexion of the limbs) used to examine infant manual asymmetries are very different from the preference and performance measures used to assess adult handedness (i.e., skilled movements such as writing, peg moving). Adults show little or no differences between sides on the elementary types of manual movements that are used to examine infant manual asymmetries. It is only when some degree of skill is required that we see differences in hand preference and performance (Provins, 1992). The earliest manifestations of these manual skills occur at about the end of the first year of life. At this point in time, the infant is capable of reaching, pointing, and performing movements that are analogous to the activities used to determine hand preference in older people. For example, Bates and her colleagues (Bates, O'Connell, Vaid, Sledge, and Oakes, 1986) reported that after pointing emerges towards the end of the first year of life, the infant is more likely to use the right hand than the left hand. Also, studies that have examined infants' performance on bimanual tasks such as a nut-and-bolt task have found that towards the end of the first year, the majority of infants (i.e., two thirds or more) turn the bolt with their right hand while holding the nut with their left hand (Cornwell, Harris, and Fitzgerald, 1991; Ramsay, 1980).

With the transition from infancy to childhood, there is a significant improvement in all motor skills. The inconsistencies in lateral hand preference shown by infants decrease and children show more stable hand preference. Cross-sectional studies that have examined hand preference in preschool and school age children suggest that there is an increase in right-hand preference with age (e.g., Belmont and Birch, 1965; Bruml, 1972; DeAgostini, Pare, Goudot and Dellatolas, 1992). For example, DeAgostini et al. (1992) reported that there was a greater proportion of mixed-handed children at 3 years of age than at 6 years of age. Further, the decreasing percentage of mixed-handed children from 3 to 6 years of age was completely accounted for by an increase in right-handed children. Thus, a certain number of children classified as mixed-handed at age 3 were reclassified as right-handed at 6 years of age. Other investigators have also reported increasing proportions of right-handers in preschool populations (Curt, Maccario, and Dellatolas, 1992). Studies that have investigated manual preferences in older children have also reported an increase in right-hand preference with age (Burml, 1972; Belmont and Birch, 1965; Maehara, Negishi, Tsai, Iizuka, Otsuki, Suzuki, Takahashi, and Sumiyoshi, 1988). However, other studies have not observed an age effect for manual preference (Rymer, Kameyama, Niwa, Hiramatsu, and Saitoh, 1984).

The few longitudinal studies that have investigated the development of handedness from infancy to childhood have reported a gradual increase in stable hand preference with age (Fennell, Satz, and Morris, 1983; Gesell and Ames, 1947). Further, both cross-sectional (Bruml, 1972) and longitudinal studies (Fennell et al., 1983; Gaillard and Satz, 1990) have found that children identified as left-handed show more instability of handedness than right-handed children as indexed by the use of different hands both across and within tasks. Specifically, Fennell et al. (1983) found that in their sample of children with reading difficulties, hand preference at age 5 predicted handedness scores at age 11 for 97% of the right-handers compared to only 74% of the left-handers. Of the children classified as "mixed-handed" at age 5, only 4% remained so at age 11 years, with the majority becoming right-handed.

Although studies that have investigated hand preference in children suggest that there is an increase in the stability of hand preference from early childhood to adolescence, cross-sectional studies of hand performance indicate that there is stability in both direction and degree of handedness as early as 3 years of age (Harris, 1992). Most studies that have investigated asymmetries in hand performance in preschool and school age children have found little evidence for developmental change (Annett, 1970; Denckla, 1973, 1974; Peters and Durding, 1978). For example, on a peg-moving task, Annett (1970) reported that the majority of children at all ages did better with their right hand. Further, although overall performance improved with age, age was not a significant factor in right-left differences between the hands in terms of speed of peg-moving. However, the results of a recent study by DeAgostini et al. (1992) suggest that the impact of age on right-left hand performance is related to the task. As with previous studies, these investigators found that on a peg-moving task, the preferred hand advantage did not increase with age. However, on a graphic task similar to that used by Tapley and Bryden (1985), preferred hand advantage clearly increased from 3 to 6 years of age. These investigators suggested that these differences in task performance could be explained by the influence of training. The period between 3 and 6 years of age is a training period for pencil manipulation in children, whereas there is no specific training for peg-moving during this time period.

Studies that have investigated sex differences in handedness have repeatedly found a higher prevalence of mixed or left-handedness in boys compared to girls (Annett, 1970; Annett and Kilshaw, 1983, Brito, Lins, Paumgartten, and Brito, 1992; DeAgostini et al., 1992; Hardyck, Goldman, and Petrinovich, 1975). This is consistent with findings reported in the adult literature (Bryden, 1977; Porac and Coren, 1981). Why there are more left-handed males than females is not known; however, Geschwind and Galaburda (1985) have suggested that hormonal factors acting *in utero* may play a role in cerebral lateralization and handedness.

4. MANUAL ASYMMETRIES IN CHILDREN WITH DEVELOPMENTAL DISABILITIES

The idea of a link between handedness and developmental disabilities is not new. Orton (1937) suggested that a lack of strong hand preference in children may indicate underlying confusion of cerebral dominance that results in an increased risk of specific reading problems and stuttering in children. Theories that implicate a lack of strong cerebral lateralization have remained popular as explanations for reading disability, developmental language disorders, and other types of developmental disabilities (i.e., autism, mental retardation, clumsiness) (e.g., Geschwind and Galaburda, 1985). Further, handedness has been viewed as an indirect index of this lack of cerebral lateralization of function. The following sections of this chapter will present research that has investigated manual asymmetries in different populations of children with developmental disabilities.

4.1 MANUAL ASYMMETRIES IN READING AND LANGUAGE DISORDERS

The relationship between reading and language disorders and left-handedness has been the subject of a number of studies. However, the results of these studies have been inconsistent. For example, in the case of reading disorders, some studies have reported a higher percentage of left-handers among retarded readers compared to normal controls (e.g., Annett, 1985; Obrzut and Atkinson, 1993), while other studies have not found an elevated incidence of left-handedness in poor readers (e.g., Bishop, 1984; Hugdahl, Synnevag, and Satz, 1990; Satz and Fletcher, 1987). Satz and Fletcher (1987) argued that the relationship between left-handedness and dyslexia that is part of the lore of the learning disability literature is a "myth" based on anecdotal evidence or small clinical samples where selection bias is high. Bishop (1990b) in her review of the literature on handedness and developmental disorders states that many of the studies that have investigated the relationship between poor reading and handedness have only been concerned with the relationship between reading ability and handedness. They have not specifically investigated the relationship between dyslexia (i.e., specific reading disability) and handedness. Her summary of the data from 25 studies that have investigated the association between handedness and specific reading disability suggested that there was no real difference in handedness between dyslexic and control children. She noted, however, that her data were heavily influenced by the large British National Child Development Study (Bishop, 1984) which found no difference in the incidence of left-handedness between dyslexics and normal controls. When the 24 remaining studies were examined, the overall rate of left-handedness was found to be 11.2% in dyslexics and 5.8% in control subjects. Recently, Eglington and Annett (1994) reanalyzed these studies using a meta-analysis procedure. Results showed that there was a small but reliable increase in the proportion of nonrighthanders among dyslexics. Given these conflicting data, it is difficult to come to any conclusions concerning the relationship between hand preference and dyslexia. However, Bishop's (1990a) and Eglington and Annett's (1994) reviews do suggest that the proportion of nonrighthanders is higher in children with specific reading problems.

Many children who ultimately have difficulty learning to read show early developmental language disorders (Tallal and Katz, 1989). Therefore, one may predict that these children will display a higher level of nonrighthandedness than would be expected in the normal population. However, recent studies that have investigated the relationship between developmental language disorders and handedness have reported no differences in hand preference between children with developmental language disorders and normal controls (Bishop, 1990a; Neils and Aram, 1986). It is possible that the lack of evidence for an increase in nonrighthandedness among children with developmental language disorders may be due to the fact that developmental language disorders are often detected in very young children and the techniques for measuring handedness in these children are quite crude or idiosyncratic (Bryden, McManus and Bulman-Fleming, 1994). A second reason for the lack of significant findings may be due to the fact that children with language problems are quite a heterogeneous group (Bishop, 1990a). Studies that have attempted to look at subgroups of children with developmental language problems have found that left-handedness appears to be associated with a subgroup of language-impaired children with severe difficulties in speech sound production (Morley, 1972; Neils and Aram, 1986).

Although many studies have examined the relationships of hand preference, dyslexia, and developmental language disorders, fewer studies have specifically looked at the relationships between these disorders and hand skill. Studies that have looked at peg-moving speed in dyslexics and in children with developmental language disorders have reported no significant differences in asymmetries in hand performance compared to normal controls (Annett and Kilshaw, 1984; Bishop, 1990a; Bishop and Edmundson, 1987, Powell and Bishop, 1992). However, Bishop (1990a) noted that in her language-impaired sample, the skill of both hands was poorer in children with persisting language difficulties than it was in normal controls and in children whose specific language difficulties had resolved. Of note is the finding that both dyslexics and children with developmental language disorders appeared to have difficulties on tasks involving rate of movement (Johnston, Stark, Mellitis, and Tallal, 1981; Wolff, Cohen, and Drake, 1984). Studies by Wolff and his colleagues (Klicpera, Wolff, and Drake, 1981; Rousselle and Wolff, 1991; Wolff et al., 1984, Wolff, Michel, Drake, and Ovrut, 1990) have also found that dyslexics do well on both unimanual and bimanual synchronous motor tasks, but have greater difficulty with bimanual asymmetrical coordination tasks. Since no performance differences were found between the right and the left hand, Wolff et al. (1990) concluded the difficulties in bimanual coordination seen in dyslexia are associated with a reduced efficiency in interhemispheric transfer of information.

4.2 MANUAL ASYMMETRIES IN AUTISM AND MENTAL RETARDATION

Studies that have investigated the relationship between handedness and autism have reported that autistic children show an increased incidence of left-handedness (approximately 18%) (Bryson, Porac, and Smith, 1990; Fein, Humes, Kaplan, Lucci, and Waterhouse, 1984; Gillberg, 1983) and increased incidence of lack of hand preference (approximately 36%) (Fein et al., 1984; Satz, Soper, Orsini, Henry, and Zvi, 1985; Soper, Satz, Orsini, Henry, Zvi, and Schulman, 1986). This lack of hand preference has been called "ambiguous handedness" and refers to an inconsistency in hand preference for a particular activity across repeated testings (Satz et al., 1985; Soper et al., 1986). Satz and his colleagues argue that many autistic children have simply not developed any hand preference and thus are less strongly right-handed than normal children. Further, three recent studies have reported that autistic children who display this pattern of ambiguous handedness represent a more cognitively impaired group compared to autistic children who display consistent hand preferences (Fein, Waterhouse, Lucci, Pennington, and Humes, 1985; Soper et al., 1986; Tsai, 1982).

While few studies have investigated hand performance in autistic children, McManus, Murray, Doyle, and Baron-Cohen (1992) did not find a significant difference in performance between autistic and normal comparison children on Annett's peg-moving task. Unlike normal comparison children and children with mental retardation who demonstrated a high level of concordance between hand preference and hand skill (i.e., 90 and 92%, respectively), children with autism showed a significantly lower level of concordance of preference and skill (i.e., 50%). This dissociation between hand preference and hand skill is quite unusual when compared to other populations and suggests that handedness in children with autism is different from that of normal comparison children and children with mental retardation. Further, on the basis of these data, McManus et al. propose a developmental model of handedness in which the development of hand preference precedes the development of hand skill. In normal children, the development of skill asymmetry occurs as a secondary consequence of the establishment of hand preference. In children with autism, however, this developmental sequence is disrupted and although hand preference is established it does not result in concordant hand skill asymmetries.

Among children with mental retardation, left-handedness also appears to be more frequent than among normal comparison children. Studies have reported that the percentage of left-handers among children with mental retardation is about double that of the normal population (e.g., Batheja and McManus, 1985; Bradshaw-McAnulty, Hicks, and Kinsbourne, 1984; Ross, Lipper, and Auld, 1987). For example, Ross et al. (1987) reported that in a group of 4-year-old children with IQs under 85, 19% were left-handed compared to 11% of a group of children with normal IQs. When severity of mental retardation has been investigated, a different picture begins to emerge for this population. Specifically, the increased percentage of left-handers in the population of children with mental retardation appeared to be due to an increase in the number of left-handers in the more severely retarded individuals. Among the mild or moderately retarded, the percentage of left-handers was found to be similar to that found in the normal population (Bradshaw-McAnutly et al., 1984; Hicks and Barton, 1975). The question that must be asked then is whether the increased levels of left-handedness reported in the more severely retarded children are due to an increased level of left hand preference or due to an inconsistency in hand preference or "ambiguous handedness." The results of recent studies suggests that an increased incidence in "ambiguous handedness" among severely retarded individuals may account for the reports of increased levels of left-handedness in the mentally retarded population (Bishop, 1990b; Soper, Satz, Orsini, Van Gorp, and Green, 1987).

4.3 MANUAL ASYMMETRIES IN DEVELOPMENTAL COORDINATION DISORDER

Mixed-hand preference, poorly established hand preference, and pathological left-handedness have all been linked with clumsiness (Armitage and Larkin, 1993). However, examination of the literature indicates that very little research has specifically investigated manual asymmetries in children with motor problems. The lack of research with this group of children may be due to the fact that motor problems are often accompanied by a wide range of impairments such as language, learning, and attention problems (Henderson, 1987). Thus, developmental motor problems are often viewed as difficulties that are secondary to the language, learning, or attentional impairments, and their relationship to handedness has not been investigated.

Investigators in the field of learning disabilities have claimed that left-lateralized children tend to have more motor and perceptual-motor problems (Hallahan and Kaufman, 1977). Further, teacher reports have supported this view (Calnan and Richardson, 1976). However, the few studies that have examined the relationship between handedness and motor skills have not reported consistent results. Flick (1966) compared the performance of left- and right-handed 4-year-olds on five perceptual-motor tests and reported that left-handers obtained lower scores than right-handers. Conversely, Tan (1985) reported that consistent left-handers and right-handers who were 4 years of age did not differ in performance on the Preschool Fine Motor Scale of the McCarthy Scales (McCarthy, 1972). However, children who displayed a lack of definite hand preference obtained significantly lower scores on this measure of motor ability. Similar findings have been reported by other investigators (Gottfried and Bathurst, 1983; Kaufman, Zalma, and Kaufman, 1978) and suggest that children who establish handedness early whether it is right- or left-handedness are better coordinated than those who establish it later or not at all. A recent study by Gabbard, Hart, and Kanipe (1993) tested this assumption. They classified 4- to 6-year-olds as either consistent or inconsistent in their hand preference and tested fine motor performance using a finger tapping task. Results revealed no significant difference between groups in finger tapping performance. Contrary to the previous reports, children with consistent and inconsistent hand preferences did not differ in motor behavior as revealed by their performance on the finger tapping task.

What may account for the inconsistencies in the findings of the above studies? One possible explanation may be differences in the tasks used to assess motor behavior. Specifically, the studies of Gottfried and Bathurst (1983), Kaufman et al. (1978), and Tan (1985) assessed gross- and fine-motor activities that required the use of relatively large groups of muscles and considerable eye-hand coordination, while the motor task used by Gabbard et al. (1993) demanded the use of a relatively small group of muscles and little ocular control. Thus, the findings of the above studies suggest that motor differences may exist between children with and without definite hand preferences on motor tasks that demand the use of relatively large groups of muscles and considerable eye-hand coordination. Whether children with developmental coordination disorders are more likely to display inconsistent hand preference relative to other comparison groups of children is an area in need of further study.

Examination of the literature on children with developmental coordination disorder reveals that few studies have specifically investigated manual preferences in this group of children. Further, many of the studies that have investigated the performance of children with developmental coordination disorders on motor and nonmotor tasks have not reported hand preference (e.g., Henderson and Hall, 1982; Hoare, 1994). Studies that have reported on the hand preference of children with developmental coordination disorder (i.e., clumsy children) have found that the incidence of left-handedness among this population is not significantly different from normal comparison groups (Armitage and Larkin, 1993; Dewey and Kaplan, 1992; Gubbay, 1975; Hoare, 1991). However, Gillberg and Rasmussen (1982) reported an increased incidence of left-handedness in their "minimal brain dysfunction" (MBD) group, which was composed of children who were both clumsy and showed signs of attention deficit (i.e., 21%), compared to their normal comparison group (i.e., 7%). They also reported that a small group of children (n = 7) with fine or gross motor dysfunction or perceptual dysfunction ("minimal perceptual dysfunction"; MPD) did not display an increased incidence of left-handedness. Thus, the findings of the above studies suggest that left-handedness may be associated with a specific subgroup of children with developmental coordination disorder who may also display attentional deficits. However, further research on manual preferences in children with developmental coordination disorder is needed to determine if these different subgroups do display significant differences in manual preferences.

The few studies that have investigated hand skill asymmetries in children with developmental coordination disorder have consistently reported that these children do not display significant manual skill asymmetries compared to normal comparison children (Dewey, 1990; Dewey and Kaplan, 1992; Geuze and Kalverboer, 1994). However, Dewey (1990) did find that on tests that measure the speed of performance of repetitive and alternating movements, children with developmental coordination disorder were significantly slower with both their preferred and nonpreferred hands than normal control children except on the hand pronation-supination test (see Table 10.1). Similarly, Dewey and Kaplan (1992) found that children with developmental motor deficits performed nonrepresentational limb gestures less well with both their preferred and nonpreferred hands. Geuze and Kalverboer (1992) in their investigation of timing problems in "clumsy" children reported that these children did not display any lateralized performance differences on unimanual, alternating bimanual or asymmetrical bimanual tapping tasks.

Table 10.1 Means and Standard Deviations for the Preferred and Nonpreferred Hand

	Motor Problem				Normal Comparison			
	Preferred		Nonpreferred		Preferred		Nonpreferred	
	Mean	SD	Mean	SD	Mean	SD	Mean	SD
Repetitive Finger Taps	6.61	2.37	7.08	2.52	5.27	.91	5.70	1.13
Successive Finger Opposition	13.14	4.09	12.78	3.76	9.51	2.39	9.92	3.17
Repetitive Hand Taps	5.51	1.67	6.16	1.70	4.67	.89	5.17	.91
Hand Pronation-Supination	7.71	1.85	7.94	1.81	6.58	1.29	7.47	4.89

Note: The above numbers are time in seconds to produce 20 movements.

However, compared to a group of dyslexics and a group of children without reading and motor problems, the "clumsy" children showed a slight increase in timing variability across all tasks.

4.4 SUMMARY

The literature on children with developmental disabilities does not provide us with a consistent picture concerning manual asymmetries in these clinically defined groups. Research with children with developmental dyslexia suggests that the proportion of nonrighthanders may be higher in children with specific reading problems; however, this is not a consistently reported finding. In children with developmental language disorders, the findings are even less clear. Overall, the studies have revealed no differences in hand preference between children with language disorders and normal comparison children, though there is some evidence to suggest that an increased prevalence of left-handedness may be associated with a subgroup of children with severe difficulties in speech sound production. With autistic and mentally retarded children, the research shows an increased incidence of left-handedness and lack of hand preference. However, in both of these populations the increased levels of left-handedness and/or "ambiguous handedness" are associated with more severe cognitive impairments. Finally, among children with developmental coordination disorder, a higher incidence of left-handedness has not been found in clinical populations. Further, studies that have examined the performance of these children on motor tasks have not found any lateralized performance differences. Thus, the results of these studies suggest that with some groups of children with developmental disabilities there may be an increased incidence of left-handedness. However, this relationship is not as clear and consistent as has been suggested by some theorists.

5. FUTURE DIRECTIONS

This chapter has examined research on the development of manual asymmetries in children and on manual asymmetries in children with developmental disabilities. The results of these studies provide interesting suggestions for future research. One area of research that needs further investigation is the question of what develops first hand preference asymmetries or hand performance asymmetries. McManus et al. (1992) presents a developmental model of handedness in which he proposes that hand preference asymmetries precede performance asymmetries. According to his model, the normal sequence of laterality development involves three sequential stages: (1) an initial stage of simple turning tendencies, (2) a period of "chaotic lateralization," and (3) the formation of hand preference. Practice of a skill with either hand will result in improved performance of that skill. However, hand preference asymmetry will result in the child using their preferred hand to practice a skill more frequently causing the manual skill of the preferred hand to be enhanced relative to the nonpreferred hand. As 90% of the adult population are right-handed in that they prefer to use the right hand for carrying out actions (McManus et al., 1992), a preference before performance model suggests that there is some hard-wired mechanism that increases the probability of preferring the right hand. One possible mechanism may be related to the fact that speech/language is in most cases lateralized to the left hemisphere. This might result in increased activation of the left hemisphere as language develops which in turn may result in an increase in the propensity to use the right hand. This sequence of development would suggest that hand preference and language would emerge at about the same time. The fact that at approximately 1 year of age we begin to see the emergence of language (Lenneberg, 1967) and the development of consistent manual preferences (Bates et al., 1986; Cornwell et al., 1991; Ramsay, 1980) provides some support for the idea that hand preference asymmetries precede performance asymmetries. Longitudinal studies which examine the development of both manual preference asymmetries and manual skill asymmetries in infants will assist us in determining the causal relationship between hand preference and hand skill. Further, prospective longitudinal studies which examine the relationship between language development, manual preference, and manual skill in normal and disabled populations (i.e., speech and language disordered, dyslexics, dyspraxic, autistic, mentally retarded) may provide us with some insight concerning the neurodevelopmental changes that affect the emergence of hand preference and manual skill.

Typically it has been found that in children and adults hand preference asymmetries are highly concordant with hand performance asymmetries (McManus et al., 1992). In other words, the preferred hand is also the more skilled hand for performing motor tasks. However, there is some suggestion in the research literature that the relationship between manual preference asymmetries and manual performance asymmetries may depend upon the nature of the motor task (Gabbard et al., 1993). It is possible that manual preference/performance asymmetries are specific to tasks that involve the use of tools (e.g., writing with a pen, cutting with scissors). In motor tasks that do not involve the use of tools, such as finger tapping or playing the piano, it is possible that children still may indicate a specific manual preference; however, this preference may not be concordant with hand performance asymmetries. The relationship between preference asymmetries and performance asymmetries may also vary as a function of both task demands and the age of the child (Denckla and Roeltgen, 1992). It is possible that as a child matures, asymmetries in skill performance with the preferred hand may disappear on specific tasks. Thus, future research which investigates the relationship between hand preference asymmetries and hand performance asymmetries needs to take into account the type of tasks that are being used, the age of the child performing the tasks, and how these variables interact to affect performance.

The research literature suggests that in some groups of children with developmental disabilities, there may be an increased incidence of left-handedness or ambiguous handedness. Further, research suggests that among children with autism and children with mental retardation, the increased incidence of left-handedness or ambiguous handedness appears to be found in the more cognitively impaired children (Bradshaw-McAnutly et al., 1984; Fein et al., 1985; Hicks and Barton, 1975; Soper et al., 1986; Tsai, 1982). It may be of interest for future research to investigate the relationship between severity of the disability, hand preference asymmetries and hand performance asymmetries. It is possible that such research may be better able to identify specific populations that display a higher incidence of left-handedness. For example, such research may reveal that among children with speech and language disorders, only a subgroup of children with severe language disorders of a specific type display a higher incidence of left-handedness. Future research should also attempt to clarify differences between developmentally disabled children who display left-hand preference/performance asymmetries and those that display ambiguous handedness or an inconsistency in hand preference/performance. The findings of the present research suggest that not showing any consistent asymmetry in manual preference or manual performance may be indicative of a more severe disability. However, more research with different populations of developmentally disabled children is needed to clarify this issue.

ACKNOWLEDGMENT

Support for this chapter was provided by the Alberta Children's Hospital Foundation.

REFERENCES

Annett, M.A. (1970). The classification of hand preference by association analysis. *Br. J. Psychol.*, 61, 303.

Annett, M.A. (1985). *Left, Right, Hand and Brain: The Right Shift Theory.* London, Erlbaum.

Annett, M.A. and Kilshaw, D. (1983). Right-and left-hand skill II: estimating the parameters of the distribution of L-R differences in males and females. *Br. J. Psychol.*, 74, 269.

Annett, M.A. and Kilshaw, D. (1984). Lateral preference and skill in dyslexics: implications of the right shift theory. *J. Child Psychol. Psych.*, 25, 357.

Aram, D.M., Elkelman, B., and Satz, P. (1986). Tropic changes following early unilateral injury to the brain. *Dev. Med. Child Neurol.*, 28, 165.

Armitage, M. and Larkin, D. (1993). Laterality, motor asymmetry and clumsiness in children. *Hum. Move. Sci.*, 12, 155.

Bakan, P., Dibb, G., and Reed, P. (1973). Handedness and birth stress. *Neuropsychologia*, 11, 363.

Barden, H.S. (1980). Fluctuating dental asymmetry: a measure of developmental instability in Down's Syndrome. *Am. J. Phys. Anthropol.*, 52, 169.

Bates, E., O'Connell, B., Vaid, J., Sledge, P., and Oakes, L. (1986). Language and hand preference in early development. *Dev. Neuropsychol.*, 2, 1.

Batheja, M. and McManus, I.C. (1985). Handedness in the mentally handicapped. *Dev. Med. Child Neurol.*, 27, 63.

Beaton, A. (1985). Leftside Rightside: A Review of Laterality Research. New Haven, Yale University Press.

Belmont, L. and Birch, H.G. (1965). Lateral dominance, lateral awareness, and reading disability. *Child Develop.*, 36, 57.

Bishop, D.V.M. (1984). Using nonpreferred hand skill to investigate pathological left-handedness in an unselected population. *Dev. Med. Child Neurol.*, 26, 214.

Bishop, D.V.M. (1990a). Handedness, clumsiness and developmental language disorders. *Neuropsychologia*, 28,681.

Bishop, D.V.M. (1990b). *Handedness and Developmental Disorder.* Oxford: Blackwell.

Bishop, D.V.M. and Edmundson, A. (1987). Specific language impairment as a maturational lag: Evidence from longitudinal data on language and motor development. *Dev. Med. Child Neurol.*, 29, 442.

Brito, G.N.O., Lins, M.F.C., Paumgartten, F.J.R., and Brito, L.S.O., (1992). Hand preference in 4-7-year-old children: an analysis with the Edinburgh Inventory in Brazil. *Dev. Neuropsychol.*, 8, 59.

Bradshaw-McAnutly, G., Hicks, R.E., and Kinsbourne, M. (1984). Pathological left-handedness and family sinistrality in relation to degree of mental retardation. *Brain Cognit.*, 3, 349.

Bruml, H. (1972). Age changes in preference and skill measures of handedness. *Percept. Motor Skills*, 34, 3.

Bryden, M.P. (1977). Measuring handedness with questionnaires. *Neuropsychologia*, 15, 617.

Bryden, M.P., MacRae, L., and Steenhuis, R.E. (1991). Hand preference in school children. *Dev. Neuropsychol.*, 7, 477.

Bryden, M.P., McManus, I.C., and Bulman-Fleming, M.B. (1994). Evaluating the empirical support for the Geschwind-Behan-Galaburda model of cerebral lateralization. *Brain Cognit.*, 26, 103.

Bryson, S.E., Porac, C., and Smith, I.M. (1990). Lateral preferences in autistic children. *Can. Psychol.*, 31, 369.

Butterworth, G. and Hopkins, B. (1988). Hand-mouth coordination in the new-born baby. *Br. J. Dev. Psychol.*, 6, 303.

Calnan, M. and Richardson, K. (1976). Developmental correlates of handedness in a national sample of 11-year-olds. *Ann. Hum. Biol.*, 3, 329.

Caplan, P.J. and Kinsbourne, M. (1976). Baby drops the rattle: asymmetry of duration of grasp by infants. *Child Dev.*, 47, 532.

Carlson, D.F. and Harris, L.J. (1985). Development of the infant's hand preference for visually directed reaching: Preliminary report of a longitudinal study. *Inf. Ment. Health J.*, 6, 158.

Clarke, G.M., Brand, G.W., and Whitten, M.J. (1986). Fluctuating asymmetry: a technique for measuring developmental stress caused by inbreeding. *Aust. J. Biol. Sci.*, 39, 145.

Cohen, M.E. and Duffner, P.E. (1981). Prognostic indicators of hemiparetic cerebral palsy. *Ann. Neurol.*, 9, 353.

Colburne, K.A. Kaplan, B.J., Crawford, S.G. and McLeod, D.R. (1993). Hand Asymmetry: its relationship to nonrighthandedness. *J. Clin. Exp. Neuropsychol.*, 15, 67.

Coren, S. (1994). Are fingerprints a genetic marker for handedness? *Behav. Gen.*, 24, 141.

Cornwell, K.S., Harris, L.J., and Fitzgerald, H.E. (1991). Task effects in the development of hand preference in 9-, 13-, and 20-month-old infant girls. *Dev. Neuropsychol.*, 7, 19

Coupland, S.G., McLeod, D.R., Wesenberg, R.L., and Lowry, R.B. (1985). CAMPS: Computer-automated metacarpophalangeal profile system. *Am. J. Med. Gen.*, 22, 375-381

.Crovitz, H.F. and Zener, K. (1962). A group-test for assessing hand- and eye-dominance. *Am. J. Psychol.*, 73, 271.

Curt, F., Maccario, J., and Dellatolas, G. (1992). Distributions of hand preference and hand skill in preschool children: theoretical implications. *Neuropsychologia*, 30, 27.

DeAgostini, M., Pare, C., Goudot, D., and Dellatolas, G. (1992). Manual preference and skill development in preschool children. *Dev. Neuropsychol.*, 8, 41.

Denckla, M.B. (1973). Development of speed in repetitive and successive finger-movements in normal children. *Dev. Med. Child Neurol.*, 15, 635.

Denckla, M.B. (1974). Development of motor coordination in normal children. *Dev. Med. Child Neurol.*, 16, 729.

Denckla, M.B. and Roeltgen, D.P. (1992). Disorders of motor function and control. In I. Rapin and S.J. Segalowitz (Eds.), *Handbook of Neuropsychology: Vol. 6. Child Neuropsychology*, Amsterdam, Elsevier, 455.

Dewey, D. (1990). *An Investigation of the Relationship Between Motor Deficits and Academic Performance.* Unpublished Doctoral Dissertation, University of Calgary, Calgary, AB, Canada.

Dewey, D. and Kaplan, B.J. (1992). Analysis of praxis task demands in the assessment of children with developmental motor deficits. *Dev. Neuropsychol.*, 8, 367.

Dewey, D., McLeod, D.R., and Kaplan, B.J. (1993). Hand asymmetry: a possible index of prenatal stress. *J. Clin. Exp. Neuropsychol.*, 15, 88.

Difranco, D., Muir, D., and Dodwell, P. (1978). Reaching in very young infants. *Perception*, 7, 385.

Eaton, W.O., McKeen, N.A., and Lam, C.S. (1988). Instrumented motor activity measurement of the young infant in the home: validity and reliability. *Inf. Behav. Dev.*, 11, 375.

Eglington, E. and Annett, M. (1994). Handedness and dyslexia: a mete-analysis. *Percept. Motor Skills*, 79, 1611.

Fein, D., Humes, M., Kaplan, E., Lucci, D., and Waterhouse, L. (1984). The question of left hemisphere dysfunction in infantile autism. *Psychol. Bull.*, 95, 258.

Fein, D., Waterhouse, L., Lucci, D., Pennington, B., and Humes, M. (1985). Handedness and cognitive functions in pervasive developmental disorders. *J. Aut. Dev. Dis.*, 15, 323.

Fennell, E.B., Satz, P., and Morris, R. (1983). The development of handedness and dichotic ear listening asymmetries in relation to school achievement: a longitudinal study. *J. Exp. Child Psychol.*, 35, 248.

Flick, G.L. (1966). Sinistrality revisited: a perceptual-motor approach. *Child Dev.*, 37, 612.

Gabbard, C., Hart, S., and Kanipe, D. (1993). Hand preference consistency and fine motor performance in young children. *Cortex*, 29, 749.

Gaillard, F. and Satz, P. (1989). Handedness and reading disability: a developmental study. *Arch. Clin. Neuropsychol.*, 4, 63.

Garn, S.M., Mayor, G.H., and Shaw, H.A. (1976). Paradoxical bilateral asymmetry in bone size and bone mass in the hand. *Am. J. Phys. Anthropol.*, 45, 209.

Geschwind, N. and Galaburda, A.M. (1985). Cerebral lateralization. *Arch. Neurol.*, 42, 428.

Gesell, A. and Ames, L.B. (1947). The development of handedness. *J. Gen. Psychol.*, 70, 155.

Geuze, R.H. and Kalverboer, A.F. (1994) Tapping a rhythm: a problem of timing for children who are clumsy and dyslexic? *Adapt. Phys. Act. Q.*, 11, 203.

Giesecke, M. (1936). The genesis of hand preference. *Monogr. Soc. Res. Child Dev.*, 1 (Serial No. 5).

Gillberg, C. (1983). Autistic children's hand preferences: Results from an epidemiological study of infantile autism. *Psych. Res.*, 10, 21.

Gillberg, C. and Rasmussen, P. (1982). Perceptual, motor and attentional deficits in seven-year-old children: Background factors. *Dev. Med. Child Neurol.*, 24, 752.

Gottfried, A.W. and Bathurst, K. (1983). Hand preference across time is related to intelligence in young girls, not boys. *Science*, 221, 1074.

Gubbay, S.S. (1975). *The Clumsy Child: A Study of Developmental Apraxic and Agnosic Ataxia.* London, W.B. Saunders.

Hallahan, D.P. and Kaufman, J.M. (1977). *Introduction to Learning Disabilities: A Psych-Behavioral Approach.* Englewood Cliffs, NJ, Prentice-Hall.

Hardyck, C., Goldman, R., and Petrinovich, L. (1975). Handedness, sex, race, and age. *Hum. Biol.*, 47, 369.

Harris, L.J. (1992). Left-handedness. In I. Rapin and S.J. Segalowitz (Eds.), *Handbook of Neuropsychology, Vol 6: Child Neuropsychology*, New York, Elsevier, 145.

Harris, L.J. and Carlson, D.F. (1988). Pathological left-handedness: an analysis of theories and evidence. In D.L. Molfese and S.J. Segalowitz (Eds.). *Brain Lateralization in Children*, New York, Guilford Press, 289.

Hawn, P.R. and Harris, L.J. (1983). Hand differences in grasp duration and reaching in two and five month old infants. In G. Young, S.J. Segalowitz, C.M. Corter, and S.E. Trehub (Eds.), *Manual Specialization and the Developing Brain*, New York, Academic, 285.

Henderson, S.E. (1987). The assessment of "clumsy" children: old and new approaches. *J. Child. Psychol. Psych.*, 28, 551.

Henderson, S.E. and Hall, D. (1982). Concomitants of clumsiness in young school children. *Dev. Med. Child Neurol.*, 24, 448.

Hicks, R.E. and Barton, A.K. (1975). A note on left-handedness and severity of mental retardation. *J. Gen. Psychol.*, 127, 323.

Hiscock, C.K., Hiscock, M., Benjamins, D., and Hillman, S. (1989). Motor asymmetries in hemiplegic children: implications for the normal and pathological development of handedness. *Dev. Neuropsychol.*, 5, 169.

Hoare. D.G. (1991). *Classification of movement dysfunction in children: Descriptive and statistical approaches.* Unpublished Doctoral Thesis, University of Western Australia.

Hoare, D. (1994). Subtypes of developmental coordination disorder. *Adapt. Phys. Act. Q.*, 11, 158.

Hoffer, N. and Kaplan, B.J. (1993). *Nonrighthandedness and Skeletal Asymmetry of the Hands.* Unpublished manuscript, University of Calgary, Department of Psychology, Calgary, AB, Canada.

Hofsten, C. von (1982). Eye-hand coordination in the newborn. *Dev. Psychobiol.*, 18, 450.

Hofsten, C. von (1984). Developmental changes in pre-reaching movements. *Dev. Psychol.*, 20, 378.

Hopkins, B., Lems, W., Janssen, B., and Butterworth, G. (1987). Postural and motor asymmetries in newlyborns. *Hum. Neurobiol.*, 6, 153.

Hugdahl, K., Synnevag, B., and Satz, P. (1990). Immune and autoimmune diseases in dyslexic children. *Neuropsychologia*, 28, 673.

Iloeje, S.O. (1988). Trophic limb changes among children with developmental apraxia. *Dev. Med. Child Neurol.*, 30, 791.

Johnston, R.B., Stark, R.E., Mellitis, E.D., and Tallal, P. (1981). Neurological status of language-impaired and normal children. *Ann. Neurol.*, 10, 159.

Kaufman, A.S., Zalma, R., and Kaufman, N.L. (1978). The relationship of hand dominance to the motor co-ordination, mental ability and right-left awareness of young normal children. *Child Dev.*, 49, 885.

Kimura, K. and Konishi, M. (1981). Handedness and laterality in some measurements of the human upper limb. *Hum. Ecol. Race Hyg.*, 47, 51.

Kinsbourne, M. and Hiscock, M. (1983). The normal and deviant development of functional lateralization of the brain. In M.M. Haith and J.J. Campos (Eds.), *Handbook of Child Psychology (4th ed.): Vol. 2. Infancy and Developmental Psychobiology*, New York, Wiley, 157.

Klicpera, C., Wolff, P.H., and Drake, C. (1981). Bimanual co-ordination in adolescent boys with reading retardation. *Dev. Med. Child Neurol.*, 23, 617.

Korczyn, A.D., Sage, J.I., and Karplus, M. (1978). Lack of limb motor asymmetry in the neonate. *J. Neurobiol.*, 9, 483.

Lenneberg, E.H. (1967). *Biological Foundations of Language*. New York, Wiley.

Livshits, G., David, L., Kobyliansky, E., Ben-Amital, D., Levi, Y., and Merlob, P. (1988). Decreased developmental stability as assessed by fluctuating asymmetry of morphometric traits in preterm infants. *Am. J. Med. Gen.*, 29, 793.

Livshits, G. and Kobyliansky, E. (1987). Dermatoglyphics traits as possible markers of developmental processes in humans. *Am. J. Med. Gen.*, 26, 111.

Malina, R.M. and Buschang, P.H. (1984). Anthropometric asymmetry in normal and mentally retarded males. *Ann. Hum. Biol.*, 11, 515.

McLeod, D.R. and Coupland, S.G. (1992). Asymmetry quantification utilizing hand radiographs. *Am. J. Med. Gen.*, 44, 321.

McLeod, D.R. and Dewey, D. (in preparation). *Asymmetry Quantification Utilizing Hand Radiographs — Pediatric Normative Data*.

McManus, I.C., Murray, B., Doyle, K., and Baron-Cohen, S. (1992). Handedness in childhood autism shows dissociation of skill and preference. *Cortex*, 28, 373.

Maehara, K., Negishi, N., Tsai, A., Iizuka, R., Otsuki, N., Suzuki, S., Takahashi, T., and Sumiyoshi, Y. (1988). Handedness in the Japanese. *Dev. Neuropsychol.*, 4, 117.

McCarthy, D. (1972). *Manual for the McCarthy Scales of Children's Abilities*. New York, Psychological Corp.

McDonnell, P.M., Anderson, V.E.S., and Abraham, A. (1983). Asymmetry and orientation of arm movements in 3 to 8 week old infants. *Inf. Behav. Dev.*, 6, 287.

Morley, M.E. (1972). *The Development of Disorders of Speech in Childhood, 3rd Edition*. Edinburgh: Churchill Livingstone.

Neils, J.R. and Aram, D.M. (1986). Handedness and the sex of children with developmental language disorders. *Brain Lang.*, 28, 53-65, 1986.

Obrzut, J.E. and Atkinson, M.H. (1993). Relations among learning disorders, handedness and immune disease. *J. Clin. Exp. Neuropsychol.*, 15, 86.

Oldfield, R.C. (1971). The assessment and analysis of handedness: the Edinburgh Inventory. *Neuropsychologia*, 9, 97.

Ortiz De Zarate, J.C. and Ortiz De Zarate, C.O. (1991). Hair whorl and handedness. *Brain Cognit.*, 16, 228.

Orton, S.T. (1937). *Reading, Writing and Speech Problems in Children*. London, Chapman and Hall.

Ottaviano, S., Guidette, V., Allemand, F., Spinetoli, B., and Seri S. (1989). Laterality of arm movement in full-term newborns. *Early Hum. Dev.*, 19, 3.

Peretz, B., Ever-Hadani, P., Casamassimo, P., Eidelman, E., Shellhart, C., and Hagerman, R. (1988). Crown size asymmetry in males with Fra (x) or Martin-Bell syndrome. *Am. J. Med. Gen.*, 30, 185.

Peters, M. (1988). Footedness: Asymmetries in foot preference and skill and neuropsychological assessment of foot movement. *Psychol. Bull.*, 103, 179.

Peters, M. and Durding, B. (1978). Handedness measured by finger-tapping: a continuous variable. *Can. J. Psychol.*, 32, 257.

Peters, M. and Durding, B. (1979). Left-handers and right-handers compared on a motor task. *J. Motor Behav.*, 11, 103.

Petrie, B.F. and Peters, M. (1980). Handedness: left/right differences in intensity of grasp response and duration of rattle holding in infants. *Inf. Behav. Dev.*, 3, 215.

Powell, R.P. and Bishop, D.V.M. (1992). Clumsiness and perceptual problems in children with specific language impairment. *Dev. Med. Child Neurol.*, 34, 755.

Porac, C. and Coren, S. (1981). *Lateral Preferences and Human Behavior*. New York: Springer-Verlag.

Poznanski, A.K. (1984). *The Hand in Radiologic Diagnosis with Gamuts and Pattern Profiles* (Vol. 1, 2nd ed.). Philadelphia, PA, W. B. Saunders.

Prechl, H.F.R. (1977). *The Neurological Examination of the Full Term Newborn Infant*. London, Heinemann.

Provins, K.A. (1992). Early infant motor asymmetries and handedness: a critical evaluation of the evidence. *Dev. Neuropsychol.*, 8, 325.

Provins, K.A., Milner, A., and Kerr, P. (1982). Asymmetry of manual preference and performance. *Percept. Motor Skills*, 54, 179.

Ramsay, D.S. (1980). Beginnings of bimanual handedness and speech in infants. *Inf. Behav. Dev.*, 3, 67.

Ross, G., Lipper, E.G., and Auld, P.A.M. (1987). Hand preference in four-year-old children: its relationship in premature birth and neurodevelopmental outcome. *Dev. Med. Child Neurol.*, 29, 615.

Rousselle, C. and Wolff, P.H. (1991). The dynamics of bimanual coordination in developmental dyslexia. *Neuropsychologia*, 29, 907.

Rymer, K., Kameyama, T., Niwa, S.I., Hiramatsu, K.I., and Saitoh, O., (1984), Hand and eye preference patterns in elementary and junior high school students. *Cortex*, 20, 441.

Satz, P. (1977). Laterality tests: An inferential problem. *Cortex*, 13, 208.

Satz, P. and Fletcher, J.M. (1987). Left-handedness and dyslexia: an old myth revisited. *J. Ped. Psychol.*, 12, 291.

Satz, P., Soper, H.V., Orsini, D.L., Henry, R.R., and Zvi, J.C. (1985). Handedness subtypes in autism. *Psych. Ann.*, 15, 447.

Satz, P., Yanowitz, J.S., and Willmore, J. (1984). Early brain damage and lateral development. In R. Bell, J. Elias, R. Green, and J. Harvey (Eds.), *Interfaces in Psychology*. Austin, University of Texas Press.

Soper, H.V., Satz, O., Orsini, D.L., Henry, R.R., Zvi, J.C., and Schulman, M. (1986). Handedness patterns in autism suggest subtypes. *J. Aut. Dev. Dis.*, 16, 155.

Soper, H.V., Satz, O., Orsini, D.L., Van Gorp, W.G., and Green, M.F. (1987). Handedness distribution in a residential population with severe or profound mental retardation. *Am. J. Ment. Def.*, 92, 94.

Steenhuis, R.E. and Bryden, M.P. (1989). Different dimensions of hand preference that relate to skilled and unskilled activities. *Cortex*, 25, 289.

Strauss, E. (1982). Manual persistence in infancy. *Cortex*, 18, 319.

Tapley, S.M. and Bryden, M.P. (1985). A group test for the assessment of performance between hands. *Neuropsychologia*, 23, 215.

Tallal, P. and Katz, W. (1989). Neuropsychological and neuroanotomical studies of developmental language/reading disorders: recent advances. In C. von Euler, I. Lundborg, and G. Lennerstraned (Eds.), *Brain and Reading*, New York, Stockton Press, 183.

Tan, L.E. (1985). Laterality and motor skills in four-year-olds. *Child Dev.*, 56, 119.

Tsai, L.Y. (1982). Handedness in autistic children and their families. *J. Aut. Dev. Dis.*, 12, 421.

Valentine, W.L. and Wagner, I. (1934). Relative arm motility in the newborn infant. *Ohio State Univ. Studies*, 12, 53.

Van Dusen, C.R. (1939). An anthropometric study of the upper extremities of children. *Hum. Biol.*, 11, 277.

Walker, T.M. and Ashcroft, M.T. (1978). The metacarpal index in Jamaican children and adults. *Br. J. Radiol.*, 51, 338.

White, L.E., Lucas, G., Richards, A., and Purves, D. (1994). Cerebral asymmetry and handedness. *Nature*, 368, 198.

Witelson, S.F. (1985). On hemispheric specialization and cerebral plasticity from birth: Mark II. In C.T. Best (Ed.), *Hemispheric Function and Collaboration in the Child*, New York, Academic, 33.

Wolanski, N. (1972). Functions of the extremities and their influence on the asymmetric structure of the body in children and young persons from different environmental conditions. *Acta Med. Auxolog.*, 4, 3.

Woolf, C.M. and Gianas, A.D. (1976). Congenital cleft lip and fluctuating dermatoglyphics asymmetry. *Am. J. Hum. Gen.*, 28, 400.

Wolff, P.H., Cohen, C. and Drake, C. (1984). Impaired motor timing control in specific reading retardation. *Neuropsychologia*, 22, 587.

Wolff, P.H., Michel, G.F., Drake, C., and Ovrut, M. (1990). Rate and timing precision of motor coordination in developmental dyslexia. *Dev. Psychol.*, 26, 349.

Yu-Yan, M., Cun-Ren, F., and Over, R. (1983). Lateral symmetry in the duration of grasp by infants. *Aust. J. Psychol.*, 35, 81.

Chapter 11

Hand Preference, Manual Asymmetries, and Limb Apraxia

Eric A. Roy

CONTENTS

1. INTRODUCTION

Limb apraxia represents an inability to perform hand gestures such as showing someone how to wave goodbye or how to slice bread. In some particularly severe forms, the patient may even be unable to actually use a knife to slice bread. This deficit has been reported in a variety of neurologic disorders (Heilman and Rothi, 1993; Roy, 1982, 1985; Roy and Square, 1994), although our discussion will focus primarily on apraxia associated with stroke lateralized to either hemisphere. The question of interest here is how apraxia relates to asymmetries in hand preference and performance. The relationship between handedness and praxis is linked in many ways with the relationship between handedness and cerebral dominance for speech and language function since apraxia and aphasia often occur together. Contemplating the nature of the relationship between handedness and apraxia, then, requires one to examine how handedness relates to aphasia and how aphasia and apraxia are linked. Further, we must consider how one measures handedness and how one can best characterize apraxic deficits.

We will begin the chapter reviewing current perspectives on apraxia. A consideration of the origins of handedness, how it is measured, and how it relates to the laterality of language will follow this review. We will then examine how praxis and handedness might be related, using as a reference point the link between handedness and cerebral dominance for speech and language function. A discussion of directions for future research will conclude the chapter.

0-8493-8999-2/96/$0.00+$.50

2. APRAXIA

Apraxia is a disorder affecting the ability to pantomime or imitate gestures. Both familiar, well known gestures involving the use of objects (e.g., brushing teeth, [transitive gestures]) or interpersonal communication (e.g., wave goodbye [intransitive, representational gestures]) and novel, meaningless hand gestures (intransitive, nonrepresentational gestures) are affected. Identifying apraxia typically involves noting the occurrence of particular types of performance errors. One of the most well known is termed a body-part-as-object error in which the hand is used as if it were the object (e.g., the extended index finger representing a toothbrush, see Haaland and Flaherty [1984], McDonald, Tate and Rigby [1994]; Rothi, Mack, Verfaillie, Brown, and Heilman [1988] and Roy and Square, [1985, 1994] for a broader discussion of errors). An impairment in gesturing cannot be termed an apraxia, however, if it results from a basic motor problem (e.g., a hemiparesis), a difficulty in simply comprehending the verbal command requesting that the patient demonstrate the gesture, an impairment in recognizing the object with which the gesture is associated, or a generalized decline in cognitive functions such as is seen in dementia (Poeck, 1986; Roy and Square, 1985).

Several different types of apraxia have been identified (see Heilman and Rothi, 1993; Mozaz, 1992; Roy, 1978, 1982, 1985), although the two most well known types are ideational and ideomotor apraxia. The distinction between these two apraxias is largely based on the pattern of performance when pantomiming as opposed to imitating gestures (see Roy, 1982 for other distinctions). In the pantomime condition the patient demonstrates how to perform a gesture (e.g., salute) or use an object (e.g., a hammer) although the tool, in the case of transitive (tool use) gestures, is not actually manipulated. In the imitation condition, the patient attempts to imitate the gesture demonstrated by the examiner. In ideational apraxia, performance is impaired when pantomiming but not when imitating the gesture. With ideomotor apraxia both pantomime and imitation performance are impaired.

This distinction in the pattern of performance is thought to reflect differences in the integrity of memory structures used in programming the movements in gesturing. In ideational apraxia, these engrams are thought to be destroyed. The patient's performance, then, is impaired in the pantomime condition when these memory structures must be accessed, but not in the imitation condition when visual gestural information is available in the examiner's demonstration. In ideomotor apraxia these memory structures are thought to be intact. The posterior brain areas thought to subserve these structures (supramarginal gyrus) as well as processes involved in the analysis of visual gestural information (occipital lobe) are thought to be disconnected from the more anterior brain areas responsible for movement control. Thus, the patient's performance is impaired both when pantomiming and imitating gestures.

2.1 MODELS OF APRAXIA

A number of approaches have been developed to understand apraxia (Duffy and Duffy, 1990; Rothi, Ochipa, and Heilman, 1991; Roy, 1983a,b). An approach developed by Roy (1983a,b; Roy and Hall, 1992; Roy and Square, 1985, 1994) proposes that apraxia may arise from disruptions to sensory/perceptual, conceptual, and/or production systems and points to the complex nature of this disorder which reflects the interface among perceptual, cognitive, and motor processes (see Figure 11.1). These disorders may arise from disruptions at various stages in the evolving gesture or sequence. Early stages associated with analyzing visual gestural information and identifying key features of tools and

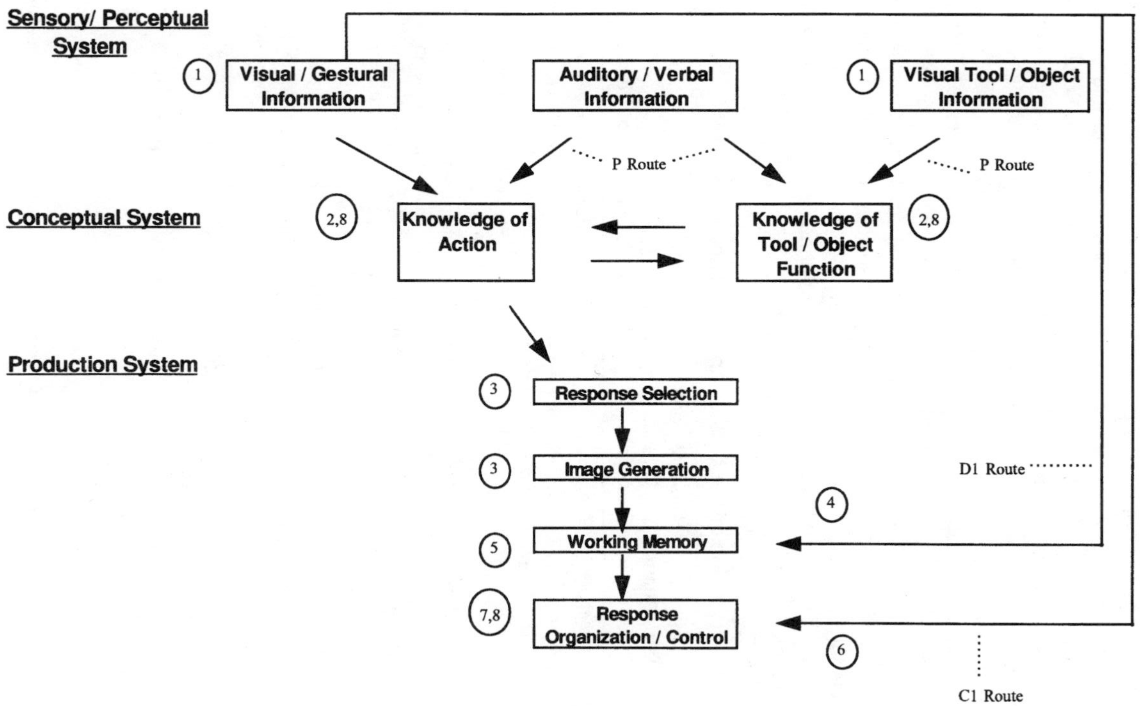

Figure 11.1 Depicts the conceptual-production system model of limb apraxia developed by Roy (Roy and Square, 1994). "P" refers to pantomime of a gesture, "DI" refers to delayed imitation, while "CI" refers to concurrent imitation (see text). The encircled numbers refer to patterns reflecting disruptions at particular stages of gesture production (see Table 11.1 and text).

objects to be used, somewhat later stages involving response selection or image generation, and still later stages associated with movement sequencing and coordination may be affected to varying degrees. Identifying which of these stages are affected requires careful task manipulation so as to place demands on particular stages (cf., Roy and Square, 1994; Roy, Square-Storer, Hogg, and Adams, 1991).

2.1.1 Patterns of Performance Predicted from the Model

According to this model, a number of patterns of performance are plausible indicators of an apraxic impairment (see Table 11.1). These patterns (see Roy and Square, 1994 for details) can be denoted by a series of letters signifying the performance conditions (pantomime [P], delayed imitation [DI], concurrent imitation [CI]) and whether performance in these conditions is intact (+) or impaired (–). Recall that in the pantomime condition the patient must generate the gesture from memory, usually in response to a verbal command (e.g., "Show how you would drive a nail into wood"). Imitation involves copying a gesture demonstrated by the examiner. In the CI condition, the examiner's demonstration continues throughout the patient's attempt to copy it. In the DI condition, the examiner ends the demonstration before the patient attempts to copy it. In this condition the patient must retain the visual gestural information from the examiner's model in working memory.

Table 11.1 Summary of Major Patterns of Apraxic Performance

Pattern Number (see Figure 1)	Apraxia Performance Pattern[1]	Gesture-Tool/ Object Recognition[1]	System Affected	Nature of Disruption
1	P+/DI–/CI–	–	Sensory/ Perceptual	Impaired ability to analyze visual gestural and tool/object information
2	P–/DI+/CI+	–	Conceptual	Impaired knowledge of action and tool/object function
3	P–/DI+/CI+	+	Production	Impaired response selection and/or image generation
4	P+/DI–/CI+	+	Production	Impaired encoding of visual gestural information into working memory
5	P–/DI–/CI+	+	Production	Impaired working memory
6	P+/DI–/CI–	+	Production	Impaired ability to use visual information in the control of movement
7	P–/DI–/CI–	+	Production	Impaired response organization and control
8	P–/DI–/CI–	–	Conceptual + Production	Impaired knowledge of action and tool/object function and impaired response organization and control

Note: [1] "–" sign means impaired; "+" sign means intact (see text of proposal for definition of impaired).

Disruptions to the sensory/perceptual system should give rise to several patterns of performance which reflect disruptions to the analysis of visual gestural and tool/object information. The hallmark of these disorders should be poor gesture and tool/object recognition and poor imitation of gestures but a preserved ability to pantomime gestures. Patients exhibiting one of these patterns (P+/DI–/CI–), for example, can generate gestures accurately from memory, suggesting that they are able to express through movement what they know about gestures. They are, however, unable to imitate gestures shown to them. Their inability to analyze the spatiotemporal characteristics of movement impacts not only on gesture recognition but also on the organization and control of movement as evident in their poor performance at concurrent imitation. The patient's poor performance at delayed imitation is a further reflection of this impairment in the analysis of visual gestural information.

Disruptions to the conceptual system should result in impaired performance to pantomime. Imitation of the gesture should be intact, however. This pattern of performance (P–/DI+/CI+) is indicative of what some have called ideational apraxia. This deficit in pantomime should be accompanied by poor performance on cognitive tasks assessing the integrity of the knowledge structures. Gesture and tool/object recognition tasks, then, should be performed poorly. Ochipa, Rothi, and Heilman (1992a) have devised a tool selection task which taps into one aspect of this knowledge, that pertaining to tool/object function. In this task, patients were presented with several tools (e.g., spoon, toothbrush, comb) and an object (e.g., a bowl of soup) and asked to use the appropriate object to carry out an action (e.g., eat soup). Ochipa et al. (1992a) identified a group of patients who chose the wrong tool (e.g., the toothbrush) but carried out the action correctly. They referred to these errors as *content* errors and contrasted them with *production* errors (see below) which reflect deficits in the actual execution of the gestural movement.

A number of patterns of performance are also indicative of disruptions in the production system. Disruptions in the early stages of gesture production, for example, reflecting response selection and image generation should be seen in the pattern alluded to above where imitation performance is intact but pantomime is impaired (P–/DI+/CI+). In this case, however, gesture and tool/object recognition will be intact, suggesting that the conceptual system is intact. These patients know what the gesture should look like and what the tool is used for but have difficulty in translating what they know into action.

Disruptions to the working memory stage of the production system may be seen in two patterns (P+/DI–/CI+ and P–/DI–/CI+) in which the patient exhibits intact gesture recognition and tool knowledge. A deficit in encoding visual gestural information into working memory should result in the first pattern (P+/DI–/CI+). The patient retains the ability to select the appropriate response and generate and retain an image of the response in working memory (P+) and to analyze visual gestural information (CI+), but has a deficit in encoding visual gestural information into working memory (DI–). According to this model, the images generated in the early stages of the production system when pantomiming and those encoded from the analysis of visual gestural information in the examiner's demonstration when imitating are both retained in working memory. Disruptions to working memory per se, then, should give rise to the second pattern (P–/DI–/CI+) where pantomime and delayed imitation are impaired but concurrent imitation is intact.

Disruptions to the later stages of the production system will be seen in two patterns (P+/DI–/CI– and P–/DI–/CI–). In contrast to the P+/DI–/CI– pattern indicative of a disruption in the sensory/perceptual system alluded to above, a disruption in the production system producing this pattern should not result in poor gesture and tool/object recognition. Patients with an impairment at this stage, then, should be capable of analyzing visual gestural information as evidenced by their ability at gesture recognition. Their poor performance on imitation indicates more an inability to use this information to organize and control movement, a stage in the production system involving communication with the sensory/perceptual system. As such, this disconnection disorder seems conceptually similar to conduction aphasia. Ochipa, Rothi, and Heilman (1992b) have described just such a case and have termed the disorder conduction apraxia.

A disruption at the latest stage in the production system will be seen in the P–/DI–/CI–pattern without impairments to gesture and tool/object recognition. Patients with a disruption at this stage know what the gesture should look like, although they are unable to produce it even when the movement patterns are demonstrated for them by the examiner. This pattern is indicative of what some have called ideomotor apraxia. This disorder might be considered a pure production disorder involving the latest stages in the production system associated with the organization and control of movement. This disorder seems similar to the motor deficits observed in Broca's aphasia.

Disruptions to both the conceptual and production systems will also give rise to the P–/DI–/CI– pattern. In this case, however, the gesture and tool/object recognition will be impaired. Not only do patients with these disruptions not know what the gesture should look like, but they are also unable to produce it even when this information is provided. Thus, these patients might be considered to have the most severe apraxia. As such, one might liken this disorder to a global aphasia.

2.1.2 Neuroanatomic Correlates of Apraxia

Using this model, it is possible to predict patterns of performance which should reflect disruptions at different stages in gesture production. How do these disruptions relate to the hand used and lesion localization? Much of the work on apraxia points to the importance of damage to the left hemisphere, particularly the parietal and prefrontal areas (e.g., Jason, 1990; Kimura, 1982). This hemisphere is thought to subserve a praxis system used to control gestural movements with both hands as damage to this hemisphere, especially in the parietal area, produces apraxia bilaterally (e.g., Kimura, 1982). Unilateral expressions of apraxia which usually affect the left hand arise primarily in the context of a right hemiparesis or callosal damage. In the first instance, the apraxia is really bilateral, but is not seen in the right hand because of the paralysis. In the case of callosal damage, the apraxia is thought to arise because the motor area in the right hemisphere controlling the left hand is disconnected from the praxis system in the left hemisphere.

A considerable number of studies, however, which have used detailed error analyses or varied the performance demands of the praxis task have questioned the exclusive role of the left hemisphere in apraxia. Some have implicated the importance of the right hemisphere, particularly the prefrontal area (e.g., Kolb and Milner, 1981), while others have suggested that each hemisphere may have its own "action system" such that damage to either hemisphere may give rise to apraxia in the contralateral hand (e.g., Pilgrim and Humphreys, 1991).

These findings suggest that gesture production involves a complex network of brain areas, each of which may subserve some stage or process. Our model strives to identify stages in gestural expression. Examination of the patterns of performance alluded to above in conjunction with analyses of the size and location of brain lesions may provide a clearer understanding of the neurobehavioral basis of apraxia.

Heilman's work (Heilman, Rothi, and Valenstein, 1982) suggests that disruptions to the conceptual system may be seen with damage to the parietal area in the left hemisphere. Visuokinesthetic engrams in the supramarginal gyrus, he argues, form the knowledge base for gesturing as he has found that apraxic patients with damage in this region are impaired at gesture recognition. In the context of this model, one might expect that patients with damage in this region should exhibit poor gesture recognition and poorer performance in the pantomime condition in which accurate performance is dependent on accessing these engrams (i.e., P–/DI+/CI+).

More anterior damage involving prefrontal, premotor, and supplementary motor areas may not affect the conceptual system. Heilman found that apraxic patients with damage in these areas were not impaired in gesture recognition. Damage in these areas may affect the production system more. In the context of this model, three groups of patients with deficits at different stages may be observed, one which is more impaired in the pantomime condition (P–/DI+/CI+), one which is more impaired in the imitation condition (P+/DI–/CI–), and the other which is equally impaired in both performance conditions (P–/DI–/CI–). All of these patients should exhibit intact gesture and tool/object recognition. These patients should exhibit a preponderance of production errors (cf., Ochipa et al., 1992a) alluded to above. Their performance should be characterized by disruptions to the spatial, temporal, and postural dimensions of performance (e.g., Haaland and Flaherty, 1984; Rothi et al., 1988; Roy and Black, 1993; Roy, Black, Blair, and Dimeck, 1995).

According to our model, the patients who are more impaired to pantomime have particular problems in the early stages of gesture production associated with response selection and image generation. Damage in these patients may be focused on the dorsolateral prefrontal and supplementary motor areas. Both of these regions have been implicated in the early stages of response organization and planning (e.g., Goldberg, 1985). The patients who are more impaired to imitation are not able to use visual gestural information to guide movement. In these patients, damage may be deep to the parietal lobe and affect the fiber tracts which provide communication between the occipital cortex and the premotor cortex. This tract, the superior longitudinal fasciculus, has been found to be important in visually guided hand movements (e.g., Paillard, 1982). Kertesz and Ferro (1984) reported one patient with damage largely confined to this tract who exhibited a profound inability to imitate gestures he was readily able to pantomime.

The group which is equally impaired in all performance conditions may have problems in the later stages of gesture production associated with response organization and control. The patients in this group may have damage located more centrally in the premotor, motor, and sensorimotor areas. These areas have been shown to affect the programming and control of movement (Paillard, 1982).

The most profound apraxia (P–/DI–/CI–) involving both deficits in gesture production and poor gesture and tool/object recognition should be associated with relatively large lesions in the context of stroke or with diffuse neuronal degeneration seen in the dementias. Indeed, using our notions of conceptual disorders in apraxia (Roy, 1983a,b; Roy and Square, 1985, 1994), Ochipa et al. (1992a) have identified such a profound apraxic disorder in patients with Alzheimer's disease.

Apraxia then appears to involve disruptions at a number of stages in gesture production, each of which may be subserved by localized regions in the cortex. Most of the research indicates that these critical regions are in the left hemisphere. Work reviewed by Jason (1990) and Roy, Brown, Winchester, Square, Hall, and Black (1993), however, suggests that this lateralization of praxis to the left hemisphere may be most pronounced in tasks which require the patient to generate the gesture from memory. Disruptions affecting the conceptual system and the early stages of the production system which involve pantomime tasks might be more likely to be lateralized to the left hemisphere. Disruptions to intermediate stages of the production system affecting working memory, however, might also exhibit the same lateralization.

The potential for studying the relationship between praxis lateralization and handedness would appear to be most fruitful for these more lateralized types of disruptions to praxis. The fact that both hands may be affected, however, raises some interesting challenges to studying this relationship. The apraxic deficit arises in the context of preexisting differences in hand performance. How does one measure and interpret this deficit given these premorbid manual asymmetries? The answer to this question will be addressed in our later discussion. Some insight, however, is provided in the work on handedness to which we now turn.

3. DIMENSIONS OF HANDEDNESS

3.1 PREFERENCE AND PERFORMANCE DIMENSIONS OF HANDEDNESS

Handedness in its most common terms refers to the hand one prefers to use for most tasks encountered in daily living. This dimension of handedness, termed hand preference, is usually assessed with self-report questionnaires (see Chapters 3 and 6). Handedness is also determined on the basis of performance measures. Most often these measures on pegboard (Annett, 1967, 1976; Annett and Kilshaw, 1983), other visual-motor (e.g., dot aiming test, Annett, 1992; Tapley and Bryden, 1985), or motor (e.g., finger tapping, see Chapter 5) tasks are used to identify which hand is more proficient (i.e., faster and/or more accurate) at a task. More recently, however, performance measures have been used to assess hand preference, reflecting the tendency to use one hand more frequently to pick up objects (Bishop, Ross, Daniels, and Bright, in press) to turn knobs on a dial (Bryden and Edmonds, 1995) or to move pegs (Bryden, Singh, Steenhuis, and Clarkson, 1994).

These two dimensions of handedness often concur. That is, the hand which one reports is preferred for a given task is indeed more proficient at that task. There are exceptions, however. For example, performance on the Annett pegboard task correlates more highly with hammering preference than with handwriting preference, while the Tapley and Bryden (1985) dot-aiming task correlates more highly with handwriting preference.

The potential for a discrepancy between preference and performance appears to relate to the multifactorial nature of each dimension of handedness as well as to the measures used. Barnsley and Rabinovitch (1970) and more recently Van Horn and McManus (1993) observed that performance differences between the hands load on several independent factors. Similarly, Steenhuis and Bryden (1989a) found that hand preference could be demarcated into factors on the basis of the skill required in performing a task. Recent work by Steenhuis and Bryden (1989b; see also Chapter 6) has looked at the relationship between hand skill as measured on a preference questionnaire with that observed in performance involving picking up or manipulating tools and objects. They observed that for left- and right-handers the frequency of both actual and self-reported hand use was dependent on the task. For example, the nonpreferred hand was used more often to pick up as opposed to manipulate (i.e., use) the tools. Generally, the concordance between preference and performance depended on the measures used, preference or proficiency, on whether the direction or degree of handedness was examined, and on whether the person was left- or right-handed.

With regard to the measurement issue, a discrepancy between preference and performance can arise to the extent that there are marked differences in measuring each dimension. The problem here centers around the notion of the direction and degree of asymmetry. Direction reflects which hand exhibits a preference or performance advantage and is a dichotomous measure, while degree of asymmetry reflects the magnitude of the preference or performance advantage and is a continuous variable. Performance measures of handedness reflect both the direction and degree of asymmetry (e.g., Steenhuis and Bryden, 1987). Hand preference measures reflect primarily the direction of asymmetry, although the degree of asymmetry can be measured depending on gradations of preference asked for on the handedness inventory. A discrepancy or a low correlation between preference and performance can occur when the measurement scales differ (e.g., degree in one dimension and direction and degree in another) or when the precision of measurement used to reflect the degree of asymmetry differs markedly. For example, a number of studies have revealed that correlations between preference and performance measures which include the direction of handedness are larger than those which look only at the degree of handedness (see Chapters 3 and 6 for details).

The ideal situation for studying the relationship between preference and performance would seem to require that both dimensions reflect degree of asymmetry to somewhat comparable levels of precision. Bryden et al. (Chapter 3) and Schacter (1993) have pointed out some of the problems with measuring the degree of asymmetry as it pertains to the preference dimension. The precision in measuring the gradations in preference will be enhanced with a greater number of response categories. For example, a 5-point scale ranging from "always use left or right hand," to "usually use left or right hand," to "use both hands equally often" is potentially more precise than a dichotomous scale reflecting simply preference for using the left or right hand. The problem here is that the category boundaries such as "always" or "usually" may not mean the same thing to all respondents. This observation indicates the inherent subjectivity and idiosyncrasy of the handedness inventory approach to measuring preference. This shortcoming of the inventory approach will necessarily place limits on the degree of precision possible in measuring preference and in the validity and reliability of the measurements obtained. Both factors will limit the potential magnitude of the relationship between preference and performance. One solution to this problem may be to employ performance-based measures of preference and incorporate these into the performance task (e.g., Bryden et al., 1994).

A number of studies have addressed the issue of degree of asymmetry in performance measures of handedness. The notion here is that certain tasks or performance measures may reveal larger hand differences than others. Hand differences in performance have been found to be larger in tasks which would appear to be more complex or require more precise control of movement. For example, the preferred hand advantage in performance is larger in a handwriting as opposed to a grip strength task (Provins and Magliaro, 1989), in an aiming as opposed to a tapping task (Flowers, 1975), and in throwing as opposed to intercepting a ball (Watson and Kimura, 1989).

Recent work by Roy, Bryden, and Bulman-Fleming (in preparation) examined hand differences in performance on the Grooved Pegboard, a test frequently used in assessing visuomotor control in clinical neuropsychology. In this study of right-handers, each trial of the task involved two phases, Place and Replace. In the Place phase, 25 small pegs were moved one at a time from a large receptacle and placed into holes on a board situated directly above the receptacle. In the Replace phase, the pegs were removed from the holes in the board one at a time and returned to the receptacle. Performance was reflected in the time in seconds to complete each phase. Subjects, all right-handers, performed two trials with each hand, half beginning with the preferred right hand. Since movements in the Place phase were thought to require more precise visuomotor control, the hypothesis was that the right hand advantage should be larger in this phase of the task.

Analyses comparing performance in the two phases revealed a significantly longer time for the Place (55 seconds) than the Replace (18 seconds) phase, indicating that the movement task in the Place phase is more demanding and precise. Comparisons of performance between the hands provided support for the hypothesis of a larger right-hand advantage in the Place phase. The right hand (51.8 seconds) was significantly faster than the left (58.7) in the Place, while in the Replace phase times for the right (18.2 seconds) and left (18.9 seconds) hands were not significantly different. One task dimension which has been of particular interest in studying the degree of performance asymmetries is the index of difficulty of a pointing or reaching task as measured by the amplitude of the movement and the size of the target (see Fitts, 1954). Using this notion of task difficulty, VanHorn and McManus (1993) systematically varied target size and movement amplitude on a series of tasks which have been used to measure handedness (e.g., Annett pegboard). They observed that differences in hand performance remained the same regardless of the task difficulty.

Work by Roy and Elliott (e.g., Roy, 1983c; Roy and Elliott, 1986, 1989; see also Chapter 7), in contrast, does reveal the impact of this (i.e., index of difficulty) and other dimensions of task complexity on the degree of performance asymmetries. Their work suggests that variables such as the speed of movement (e.g., Roy, 1983c; Roy and Elliott, 1986, 1989), the spatial mapping of visual feedback to movement (Maraj, Roy, and Elliott, 1994), and the constraints placed on spatial variability of movement (Roy, Winchester, Elliott, and Carnahan, 1995) all serve to affect the size of the right-hand advantage in a pointing task. For example, the advantage for the right hand increased as time to complete the pointing task decreased. This increased advantage arose from hand differences in the speed accuracy trade-off function where accuracy with the left hand decreased more with movement speed (Roy and Elliott, 1986).

Their work using kinematic measures also revealed that the size of the right-hand advantage depended on which dependent measure was examined. The right-hand advantage was most pronounced on the measure reflecting time in deceleration (e.g., Roy, Kalbfleisch, and Elliott, 1994). The right hand spent less time than the left in deceleration, suggesting that the right-hand, left-hemisphere system was more proficient at processing visual feedback information.

3.2 HANDEDNESS AND LATERALITY OF LANGUAGE

There are number of reasons for studying handedness. One of the most compelling is that handedness is thought to provide some insight into cerebral organization. The lateralization of speech and language function is the aspect of cerebral organization which has been the most extensively examined as it pertains to handedness. The most consistent findings across a range of studies examining the incidence of aphasia following a stroke lateralized to one cerebral hemisphere (Segalowitz and Bryden, 1983) and the effects of unilateral injections of sodium amytal (Beaton, 1995 [see Chapter 3]; Rasmussen and Milner, 1977) suggest that language deficits arise following suppression of left hemisphere function in 95% of right-handers but only 60 to 70% of left-handers. Suppression of right hemisphere function affects language function in 5% of right-handers but in 15 to 20% of left-handers. Studies of healthy adults using noninvasive techniques such as dichotic listening have generally confirmed these findings from pathology. Right-handers are much more likely to show a right ear or right visual field advantage (i.e., a left-hemisphere advantage) for language tasks than are left-handers (Bryden, 1988; Kim, 1994).

Another approach to studying the relationship of handedness to cerebral organization involves examining asymmetries of size in selected anatomical structures such as regions of the cerebral cortex (e.g., Geschwind and Galaburda, 1987) or the corpus callosum (e.g., Habib, Gayraud, Oliva, Regis, Salamon, and Khalil, 1991; Witelson, 1985). While there is much debate about the functional significance of these asymmetries, there is considerable evidence that the asymmetries are larger in right-handers (see Beaton, 1995 [see Chapter 3] and Geschwind and Galaburda, 1987 for reviews). For example, the planum temporale and the occipital horn are larger in the left hemisphere in right-handers but not left-handers. More recent work with more precise measurements techniques involving magnetic resonance imaging (MRI) seems to provide a link between structure and function. Foundas, Leonard, Gilmore, Fennell, and Heilman (1994), in a study of language lateralization, observed that 11 of their 12 subjects who were right handed had speech lateralized to the left hemisphere and had a larger planum in the left temporal lobe. The one non-right-hander had the opposite pattern, speech in the right hemisphere and a larger right temporal planum. Using functional MRI to examine asymmetries in the sensorimotor cortex, Thoma, Lewine, Yeo, Provencal, Davis, Orrison, and Hill (1995) found that the distance between thumb and fifth finger was larger in the hemisphere opposite the dominant hand as reflected in performance on the Annett pegboard.

3.3 MODELS OF HANDEDNESS AND CEREBRAL ORGANIZATION

Looking at the most extensively investigated lateralized function, language, left-handers and right-handers are not mirror images of one another with regard to cerebral organization. If they were, one would expect an equal proportion of left-handers and right-handers to have speech and language function in the hemisphere contralateral to the preferred hand. Such a finding would indicate a tight coupling between the laterality of handedness and language laterality. More left-handers than right-handers do indeed have language lateralized to the right hemisphere, suggesting that there must be some factor which leads to handedness and language functions being controlled by the same hemisphere. The fact that most people regardless of handedness have language represented in the left hemisphere, however, indicates that there must also be a factor which decouples handedness and language laterality.

A number of models of the origins of handedness have been developed (Gangestad and Yeo, 1994; Hardyk and Petrinovitch, 1977; Kimura, 1993; Porac and Coren, 1981; Yeo and Gangestad, 1993). The most powerful models, however, account for the distribution of handedness in families and, most importantly, include a mechanism for how handedness and language lateralization can be decoupled. These theories (see McManus and Bryden, 1992 for a review), which describe the genetic underpinnings of handedness and cerebral lateralization, propose that one allele (RS+ in the Annett [1985] model or D in the McManus model [McManus, 1985; McManus and Bryden, 1992]) determines both right-handedness and left-hemisphere language, while a second allele (RS– or C) leads to language and handedness being randomly lateralized. In the McManus model (McManus, 1985; McManus and Bryden, 1992), for example, the DD homozygous genotypes are all right-handed and have language in the left-hemisphere. The other homozygous genotype individuals have no systematic genetic control over their handedness. The phenotype will include both left-handers and right-handers and both left- and right-hemisphere speech in approximately equal proportions. The phenotypic manifestations of the DC heterozygotes are not specified *a priori* but are thought to be midway between the two homozygotes. This so-called additivity or semidominance should lead to a 25% chance of being left-handed, exactly midway between the chance of the DD homozygotes (0%) or CC homozygotes (50%) being left-handed. McManus (McManus, 1991; McManus and Bryden, 1992) went on to propose a sex-linked modifier gene to explain the higher incidence of left-handedness in males and the fact that left-handed mothers produce more left-handed offspring than do left-handed fathers.

In sum, handedness can be reflected in two dimensions, preference and performance. Both dimensions have been found useful for providing insight into the laterality of language. Handedness appears somewhat related to language laterality in that the hemisphere controlling the dominant hand is also dominant for language. Language laterality can, however, be decoupled from handedness as the majority of both right- and left-handers have language lateralized to the left hemisphere.

While handedness is reflected in both of these dimensions, they do not always concur. That is, hand preference does not always reflect which hand is more proficient. Part of this discrepancy arises from the fact that each dimension is multifactorial and can be measured in direction and degree of handedness. In fact, for both preference and performance there is evidence to suggest that the degree of handedness may depend on the nature of the task demands.

These observations raise some interesting questions which bear on our consideration of the relationship between handedness and praxis laterality. Some investigators suggest that the laterality of speech and language function and handedness are related because of their common dependence on a lateralized praxis control system (e.g., Kimura, 1993). Does praxis laterality then underlie the neural basis for handedness? That is, does the preferred hand enjoy a performance advantage because the hemisphere controlling this hand is also dominant for praxis? What implications do task demands have on this relationship of handedness to praxis laterality? Task demands appear to affect the magnitude of manual asymmetries in performance. They also affect the magnitude of the apraxic deficit and the degree to which the deficit is lateralized. Insight into the relationship between handedness and praxis, then, would seem to require that one is able to dissociate the apraxic deficit from the manual asymmetries present prior to the stroke which precipitates the apraxia. That is, deficits in gesture production arise in the context of pre-existing differences in hand performance and must be measured and interpreted against the background of these manual asymmetries.

4. APRAXIA AND HANDEDNESS

In our consideration as to how apraxia relates to handedness, one observation about apraxia is that it appears to affect a relatively high level system which is independent of the output system. Apraxia often affects limb, oral nonverbal, oral-verbal, and axial (whole body) motor systems, and, in the case of limb apraxia, both hands are frequently affected (e.g., Alexander, Baker, Naeser, Kaplan, and Palumbo, 1992; Kimura, 1982, 1993; Poeck, Lehmkuhl, and Willmes, 1982; Roy and Square, 1994; Roy and Square-Storer, 1990; Roy et al., 1991).

From these observations, praxis would appear to exhibit a cerebral dominance akin to that enjoyed by speech and language function. In right-handers, both praxis and speech and language function are impaired with damage to the left hemisphere and both apraxia and aphasia affect behavior no matter what the output system (e.g., speech or writing). It is not surprising, then, that aphasia and apraxia tend to occur together in right handers following damage to the left hemisphere. One view of this relationship (e.g., Geschwind, 1975) argues that apraxia arises from a disconnection between language areas of the brain subserving comprehension and those subserving the control of movement. This approach predicts that apraxia would be apparent primarily when the patient must pantomime a gesture to verbal command and much less apparent when performance is not dependent on language processes, for example, when the patient must imitate a gesture.

Liepmann (1913), one of the pioneers in the study of apraxia, observed, however, that many patients with left hemisphere stroke were also unable to imitate gestures. This observation lead Liepmann (1913), and more recently Kimura (1982, 1993), to propose that the link apraxia has with aphasia has more to do with motor control processes than language processes. According to this view, apraxia arises from disruptions to a system involved in the control of limb movements in egocentric (body-centered) space, a system which, it is argued, is also used in the control of speech.

This link between speech and limb praxis would suggest a very high co-occurrence of aphasia with limb apraxia in right handers. While there is substantial evidence for such co-occurrence (e.g., Kimura, 1993; Square-Storer, Roy, and Hogg, 1991), there are a number of notable exceptions. There are several reports of right-handers who exhibited a limb apraxia but not aphasia following left-hemisphere damage (Heilman, Gonyea, and Geschwind, 1974; Kertesz, Ferro, and Shewan, 1984; Selnes, Pestronk, Hart, and Gordon, 1991; Selnes, Risse, Rubens, and Levy, 1982). There are also a number of cases of so-called crossed aphasia in right-handers where aphasia results from right-hemisphere damage without any signs of apraxia. These observations indicate that aphasia and apraxia are not causally linked. Rather, their frequent co-occurrence suggests that the neural substrates of language and praxis are arranged so that a single lesion often affects both, possibly because of anatomical proximity. Further, handedness would appear to be as or more closely linked with praxis dominance than with language dominance. That is, when the hemisphere controlling the preferred right hand was damaged, apraxia but not aphasia was observed in a number of cases, and in several other reported cases when this hemisphere was spared in the face of aphasia with right-hemisphere damage, apraxia did not occur.

This link between language and limb praxis has also been examined in left-handers or non-right-handers. Kimura (1993) observed in her non-right-handers that praxis was more impaired with right hemisphere damage, while aphasia was more often seen with left hemisphere damage. Heilman, Coyle, Gonyea, and Geschwind (1973) also reported the case of a left-hander who developed apraxia but not aphasia with a right hemisphere lesion. This dissociation between praxis and language again questions the proposal of a common origin of these two functions. As well, these findings provide further support for the idea that handedness may be more strongly related to praxis dominance than language dominance: in some left handers, apraxia arises from right-hemisphere damage, the hemisphere controlling the preferred left hand, while speech and language functions are affected by damage to the left hemisphere.

Taken together, these findings from both left- and right-handers implying a close link between hand dominance and hemispheric dominance for praxis suggest that models of laterality may have to include genetic markers for not only language dominance and handedness but also for praxis dominance.

While damage to the right hemisphere affects limb praxis in many left-handers, Kimura (1993) observed that oral praxis was frequently affected by left hemisphere damage. In these patients, then, the commonality of apraxic deficits across movement systems with lateralized (left hemisphere) brain damage seen in right-handers breaks down such that damage to the hemisphere controlling the preferred hand results in limb apraxia only. These observations suggest that some left handers have praxis control invested in both hemispheres. In these people, the probability of limb apraxia arising from a lateralized stroke may be smaller than that for right handers and the potential for recovery might be greater. The system subserving oral praxis in the left hemisphere may have the potential to assume control of limb praxis following right hemisphere damage.

How might one identify such a subgroup of left handers? Peters' (see Chapter 5) finding with regard to consistent and inconsistent left handers may provide some insight here. Consistent left handers are those who prefer to use their left hand for both fine (i.e., hand writing) and more gross motor (i.e., ball throwing) tasks. Inconsistent left handers prefer to use their left hand for hand writing and their right hand for throwing a ball. Possibly the inconsistent left handers represent the subgroup who have praxis control represented in both hemispheres. What might be the basis for this apparent relationship between handedness and hemispheric dominance for praxis? The performance advantage enjoyed by the preferred hand may arise from the control exerted by the contralateral hemisphere through the neuroanatomical pathways (corticospinal tract) linking the hand to the hemisphere. Some evidence (e.g., Kertesz, Polk, Black, and Howell, 1992; Thoma et al., 1994) indicates that the sensorimotor cortex is larger in the hemisphere contralateral to the preferred hand. The preferred hand advantage cannot arise solely from the contralateral corticospinal pathway, however. This pathway primarily subserves control of distal (finger/hand movements) as opposed to proximal (whole arm) movements, while the preferred hand advantage is present for motor tasks regardless of whether they demand distal control (e.g., the Dot Aiming Test [Tapley and Bryden, 1985; see Chapter 3], finger tapping tasks [see Chapters 5 and 7]), or proximal control (e.g., the Annett Pegboard Test [Annett, 1976]). The preferred hand advantage, then, must arise from control exerted by the contralateral hemisphere which is subserved by brain areas other than the primary motor and sensorimotor cortices. These more anterior and posterior areas have been found to be important in giving rise to apraxia when damaged. Handedness and apraxia, then, may be linked through their joint dependence on processes subserved by these anterior and posterior brain areas in the hemisphere contralateral to the preferred hand.

Using this logic, the hemisphere contralateral to the preferred (dominant) hand could be considered dominant for praxis. Thus, in right-handers damage to the left hemisphere should give rise to apraxia, while damage to the right hemisphere should result in apraxia in left-handers. As we have seen, some evidence supports this hypothesis. If the hemisphere controlling the preferred hand is dominant for praxis, then we might expect that performance measures which underlie the preferred hand advantage should also be important measures of the apraxic deficit. Such does not appear to be the case, however.

A number of the most robust measures reflecting the performance advantage of the preferred hand are not typically affected in apraxia. Motor tasks which involve distal control such as finger tapping or rotation of a nut on a bolt (Kimura, 1979, 1993) are not performed more poorly by patients with apraxia (but see Heilman, 1975). Rather, it is only performance on more complex motor tasks (e.g., pegboard tasks) that patients with apraxia can be discriminated from those without apraxia (e.g., Haaland, Porch, and Delaney, 1980). Further, considerable evidence suggests that apraxia affects both hands, while deficits in these fine motor tasks are unilateral and affect the hand contralateral to the damaged hemisphere. Finally, damage limited to the sensorimotor areas of the cerebral cortex typically does not give rise to apraxia but rather to the deficits in fine motor control alluded to above.

What do these observations tell us about how apraxia relates to manual asymmetries in performance? If these asymmetries were based solely on hemispheric dominance for praxis, they should not exist given that the hemisphere dominant for praxis appears to control both hands (i.e., apraxia affects both hands). If one assumes some functional link between praxis laterality and the preferred hand advantage, performance differences between the hands may reflect the more direct access that the preferred hand has to the hemisphere dominant for praxis. Such a connection would likely serve to facilitate control of the preferred hand. The speed of processing the control signals may be increased, leading potentially to the shorter movement times observed for the preferred hand (e.g., Roy et al., 1994). The noise in processing might also be reduced leading to the smaller spatial variability and greater spatial accuracy observed for the preferred hand (Roy and Elliott, 1986, 1989; Roy, Winchester, et al., 1995).

Alternately, the preferred hand advantage in performance may not be linked functionally with the control of praxis. If apraxia were directly linked with the preferred hand advantage, one might expect to see the disorder only in the dominant hand. The fact that both hands are affected suggests that the systems/processes subserving praxis exert control at a higher level than those subserving the preferred hand advantage. The performance advantage for the preferred hand might then be considered to arise from more basic motor and visuomotor control processes which would be important in but independent of the control of praxis. Heilman's (1973; Heilman and Rothi, 1993) work would suggest that this component may reflect the precise control of movement which, when lost, makes movements of the hand and fingers appear clumsy and poorly coordinated.

The key to understanding the link between praxis and handedness may be to examine whether the task dimensions which serve to define the nature and degree of apraxia are similar to those which define the nature and degree of the performance advantage for the preferred hand. Studies such as those represented by Harrington and Haaland (1991, 1992), Jason (e.g., Jason, 1990), Kimura (1993) and Roy (e.g., Roy et al., 1991, 1993), which carefully manipulate task demands and examine a number of different performance measures, would be of particular importance in this regard.

While hand dominance appears to be linked in some way to hemispheric dominance for manual apraxia, it is important to recognize that manual performance asymmetries have the potential to affect the expression of the apraxic deficit. In most patients, the contralesional hand is paralyzed or weak and difficult to control. Thus, apraxia is assessed in the ipsilesional hand only. Comparisons between patients with left or right hemisphere damage, then, involve comparing left with right hand performance, respectively. Most studies of right-handers have found much poorer performance (i.e., an apraxic deficit) in the patients with left- as opposed to right-hemisphere damage. These group differences in gestural performance, however, are confounded with manual asymmetries. That is, part of the "deficit" in the left-hemisphere patients may arise from the manual asymmetries expected premorbidly, with the magnitude of this confounding effect depending on the degree of the premorbid preferred hand advantage.

Group differences in ipsilesional hand performance, then, must be interpreted in the context of the magnitude of expected premorbid manual asymmetries in performance. One approach to this type of analysis is to make indirect comparisons between the brain-damaged groups (i.e., hands) by comparing the patients' performance in each group with the performance of healthy adults using the same hand (e.g., Roy and Black, 1993; Roy, Black, et al., 1995, in press). One problem with this approach is that it is affected by the consistency with which the healthy adults in the sample examined show a performance difference between the hands. Work by Peters (see Chapter 5) suggests that there are considerable individual differences in manual asymmetries in performance which arise largely from variability in the performance of the nonpreferred hand. These observations would suggest that between subject variability is larger for the nonpreferred hand. Thus, returning to our discussion of right-handers with left-hemisphere damage, it should be more difficult to find a significant difference between the patients and the healthy adults on the nonpreferred left hand. The fact that these patients using their left hand very often do perform significantly worse than the healthy adults would seem to attest to the fact that the magnitude of the apraxic deficit is much greater than would be expected on the basis of manual asymmetries.

The effects of manual asymmetries might be more readily dissociated from those due to apraxia in those patients who are not hemiparetic and are able to use both hands. For example, in right-handers the left hemisphere is thought to be dominant for praxis and so affects the performance of both hands. If apraxia arising from left hemisphere damage is independent of manual asymmetries in performance, one would expect to see impaired performance in both hands with a preservation of the direction and degree of the premorbid right hand advantage in performance.

The need to dissociate manual asymmetries in performance from the effects of apraxia may be particularly important when gestural performance is reflected in more sophisticated, kinematic or multi-dimensional movement/error analysis systems or when tasks are more complex. That is, the advantage for the preferred hand may be observed on some performance measures on a task (e.g., movement time) but not on others (e.g., accuracy), and this advantage may increase with task complexity. Thus, the potential for confounding manual performance asymmetries with apraxic deficits may increase with the precision of the measurement system used to reflect performance and with the complexity of the task. This point is exemplified in some of our recent studies.

In this work (Roy and Black, 1993; Roy, Black, et al., 1995, in press), we have been examining disruptions to the pantomime and imitation of gestures in patients with lateralized strokes. Using a detailed error analysis system examining performance on several dimensions (hand posture, location and orientation, action and plane of movement), we observed that healthy adults were able to pantomime a series of transitive gestures equally well with either hand on each performance dimension. Imitation of less familiar nonrepresentational, intransitive gestures, however, was not done equally well by each hand. Hand posture was performed more poorly by the left hand.

This difference in the left hand performance of the healthy adults on this performance dimension affected whether an impairment was identified in the patients with left-hemisphere damage who also used their left hands. For the transitive gestures, these patients exhibited significantly poorer performance, while on the intransitive gestures no significant impairment was found. For these latter intransitive gestures, had we not made comparisons with the performance of healthy adults using the same (left) hand, we might have erroneously concluded an apraxic deficit in these patients, since they were impaired relative to the patients with right-hemisphere damage. Clearly, the difference between the two groups of patients on this dimension of performance was due more to manual asymmetries than to the lesion lateralization.

5. DIRECTIONS FOR FUTURE RESEARCH

What does our discussion suggest about future directions for research on the relationship between apraxia and handedness? One obvious direction is to examine how handedness relates to praxis laterality. With regard to hand preference, the work we reviewed on the direction of preference suggests some relationship, with right-handers showing apraxia more often with left-hemisphere damage and left-handers (e.g., Archibald, 1987; Faglioni and Basso, 1985) or non-right-handers (Kimura, 1993) incurring apraxia very often with right-hemisphere damage. The problem with some of these data is that the direction and the degree of handedness have been confounded in some studies which have examined so-called non-right-handers or adextrals (e.g., Kimura, 1993). Indeed, in her studies Kimura (1993) found that in her two subgroups of adextrals (left-handers and ambidextrous individuals), more patients in both groups exhibited apraxia with right- than left-hemisphere lesions. Right-hemisphere dominance for praxis, then, may relate more to not being right-handed than to being left-handed.

Clearly, much more work is needed to adequately address this relationship between the direction of hand preference and praxis laterality. What about the degree of hand preference? Is this measure also related to praxis laterality? Kimura's (1993) findings noted above would suggest that the greater the degree of right-hand preference, the greater the likelihood that praxis will be represented in the left hemisphere. The propensity for recovery from apraxia might then be greater for persons whose right-handedness is less pronounced. Presumably, these people would be more likely to have praxis represented to some degree in the right hemisphere.

What about left-handers? Kimura's (1993) data would suggest that left-handedness (in direction) per se is not related to praxis laterality. The frequency of right-hemisphere apraxia was higher in all of her non-right-handers regardless of whether they were classified as left-handers. While it would be unwise to make such a conclusion based on such a small number of patients, evidence from work on language laterality would suggest that such a scenario is possible. As we discussed, left-handers are much more likely to demonstrate language representation in the right hemisphere or in both hemispheres. Such could certainly be the case for praxis laterality in left-handers. Kimura's (1993) finding in her adextrals that limb praxis (right hemisphere) and oral praxis (left hemisphere) were represented in different hemispheres suggests that praxis might indeed be less clearly lateralized in left-handers. The implications of this supposed reduced lateralization needs to be examined as it pertains to the potential for recovery from apraxia. One might also want to investigate the co-occurrence of apraxia across the limb, oral verbal, and oral nonverbal movement systems. If praxis is more strongly lateralized in right-handers, one might predict that these praxis systems would all be affected and so would tend to co-occur more frequently than in left-handers. Recovery might also occur more consistently across these praxis systems in right- than left-handers.

The lateralization of praxis in left-handers may relate to the subgroup of left-handers, as we noted in our earlier discussion. The inconsistent left-handers (write with the left hand but throw a ball with the right hand) may be more likely to exhibit bilateral representation of praxis. Such individuals would more likely show an apraxia since damage to either hemisphere could potentially affect praxis. The severity and persistence of the apraxic deficits would, however, likely be less than in consistent left-handers.

Our discussion so far with regard to future directions has focused on hand preference. Asymmetries in hand performance also present some interesting directions for research as they relate to the laterality of praxis. One of the most important challenges in this work is to recognize the differences in how hand preference and hand performance asymmetries relate to praxis laterality as compared to language laterality. Hand preference measures have no impact on observed praxis or speech and language deficits following lateralized brain damage. Thus, there is some comparability in drawing inferences as to the cerebral laterality of function for praxis and language when using preference measures.

Such is not the case for performance measures of handedness. While these performance asymmetries have no direct impact on observed deficits in speech and language function, they do have the potential to affect observed apraxic deficits. The extent to which the demands of the praxis task tap into the dimensions which define a performance advantage for the preferred hand may reflect the extent to which handedness impacts on the apraxic deficits observed.

With this proposal in mind, future work should examine how the degree of hand performance asymmetries relates to the degree and laterality of apraxic deficits. For example, in right-handers as the right hand advantage increases across different tasks or task dimensions (e.g., spatial accuracy vs. time dimensions), it may be increasingly difficult to identify apraxic deficits in patients with left-hemisphere stroke. The inferior performance of their left hand relative to the right hand of patients with right-hemisphere stroke might be increasingly attributed to a premorbid disadvantage for the left hand. Recall that we saw just this effect in our work comparing pantomime and imitation performance in patients with lateralized stroke.

These observations suggest that it would be important to examine task demands in these studies. The potential for a lateralized apraxic deficit has been found to be dependent on task demands. For example, in right-handers, tasks which place demands on memory (i.e., the gesture must be generated from memory) appear to be more lateralized to the left hemisphere (e.g., Jason, 1985; Roy, 1981; Roy et al., 1993). Task demands may also affect the degree of the right hand advantage (e.g., Roy and Elliott, 1986). Thus, some of the variability in the relationship between apraxic deficits and manual asymmetries may arise from task demands. One might then expect this relationship to be most clearly examined in tasks which show the greatest right hand advantage and which are most lateralized to the left hemisphere.

Our predictions of different patterns of performance on gesture production (pantomime and imitation) and gesture and tool/object recognition tasks examined in our consideration of apraxia (see Table 11.1) is particularly relevant to this discussion of task demands. Are these patterns of performance reflecting disruptions at particular stages in gesture production all equally strongly associated with left hemisphere damage in right-handers? Possibly the disruptions to the earlier stages involving secondary memory and associated with knowledge of action and tool/object function, memory retrieval, and image generation are more strongly lateralized to the left hemisphere (cf., Jason, 1985; Roy, 1981, Roy et al., 1983). Such more lateralized disruptions might be most clearly examined as to how they relate to handedness.

This notion that different stages or processes in gesture production may be more lateralized than others is exemplified in work by Foster, Chase, Patronas, Gillespie, and Fedio (1986) examining cortical activation (using positron emission tomography) associated with gestural pantomime and imitation. They found that pantomime performance was associated with activation of the left hemisphere, while the right hemsiphere was activated when imitating a gesture. This notion also has an analogue in speech and language deficits. Aphasic deficits affecting the early stages of verbal expression seen in Broca's aphasia and those affecting language comprehension are more lateralized to the left hemisphere than are deficits affecting word finding.

A second direction for future work involves a closer examination of the neuroanatomical correlates of handedness and praxis laterality. These correlates could be investigated both structurally and functionally. The structural analyses would follow the lead established in the study of language laterality and handedness. As we observed, this work revealed, for example, that the planum temporale which has been linked with speech and language function, was larger in the left hemisphere in right-handers. One might reasonably expect that regions in the parietal and frontal lobes linked with praxis might also be larger in the left hemisphere in right-handers. Work by Habib et al. (1995) offers some tantalizing evidence in this direction. They observed that both the planum temporale and the parietal operculum (the distance from the end of the Sylvian fissure to the opercular portion of central sulcus) were larger in the left hemisphere, but only in their right-handers.

Taken together, these types of studies are important for more clearly understanding the nature of apraxia: they provide a means of dissociating manual asymmetries in performance from apraxic deficits associated with lateralized brain damage. Such studies may also afford more insight into the relationship between handedness and apraxia, information which may ultimately reveal something of the origins of handedness.

ACKNOWLEDGMENTS

Preparation of this chapter and the research reported was partially funded through grants from the Natural Sciences and Engineering Research Council of Canada, the Ontario Mental Health Foundation, and the Parkinson Foundation of Canada. Thanks to Dr. Sandra Black for her helpful comments on an earlier draft of this chapter.

REFERENCES

Alexander, M.P., Baker, F., Naeser, M., Kaplan, E., and Palumbo, C. (1992). Neuropsychological and neuroanatomical dimensions of ideomotor apraxia. *Brain*, 115, 87.

Annett, M. (1967). The binomial distribution of right, mixed and left-handedness. *Q. J. Exp. Psychol.*, 19, 327.

Annett, M. (1976). A coordination of hand preference and skill replicated. *Br. J. Psychol.*, 67, 587.

Annett, M. (1985). *Left, Right, Hand and Brain: The Right Shift Theory.* Hillsdale, NJ, Lawrence Erlbaum.

Annett, M. (1992). Five tests of hand skill. *Cortex*, 28, 583.

Annett, M. and Kilshaw, D. (1983). Right-and left-hand skill II: estimating the parameters of the distribution of R-L differences in males and females. *Br. J. Psychol.*, 74, 269.

Archibald, Y.M. (1987). Persisting apraxia in two left-handed aphasic patients with right-hemisphere lesions. *Brain Cognit.*, 6, 412.

Barnsley, R.H. and Rabinovitch, M.S. (1970). Proficiency vs. stated preference. *Percept. Motor Skills*, 30, 343.

Bishop, D.V.M., Ross, V.A., Daniels, M.S., and Bright, P. (in press). Reaching for objects on the left and right: a new approach to quantifying hand preference. *Br. J. Psychol.*.

Bryden, M.P. (1988). Correlates of the dichotic right-ear effect. *Cortex*, 24, 313.

Bryden, M.P. and Edmonds, A. (1995). An objective measure of hand preference. *J. Int. Neuropsychol. Soc.*, 1, 322.

Bryden, M. P., Singh, M., Steenhuis, R.E., and Clarkson, K. L. (1994). A behavioral measure of hand preference as opposed to hand skill. *Neuropsychologia*, 32, 991.

Brown, J.W. and Wislon, F.R. (1973). Crossed aphasia in a dextral. *Neurology*, 23, 907.

Duffy, R.J. and Duffy, J.R. (1990). The relationship between pantomime expression and recognition in aphasia: The search for causes. In G.E. Hammond (Ed.), *Cerebral Control of Speech and Limb Movements*, Amsterdam, North Holland, 417.

Faglioni, P. and Basso, A. (1985). Historical perspectives on neuroanatomical correlates of limb apraxia. In E.A. Roy (Ed.), *Neuropsychological Studies of Apraxia and Related Disorders*, Amsterdam, North Holland, 3.

Fitts, P.M. (1954). The information processing capacity of the human motor system in controlling the amplitude of movement. *J. Exp. Psychol.*, 47, 381.

Flowers, K. (1975). Handedness and controlled movement. *Br. J. Psychol.*, 66, 39.

Foster, N.L., Chase, T.N., Patronas, N.J., Gillespie, M.M., and Fedio, P. (1986). Cerebral mapping of apraxia in Alzheimer's disease by position emission tomography. *Ann. Neurol.*, 19, 139.

Foundas, A.L., Leonard, C.M., Gilmore, R., Fennell, E., and Heilman, K.M. (1994). Planum temporale asymmetry and language dominance. *Neuropsychologia*, 32, 1225.

Gangestad, S.W. and Yeo, R. (1994). Parental handedness and relative hand skill: a test of the developmental instability model. *Neuropsychology*, 8, 572.

Geschwind, N. (1975). The apraxias: neural mechanisms of disordered learned movement. *Am. Sci.*, 63, 188.

Geschwind, N. and Galaburda, A.M. (1987). *Cerebral Lateralization*. Cambridge, MA, M.I.T. Press.

Goldberg, G. (1985). Supplementary motor area structure and function: research and hypotheses. *Behav. Brain Sci.*, 8, 567.

Haaland, K.Y. and Flaherty, D. (1984). The different types of limb apraxia errors made by patients with left or right hemisphere damage. *Brain Cognit.*, 3, 370.

Haaland, K., Porch, B.E., and Delaney, H.D. (1980). Limb apraxia and motor performance. *Brain Lang.*, 9, 315.

Harrington, D.L. and Haaland, K.Y. (1991). Hemispheric specialization for movement sequencing: abnormalities in levels of programming. *Neuropsychologia*, 29, 147.

Harrington, D.L. and Haaland, K.Y. (1992). Motor sequencing with left hemisphere damage. *Brain*, 115, 857.

Habib, M., Gayraud, D., Oliva, A., Regis, J., Salamon, G., and Khalil, R. (1991). Effects of handedness and sex on the morphology of the corpus callosum: a study with brain magnetic resonance imaging. *Brain Cognit.*, 16, 41.

Habib, M., Robichon, F., Lévrier, O., Khalil, R., and Salamon, G. (1995). Diverging asymmetries of temporo-parietal cortical areas: a reappraisal of Geschwind/Galaburda theory. *Brain Lang.*, 48, 238.

Hardyck, C. and Petrinovitch, L.F. (1977). Left-handedness. *Psychol. Bull.*, 84, 385.

Heilman, K.M. (1975). A tapping test in apraxia. *Cortex*, 11, 259.

Heilman, K. and Rothi, L.J.G. (1993). Apraxia. In K. Heilman and E. Valenstein (Eds.), *Clinical Neuropsychology* (3rd Edition, pp. 131-150) New York, Oxford University Press.

Heilman, K.M., Gonyea, E.F., and Geschwind, N. (1974). Apraxia and agraphia in a right-hander. *Cortex*, 10, 284.

Heilman, K.M., Rothi, L.J., and Valenstein, E. (1982). Two forms of ideomotor apraxia. *Neurology (NY)*, 32, 342.

Heilman, K.M., Coyle, J.M., Gonyea, E.F., and Geschwind, N. (1973). Apraxia and agraphia in a left-hander. *Brain*, 96, 21.

Jason, G. (1983). Hemispheric asymmetries in motor function: I. Left hemisphere specialization for memory but not performance. *Neuropsychologia*, 21, 35.

Jason, G. (1985). Manual sequence learning after focal cortical lesions. *Neuropsychologia*, 23, 35.

Jason, G. (1990). Disorders of motor function following cortical lesions: review and theoretical considerations. In G.R. Hammond (Ed.), *Cerebral Control of Speech and Limb Movements*, Amsterdam, North Holland, 141.

Kertesz, A., Ferro, J.M., and Shewan, C. (1984). Apraxia and aphasia: the functional anatomical basis for the dissociation. *Neurology*, 30, 40.

Kim, H. (1994). Distributions of hemispheric asymmetry in left-handers and right-handers: data from perceptual asymmetry studies. *Neuropsychology*, 8, 148.

Kimura, D. (1979). Neuromotor mechanisms in the evolution of human communication. In H.D. Steklis and M.J. Raleigh (Eds.), *Neurobiology of Social Communication in Primates*, New York, Academic Press, 197.

Kimura, D. (1982) Left-hemisphere control of oral and brachial movements and their relationship to communication. *Phil. Trans. R. Soc. of London,* B298, 135.

Kolb, B. and Milner, B. (1981). Performance of complex arm and facial movements after focal brain lesions. *Neuropsychologia*, 14, 491.

Liepmann, H.K. (1913). Motor aphasia, anarthria, and apraxia. *Transactions of the 17th International Congress of Medicine, Section XI, Part II* (97–106).

Maraj, B.K.V., Roy, E.A., Elliott, D., and Lyons, J. (1994). The influence of spatial mapping on manual asymmetries. Paper read at the annual meeting of the North American Society for the Psychology of Sport and Physical Activity. Florida, June.

McDonald, S., Tate, R.L., and Rigby, J. (1994). Error types in ideomotor apraxia: a qualitative analysis. *Brain Cognit.*, 25, 250.

McManus, I.C. (1985). Handedness, language dominance and aphasia: a genetic model. *Psychol. Med.*, Monograph Supplement 8.

McManus, I.C. (1991) The inheritance of left-handedness. In J. March (Ed.), *Biological Asymmetry and Handedness (Ciba Foundation Symposium 162)*, Chichester, John Wiley, 251.

McManus, I.C. and Bryden, M.P. (1992). The genetics of handedness and cerebral lateralization. In I. Rapin and S.J. Segalowitz (Eds.), *Handbook of Neuropsychology, Vol. 6*, Amsterdam, North-Holland, 115.

Mozaz, M.J. (1992). Ideational and ideomotor apraxia: a qualitative analysis. *Behav. Neurol.*, 5, 11.

Ochipa, C., Rothi, L.J., and Heilman, K.M. (1992a). Conceptual apraxia in Alzheimer's disease. *Brain*, 115, 1061.

Ochipa, C., Rothi, L.J., and Heilman, K.M. (1992b). Conduction apraxia. *J. Neurol., Neurosurg. Psych.*, 57, 1241.

Pilgrim, E. and Humphreys, G.W. (1991). Impairment of action to visual objects in a case of ideomotor apraxia. *Cog. Neuropsychol.*, 8, 459.

Poeck, K. (1986). The clinical examination for motor apraxia. *Neuropsychologia*, 24, 129.

Poeck, K., Lehmkuhl, G., and Willmes, K. (1982). Axial movements in ideomotor apraxia. *J. Neurol., Neurosurg. Psych.*, 45, 1125.

Poizner, H. and Kegl, J. (1992). Neural basis of language and motor behavior: perspectives from American Sign Language. *Aphasiology*, 6, 219.

Poizner, H., Mack, L., Verfaellie, M., Rothi, L.J.G., and Heilman, M. (1990). Three-dimensional computergraphic analysis of apraxia: neural representations of learned movement. *Brain 113*, 85.

Porac, C. and Coren, S. (1981). *Lateral Preferences and Human Behavior.* New York, Springer-Verlag.

Provins, K. A. and Magliaro, J. (1989). Skill, strength, handedness, and fatigue. *J. Motor Behav.*, 21, 113.

Rasmussen, T. and Milner, B. (1977). The role of early left-brain injury in determining lateralization of cerebral speech functions. *Ann. N. Y. Acad. Sci.*, 299, 355.

Rothi, L.J.G., Ochipa, C., and Heilman, K.M. (1991). Cognitive neuropsychological model of limb praxis. *Cog. Neuropsychol.*, 8, 443.

Rothi, L.J.G., Mack, L., Verfaillie, M., Brown, P., and Heilman, K.M. (1988). Ideomotor apraxia: Error pattern analysis. *Aphasiology*, 2, 381.

Roy, E.A. (1978). Apraxia: a new look at an old syndrome. *J. Hum. Move. Stud.*, 4, 191.

Roy, E.A. (1981). Action sequencing and lateralized cerebral damage: evidence for asymmetries in control. In J. Long and A. Baddeley (Eds.), *Attention and Performance IX*, NJ, L. Erlbaum, 487.

Roy, E.A. (1982). Action and performance. In A. Ellis (Ed.), *Normality and Pathology in Cognitive Function*, New York, Academic Press, 265.

Roy, E.A. (1983a). Current perspectives on disruptions to limb praxis. *J. Am. Phys. Ther. Assoc.*, 63, 1998.

Roy, E.A. (1983b). Neuropsychological perspectives on apraxia and related action sequencing disorders. In R. Magill (Ed.), *Advances in Psychology, Volume 12, Memory and Control of Action*, Amsterdam, North Holland, 293.

Roy, E.A. (1983c). Manual performance asymmetries and motor control processes: subject generated changes in response parameters. *Hum. Move. Sci.*, 2, 271.

Roy, E.A. (Ed., 1985). *Advances in Psychology, Volume 23, Neuropsychological Studies of Apraxia and Related Disorders*, Amsterdam, North Holland.

Roy, E.A. and Black, S. (1993). Movement characteristics in limb apraxia. *J. Clin. Exp. Neuropsychol.*, 19, 246.

Roy, E.A., Black, S., Blair, N., and Dimeck, P. (1995) Deficits in Gestural pantomime: error analysis and lesion localization. Submitted manuscript.

Roy, E.A. and Elliott, D. (1986). Manual Asymmetries in visually directed aiming. *Can. J. Psychol.*, 40, 109.

Roy, E.A. and Elliott, D. (1989). Manual asymmetries in aimed movements. *Q. J. Exp. Psychol.: Human Experimental Psychology*, 41A, 501.

Roy, E.A. and Hall, C. (1992). Limb apraxia: a process approach. In L. Proteau and D. Elliott (Eds.), *Vision and Motor Control*, Amsterdam, North-Holland, 261.

Roy, E.A. and Square, P.A. (1985). Common considerations in the study of limb, verbal and oral apraxia. In E.A. Roy (Ed.), *Advances in Psychology, Volume 23, Neuropsychological Studies of Apraxia and Related Disorders*, Amsterdam, North-Holland, 111.

Roy, E.A. and Square-Storer, P.A. (1990). Evidence for common expressions of apraxia. In G.R. Hammond (Ed.), *Cerebral Control of Speech and Limb Movements*, Amsterdam, North-Holland, 477.

Roy, E.A., Brown, L., and Hardie, M. (1993). Movement variability in limb gesturing. In K. Newell and D. Corcos (Eds.), *Variability in Motor Performance*, Champaign, IL, Human Kinetics Publishers, 449.

Roy, E.A., Brown, L., and Winchester, T. (1992). Kinematic analyses of limb gesturing. *J. Clin. Exp. Neuropsychol.*, 14, 62.

Roy, E.A., Bryden, M.P., and Bulman-Fleming, B. (1996). Task demands and manual asymmetries in pegboard performance. Submitted manuscript.

Roy, E.A., Kalbfleisch, L., and Elliott, D. (1994). Kinematic analyses of manual asymmetries in visual aiming movement. *Brain Cognit.*, 24, 289.

Roy, E.A., Black, S, Winchester, T., and Barbour, K. (in press). Gestural imitation following stroke. *Brain Cognit.*.

Roy, E.A., Square, P.A., Adams, S., and Friesen, H. (1985). Error/movement notation systems in apraxia. *Rech. Semiot./Semiot. Inq.*, 5, 402.

Roy, E.A., Square-Storer, P.A., Hogg, S., and Adams, S. (1991). Analysis of task demands in apraxia. *Int. J. Neurosci.*, 56, 177.

Roy, E.A., Winchester, T, Elliott, D., and Carnahan, H. (1995). Manual asymmetries in visual aiming movements: the effect of spatial variability. *J. Int. Neuropsychol. Soc.*, 1, 133.

Roy, E.A., Brown, L., Winchester, T., Square, P., Hall, C., and Black, S. (1993). Memory processes and gestural performance in apraxia. *Adapt. Phys. Act. Q.*, 10, 293.

Schacter, S.C. (1993). Studies of handedness and anomalous dominance: problems and progress. In A.M. Galaburda (Ed.), *Dyslexia and Development: Neurobiological Aspects of Extra-ordinary Brains*, Cambridge, MA, Harvard University Press, 269.

Segalowitz, S.J. and Bryden, M.P. (1983). Individual differences in hemispheric representation of language. In S.J. Segalowitz (Ed.), *Language Functions and Brain Organization*, New York, Academic Press, 341.

Selnes, O.A., Pestronk, A., Hart, J., and Gordon, B. (1991). Limb apraxia without aphasia from a left sided lesion in a right handed patient. *J. Neurol., Neurosurg. Psych.*, 54, 734.

Selnes, O.A., Risse, G.L., Rubens, A.B., and Levy, R. (1982). Transient aphasia with persistent apraxia. Uncommon sequelae of massive left hemisphere stroke. *Arch. Neurol.*, 39, 122.

Square-Storer, P.A., Roy, E.A., and Hogg, S. (1990). Aphasia and apraxia. In G.R. Hammond (Ed.), *Cerebral Control of Speech and Limb Movements*, Amsterdam, North-Holland, 477.

Steenhuis, R. E. and Bryden, M. P. (1987). Handedness: a matter of direction and degree. *Can. Psychol.*, 28, N 586.

Steenhuis, R. E. and Bryden, M. P. (1989a). Different dimensions of hand preference that relate to skilled and unskilled activities. *Cortex*, 25, 289.

Steenhuis, R.E. and Bryden, M.P. (1989b). Hand preference and performance: right-handers, left-handers, and left-handers who are not consistently left-handed. *J. Clin. Exp. Neuropsychol.*, 11, 37.

Tapley, S.M. and Bryden, M.P. (1985). A group test for the assessment of performance between the hands. *Neuropsychologia*, 23, 215.

Van Horn, J.D. and McManus, I.C. (1993). Task difficulty and hand differences in peg moving, circle marking, and square tracing. Unpublished manuscript, University College, London.

Wang, L. and Goodglass, H. (1992). Pantomime, praxis and aphasia. *Brain Lang*., 42, 402.

Watson, N.V. and Kimura, D. (1989). Right-hand superiority for throwing but not for intercepting. *Neuropsychologia*, 27, 1399.

Witelson, S.F. (1985). The brain connection: the corpus callosum is larger in left-handers. *Science*, 229, 665.

Yeo, R. and Gangestad, S.W. (1993). Developmental origins of variation in human hand preference. *Genetica*, 89, 281.

INDEX

INDEX

A

B

C

D

E

F

G

H

I

K

L

M

N

O

P

R

S

T

U

V

W

Z